AF764495

Exam Preparatory Manual for Nurses

ANATOMY AND PHYSIOLOGY

Exam Preparatory Manual for Nurses
ANATOMY AND PHYSIOLOGY

Suma HY MBBS MD
Additional Professor
Department of Anatomy
Jawaharlal Institute of Postgraduate
Medical Education and Research
Puducherry, India

Co-authors

Sulochana Sakthivel MBBS MS PhD
Associate Professor
Department of Anatomy
Jawaharlal Institute of Postgraduate
Medical Education and Research
Puducherry, India

Suman Verma MBBS MD
Associate Professor
Department of Anatomy
Jawaharlal Institute of Postgraduate
Medical Education and Research
Puducherry, India

S Velkumary MBBS MD
Additional Professor
Department of Physiology
Jawaharlal Institute of Postgraduate
Medical Education and Research
Puducherry, India

Y Dhanalakshmi MBBS MD
Additional Professor
Department of Physiology
Jawaharlal Institute of Postgraduate
Medical Education and Research
Puducherry, India

Foreword
Roopa Kulkarni

JAYPEE
JAYPEE BROTHERS MEDICAL PUBLISHERS
The Health Sciences Publisher
New Delhi | London

Jaypee Brothers Medical Publishers (P) Ltd

Headquarters
EMCA House
23/23-B, Ansari Road, Daryaganj
New Delhi - 110 002, India
Landline: +91-11-23272143, +91-11-23272703
+91-11-23282021, +91-11-23245672
E-mail: jaypee@jaypeebrothers.com

Corporate Office
4838/24, Ansari Road, Daryaganj
New Delhi 110 002, India
Phone: +91-11-43574357
Fax: +91-11-43574314
E-mail: jaypee@jaypeebrothers.com

Overseas Office
J.P. Medical Ltd
83 Victoria Street, London
SW1H 0HW (UK)
Phone: +44 20 3170 8910
E-mail: info@jpmedpub.com

EU GPSR Authorised Representative
Logos Europe, 9 rue Nicolas Poussin
17000, La Rochelle, France
Phone: +33 (0) 6 67 93 73 78
E-mail: contact@logoseurope.eu

Website: www.jaypeebrothers.com
Website: www.jaypeedigital.com

Exam Preparatory Manual for Nurses—Anatomy and Physiology

First Edition: 2022
Reprint: **2026**

ISBN 978-93-89587-52-4

Printed in India

Foreword

It is indeed a great pleasure to write a foreword for the book titled *Exam Preparatory Manual for Nurses—Anatomy and Physiology* written by Dr Suma HY and her colleagues.

This book is intended to cater to the nursing and paramedical students. The chapters are written meticulously and the questions are specific and the answers are precise. The human anatomy and physiology form the foundation of medical knowledge. The book is felt essential, since it will help in last minute revision of these subjects.

In any good hospital, the reputation of the hospital and the doctor depends on well trained and skilled nursing and supporting staffs, who are there for the in-patients all the time. For the same reason, sound knowledge of the anatomy and physiology of the human body is essential. There are plenty of books available in these subjects. The syllabus given for their course is too vast and the duration of the first year is not sufficient for the students to understand, compile and concise answers. The syllabus is almost on par with MBBS Phase I students. Apart from that they also have to attend hospital duties as part of their training. They also have to study various other subjects as well. Therefore, the students get limited time to understand, revise, compile and write in the examinations.

I, congratulate Dr Suma HY and her colleagues for thinking in this way to help the students to understand the subject better and also will be able to write in the examination to the full satisfaction of the student and the examiner. Each chapter has questions and answers which are very appropriate and meticulously written. The explanation is very simple, straightforward, and easy-to-understand and write in the examination.

I wish her all the best and wish that maximum number of students get the benefit from the book.

Roopa Kulkarni MBBS MS
Principal and Professor (Retired)
Department of Anatomy
KVG Medical College
Sullia, Karnataka, India

Preface

Exam Preparatory Manual for Nurses—Anatomy and Physiology has been written for the nursing students from the point of view of examination. It will also be beneficial for paramedical students.

The text is in question and answer format. Answers are pointwise, supplemented with figures and tables wherever necessary. The tables and flowcharts summarize important and complex information of the subjects. It will be helpful to students to score well in examinations.

The questions have been collected from various universities, medical and nursing colleges.

Nursing students have more number of subjects during their first year, anatomy and physiology being felt as tough. The book is very useful during examinations and last minute preparations.

As an author, I have tried best to make the book easy-to-follow and reproduce the same during examinations. We have tried to make the subjects easy-to-understand and interesting to read. I welcome comments and suggestions from the students, and teachers as well. This will help to improve the book in future.

Suma HY

Acknowledgments

I thank my co-authors Dr Sulochana Sakthivel, Dr Suman Verma, Dr Velkumary, Dr Y Dhanalakshmi, who dedicated their time for contributing to the book.

I wish to dedicate this to my students who have been the source of inspiration to bring out such a book.

I am greatly indebted to Dr Parkash Chand, Senior Professor, Department of Anatomy, Jawaharlal Institute of Postgraduate Medical Education and Research (JIPMER), Puducherry, who supported us to carry out such works during his tenure as Head of the Department. I sincerely thank my colleagues in the Department of Anatomy, JIPMER, for their cooperation.

I am greatful to Dr Sivakumar M, Head, Department of Anatomy, JIPMER, for his constant support and encouragement.

I extend my sincere gratitude to Dr K Aravindhan, Professor, Department of Anatomy, JIPMER, for his support.

I acknowledge supports of Dr Sarasu J, V Gladwin, Raveendranath V, Dharmaraj T, Yogesh S, Rajasekar SSSN in the Department of Anatomy, JIPMER.

I wish to remember Dr Roopa Kulkarni, my guide and Dr RN Kulkarni at MS Ramaiah Medical College, for being source of inspiration throughout my career.

I thank Mrs Ruby Sharma, for her support throughout the preparation of the book.

My sincere regards to my husband and my children—Rishika and Keerthan, for their moral support.

Syllabus for I BSc Nursing in the Subject of Anatomy

Unit I

- Human cell
- Tissues—definition, types, characteristics, classification, location, functions, and formation.
- Membranes and glands—classification and structure.

Unit II

Skeletal System

- Bones—types, axial and appendicular skeleton
- Bone formation and growth
- Description of bones
- Joints classification and structure

Unit III

Muscular System

- Types and structure of muscles
- Muscle groups

Unit IV

Nervous System

- Structure of neuroglia and neurons
- Somatic nervous system—brain, spinal cord, cranial nerves, spinal nerves, peripheral nerves
- Autonomic nervous system—structure and location

Unit V

Sensory Organs

- Structure of sensory organs—skin, eye, ear, nose, tongue

Unit VI

- Circulatory system
  - Structure of blood vessels
  - Structure of heart
  - Arteries
  - Veins
  - Types of circulation

- Lymphatic system
  - Lymphatic vessels and lymph
  - Lymphatic tissues—thymus, lymph nodes, spleen, lymphatic nodules

Unit VII

Respiratory System
- Muscles of respiration
- Structure of the organs of respiration.

Unit VIII

Digestive System
Structure of alimentary tract and accessory organs of digestion.

Unit IX

Excretory System
Structure of organs of urinary (excretory) system—kidneys, ureter, urinary bladder, urethra.

Unit X

Reproductive System
- Structure of male reproductive organs
- Structure of female reproductive organs
- Structure of breast

Unit XI

Endocrine System
Structure and functions of endocrine organs—pituitary, pancreas, thyroid, parathyroid, thymus and adrenal glands.

Contents

SECTION 1

ANATOMY

Section Outline

1. Introduction to Human Anatomy
2. Cell and its Components, and Cell Division
3. Epithelial Tissue
4. Connective Tissue
5. Bone and Cartilage
6. Joints
7. Muscle Tissue
8. Integumentary System
9. Nervous System
10. Special Senses
11. Cardiovascular System
12. Respiratory System
13. Digestive System
14. Urinary System
15. Reproductive System
16. Endocrine System

1

CHAPTER

Introduction to Human Anatomy

SHORT ANSWERS 2 MARKS

1. Name the different levels of organization of the human body.

Ans. The levels are:

- Atoms—carbon, hydrogen, oxygen, nitrogen, phosphorous
- Molecule—DNA
- Cellular level—like a liver cell
- Tissue level, e.g., muscle tissue
- Organ level, e.g., heart
- System, e.g., cardiovascular system

2. Name the systems in the body.

Ans. The systems are as follows:

- Integumentary system
- Skeletal system
- Muscular system
- Nervous system
- Endocrine system
- Cardiovascular system
- Lymphatic system
- Respiratory system
- Digestive system
- Reproductive system
- Urinary system

3. List the important life processes.

Ans. These life processes help us to differentiate living from non-living things. Cessation of any of these leads to death of the organism.

- Metabolism
- Responsiveness
- Movement
- Growth
- Differentiation
- Reproduction

4. Name the basic tissues of the body.

Ans. Tissue is made of many similar cells that perform specific function. The various tissues of the body are divided into four major groups:

a. **Epithelial tissue**—is found covering skin, lining of organs, blood and lymph vessels, body cavities. It is for protection and secretion.
b. **Connective tissue**—this connects and supports most parts of the body
c. **Muscular tissue**—it produces movements through its ability to bring about contraction. It can be skeletal, smooth or cardiac muscle
d. **Nervous tissue**—this is found in brain, spinal cord and nerves. It is capable of transmitting information through nerve impulses. It is also responsible for our response to various stimuli and thought process.

5. What is anatomical position?

Ans. In the anatomical position, the subject stands erect, eyes looking at the horizon, upper limb by the sides, palm facing forwards, lower limbs being parallel and foot facing forward. It is used as a standard reference when body parts are described relative to each other, and also ensures uniformity.

6. Name the anatomical planes.

Ans. These imaginary flat surfaces pass through the body in various directions. They are useful in describing the structural relations of various parts of the body. They are:

a. **Median plane**—passes longitudinally and divides the body into right and left halves.
b. **Sagittal plane**—any vertical plane running parallel to the median plane.
c. **Frontal (coronal)**—any vertical plane passing through the body at right angles to the median plane. It divides the body into anterior and posterior parts.
d. **Transverse plane (cross-sectional)**—any horizontal plane passing through the body at right angles to median and frontal planes. It divides the body into upper and lower parts.
e. **Oblique plane**—this plane passes through the body or organ at an oblique angle (any angle other than 90° angle).

7. What is embryology?

Ans. The study of development which occurs from conception till birth is called embryology. Developmental biology encompasses the development of an individual from fertilization till death.

8. Enumerate the main directional terms used in anatomy.

(Any 4 will be asked for 2 Marks)

Ans. Directional terms describe the position of one body part relative to the other.

a. **Superior (cranial)**—structure nearer to the head (skull)
b. **Inferior (caudal)**—structure near to the sole of foot
c. **Posterior (dorsal)**—this denotes back surface of the body
d. **Anterior (ventral)**—this denotes front surface of the body
e. **Medial**—structure nearer to the median plane
f. **Lateral**—structure farther from the median plane
g. **Dorsum**—superior surface any part projecting anteriorly from the body

h. **Sole**—inferior aspect of the foot
i. **Superficial**—anything related towards the surface of the body
j. **Deep**—any structure related away from the surface of the body
k. **Proximal**—any structure nearer to the trunk
l. **Distal**—any structure away from the trunk

Terms of Laterality

a. **Bilateral**—paired structures having right and left members
b. **Unilateral**—those occurring on one side of the body
c. **Ipsilateral**—something occurring on the same side of the body as another structure
d. **Contralateral**—something occurring on the opposite side of the body in relation to another structure

2

CHAPTER

Cell and its Components, and Cell Division

SHORT ESSAYS 5 MARKS

1. Draw neat labeled diagram of human cell.

Ans. *Refer* **Figure 2.1.**

2. Describe the various components and functions of a human cell.

Ans. The cell consists of three main components—plasma membrane, cytoplasm and the nucleus. The cytoplasm contains various organelles.

1. **Plasma membrane**—also called cell membrane, separates the interior of the cell from its external environment.
   - It consists of lipid and proteins arranged in form of fluid mosaic model.
   - The lipid bilayer composed of phospholipids, cholesterol and glycolipids.
2. **Cytoplasm**—all the contents between plasma membrane and nucleus constitute cytoplasm. It has cytosol and organelles.
   - **Cytosol**—is the fluid portion, forms 55% of the cell volume. It contains 75–90% water with dissolved and suspended components. These include ions, glucose, amino acids, fatty acids, proteins, lipids, ATP and waste products. Storage molecules like lipid and glycogen granules are also present.

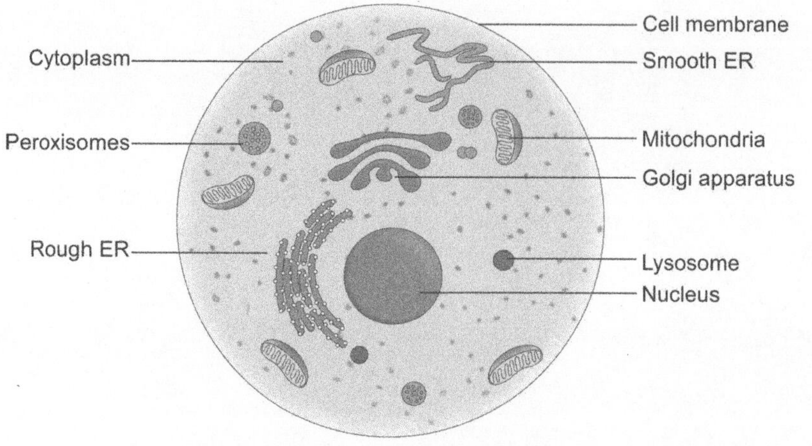

Fig. 2.1: Schematic diagram of human cell.
(ER: endoplasmic retinaculum)

- **Cytoskeleton:** Consists of network of protein filaments distributed throughout the cytoplasm. They include microfilaments, intermediate filaments and microtubules.
- **Cellular organelles:** These are small structures with specific function.
  1. **Ribosomes—**are granules composed of RNA. They are located in cytoplasm and attached to endoplasmic retinaculum. They are sites of protein synthesis.
  2. **Endoplasmic retinaculum (ER)**—are flattened membranous sacs or tubules. It is of two types—rough and smooth. *Rough ER* with ribosomes attached involved in protein synthesis, e.g., glycoproteins and phospholipids. *Smooth ER* is without ribosomes, but is rich in enzymes involved in fatty acid and steroid synthesis, e.g., estrogens and testosterone. It helps in detoxification of drugs.
  3. **Golgi complex—**it is cup-like organelle made of membranous cisterns. It is closely associated with rough endoplasmic reticulum (RER). It *modifies, sorts and packs the proteins* synthesized by ribosomes.
  4. **Lysosomes**—they are membrane enclosed structures. It contains digestive and hydrolytic enzymes. It breaks down wide variety of molecules. It also helps to recycle worn-out cell structures. It is responsible for autophagy—digestion of the cell itself.
  5. **Peroxisomes**—are smaller than lysosomes, contain oxidative enzymes. It is important in metabolism of amino acid and fatty acids. It oxidizes toxic substances, such as alcohol, protects other parts of cell from harmful effects of hydrogen peroxide.
  6. **Proteasomes**—similar to peroxisomes, but smaller contain proteases. It degrades faulty, damaged proteins.
  7. **Mitochondria**—are small, thread like, membrane bound structures. They generate ATP via aerobic respiration, hence called power house of the cell. It consists of outer and inner membranes. The inner one is thrown into folds called cristae, which house enzymes required for aerobic phase of cellular respiration. They can self-replicate. They have own DNA. They are significant in apoptosis.

3. **Nucleus**—is a spherical or oval structure present in the center of the cell. It is bound by outer and inner nuclear layer, interrupted by nuclear pores. Interior has nucleoplasm. Nucleoli present in it synthesize ribosomes. The chromosomes are present in the form of chromatin network along with some RNA and proteins. The genes in them are responsible for heredity as well as control the functioning of the cell.

3. Explain about the cytoskeleton of a cell.

Ans. Cytoskeleton is a network of protein filaments distributed throughout the cytoplasm. It includes microfilaments, intermediate filaments and microtubules **(Fig. 2.2)**.

Microfilaments:

- Composed of ***actin and myosin*** filaments
- Located at the edge of the cell
- Provide mechanical support—shape and strength to the cells
- Help in *movements as in*—cell division, locomotion, muscle contraction, during migration of the embryonic cells, WBCs migration during infection, etc.

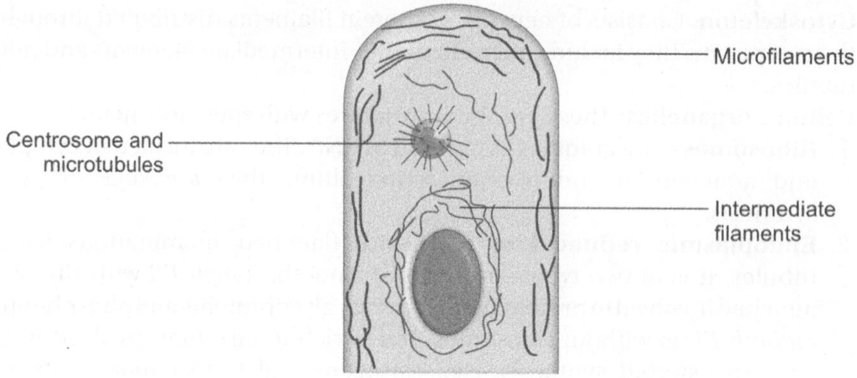

Fig. 2.2: Cytoskeleton of the cell.

- Forms the core of microvilli—these are finger-like projections of the plasma membrane. They are nonmotile. *Microvilli* helps to increase surface area for absorption, e.g., in intestines.

Intermediate filaments:

- They are found in parts of the cell subjected to mechanical stress.
- Provide support to organelles like nucleus.
- Help in cell attachment.

Microtubules:

- They are long, unbranched tubular structures.
- Made of tubulin protein.
- It is assembled by an organelle called centrosome.
- Microtubules provide shape to the cell
- Involved in movements of—secretory vesicles, chromosomes during cell division, cilia and flagella.

4. Plasma membrane.

Ans. Plasma membrane is a layer which separates the internal environment of the cell from its exterior.

- It consists of lipid and proteins arranged in fluid mosaic model.
- The lipid bilayer composed of—phospholipids, cholesterol and glycolipids.
- Lipids are amphipathic that is they have a polar and nonpolar ends.
  - Polar part—phosphate containing head—is hydrophilic.
  - Nonpolar part—two long-fatty acid tails—are hydrophobic.
- Membrane proteins are:
  - Integral proteins—are transmembrane proteins. Includes ion channels, carriers, receptors, enzymes
  - Peripheral proteins—are attached to the polar heads of the membrane. They provide support, anchor integral proteins, and movements.

5. Describe meiosis.

Ans. • Reproductive cell division.

- Occurs in germ cells of ovary and testis to form gametes.
- Number of chromosomes is reduced to half (reduction cell division).
- Haploid cells are produced.
- Two stages: Meiosis I and meiosis II **(Fig. 2.3)**.

Meiosis I

Four phases—prophase I, metaphase I, anaphase I and telophase I.

1. **Prophase I**—long phase. Chromosomes condense, nuclear membrane and nucleoli disappear. Mitotic spindle forms. Chromatids of homologous chromosomes form a **tetrad** and part of chromatids is exchanged in an event called as **crossing-over**.
2. **Metaphase I**—tetrads are arranged along equator of cell.
3. **Anaphase I**—homologous chromosomes separate. Mitotic spindle moves chromosomes to opposite poles.
4. **Telophase I**—nuclear membrane is formed. Two daughter cells with haploid number of chromosomes are formed.

Meiosis II

- **Prophase II**—chromosomes are dense. Nuclear membrane disappears.
- **Metaphase II**—chromatid pairs arrange at equator.
- **Anaphase II**—centromere divides and chromatids are separated. Chromatids move to opposite poles due to the pull of mitotic spindle.
- **Telophase II**—after nuclear membrane formation, each cell splits to form two daughter cells.

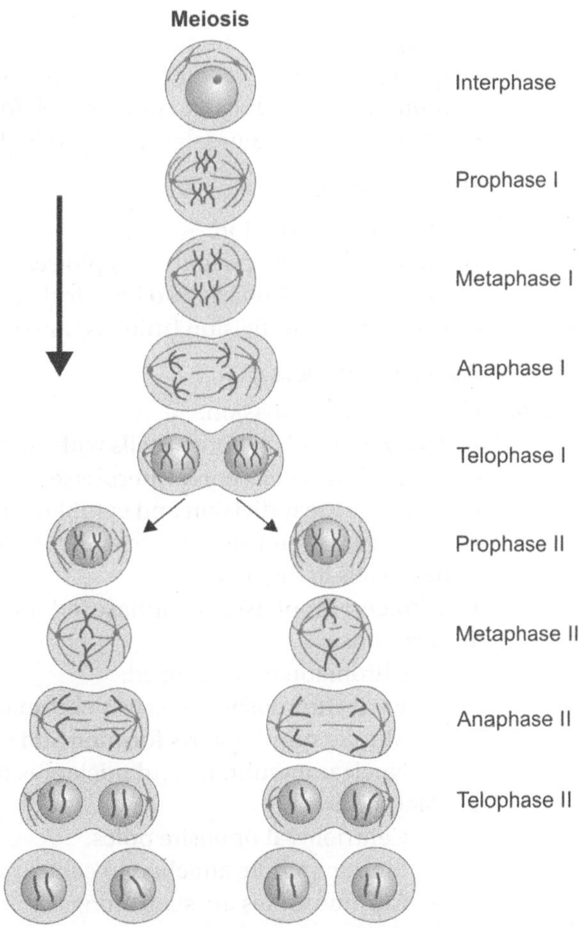

Fig. 2.3: Stages of meiosis.

6. Stages of cell cycle.

Ans.
- Cell cycle of a somatic cell consists of events of replication and cell division.
- Two stages are seen in a cell cycle: **interphase** and **mitotic phase (Fig. 2.4)**.

Interphase:

- Active metabolic state.
- Cell duplicates genetic material and produces other cell components.
- Three phases in sequence: **G1, S and G2.**
- S phase is for DNA synthesis.

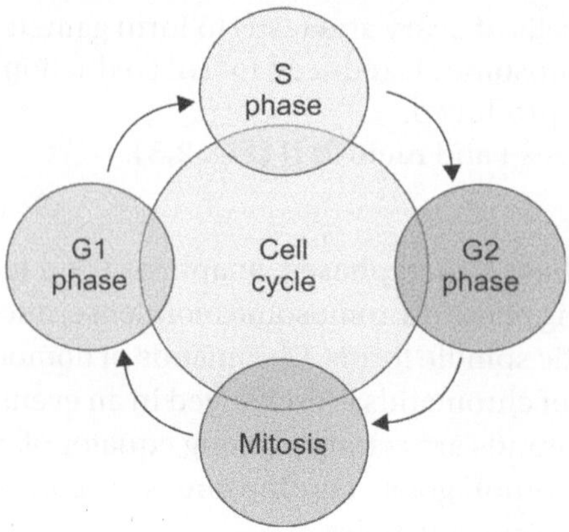

Fig. 2.4: Cell cycle.

- Dividing cells enter S phase after G1 and nondividing cells like nerve cells enter G0 phase after G1.
- After S phase, cell enters G2 and then goes to mitotic (M) phase.
- During G1, more cell organelles are added and centrosomes multiply. In G2, cell proteins are produced to prepare cell for mitotic division.
- DNA in S phase separates into two single strands and new DNA is synthesized.

Mitotic phase:

- Phase of cell division.
- After interphase, cell enters M phase.
- At the end of M phase, two identical cells are formed.
- Parts—nuclear division (mitosis) and cytoplasmic division (cytokinesis).

7. Describe mitosis.

Ans.
- Somatic cells division.
- Two genetically identical cells with 46 chromosomes are formed.
- After mitosis, cells enter interphase.
- Parts—nuclear division and cytoplasmic division (cytokinesis).
- Significance—forms new cells for growth of the organism and for replacing the dead cells in the body.

Four stages: Prophase, metaphase, telophase and anaphase **(Fig. 2.5):**

1. **Prophase:**
   - Chromatin is condensed.
   - Each chromosome has two chromatids attached at centromere.
   - Mitotic spindle starts forming and centrosomes move to poles.
   - Nuclear membrane and nucleolus disappear.
2. **Metaphase:**
   - Centrioles at opposite poles.
   - Mitotic spindle attached to centromere of chromosomes.
   - Chromosomes are seen along the equator of cell.

3. **Anaphase**:
   - Centromere divides.
   - Mitotic spindle pulls chromatids of each pair to opposite pole.
   - Cytokinesis starts.
4. **Telophase:**
   - Last phase
   - Nuclear membrane is formed and nucleoli appear.
   - Chromosomes uncoil.
   - Mitotic spindle disappears.
   - Cytokinesis is completed.
   - Two genetically identical cells are formed.

Cytokinesis—starts in the anaphase. A depression is formed on cell surface midway between poles. This depression becomes gradually deep towards the center of cell so that cytoplasm is divided into two.

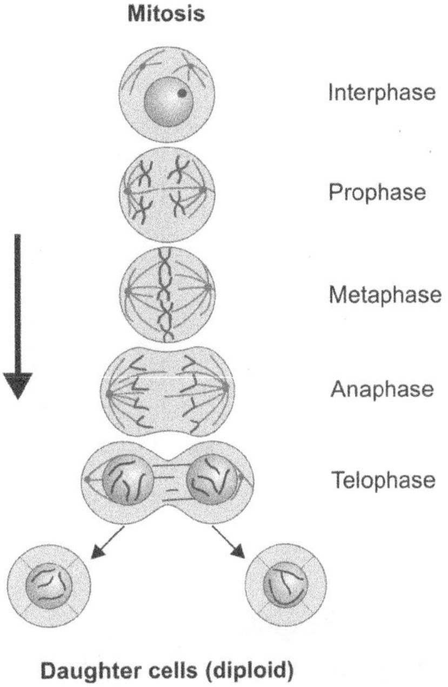

Fig 2.5: Stages of mitosis.

8. List the differences between mitosis and meiosis.

Ans. **Table 2.1.**

Table 2.1: Differences between mitosis and meiosis.

Sl. No.	Mitosis	Meiosis
1.	Somatic cell division (occurs in somatic cells)	Reproductive cell division (occurs in germ cells)
2.	Forms new somatic cells	Forms gametes
3.	Number of chromosomes same in daughter cells, 46	Number of chromosomes is half in daughter cells, 23
4.	One division	Two division
5.	Two daughter cells	Four daughter cells
6.	No tetrads	Tetrads form
7.	No chiasma formation	Chiasma formation for genetic material exchange
8.	Daughter cells genetically identical	Daughter cells not genetically identical

SHORT ANSWERS 2 MARKS

9. Cilia (Fig. 2.6A).

Ans.
- Cilia are motile hair-like projections of cell surface.
- It is composed of 20 microtubules surrounded by plasma membrane.
- Each cilium is anchored to the basal body at the apical portion of the cell.
- Its steady movement is responsible *for movement of fluid along cell surface.*
- Location: Respiratory passages, fallopian tube.

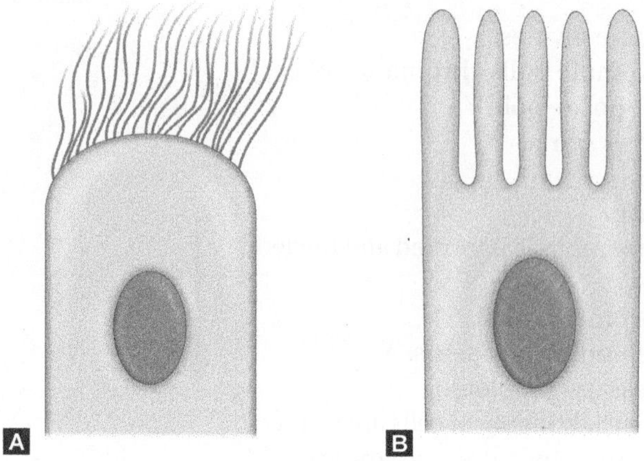

Figs. 2.6A and B: (A) Cilia are hair-like projections; (B) Microvilli are finger-like projections of the plasma membrane.

10. Flagella.

Ans.
- Flagella are long hair-like projections of cell surface. They are similar to cilia, but are longer.
- The core is composed of microtubules.
- *Capable of moving an entire cell.*
- Location: Tail of the human sperm.

11. Microvilli (Fig 2.6B).

Ans.
- Microvilli are finger-like projections of the plasma membrane. They are non-motile.
- *Microvilli* helps to increase surface area for absorption, e.g., in intestines.
- Contain core of actin filaments.

12. Define cell division. Name types of cell division and their importance.

Ans. Cell division—the process in which the parent cell divides and forms new daughter cells.

Types:
- **Mitosis**—somatic cell division, important for tissue growth to produce new cells and replace the dead ones. Number of chromosomes remains the same.
- **Meiosis**—reproductive cell division, important for production of gametes. Number of chromosomes becomes half.

13. Name the steps (stages) of mitosis and meiosis.

Ans. Mitosis:
- Prophase
- Metaphase
- Anaphase
- Telophase

Meiosis

- Prophase I and II
- Metaphase I and II
- Anaphase I and II
- Telophase I and II

14. Effect of drugs on mitosis.

Ans.
- **Cancer drugs**—cancer occurs due to uncontrolled cell division which forms a tumor. Anticancer drugs used in chemotherapy, inhibit the mitotic spindle formation and prevent cell division. By this mechanism, anticancer drugs stop the progress of cancer.
- **Colchicine**—used in karyotyping. It arrests the dividing cells in metaphase by preventing the mitotic spindle formation. Since chromosomes are condensed in metaphase, this makes it easy to study their structure in a karyotype.

15. Crossing-over.

Ans.
- Takes place in prophase I of meiosis.
- Exchange of genetic material between nonsister chromatids of homologous chromosomes is called as crossing-over.
- Significance—gametes formed are genetically different from parent cell due to crossing-over. The **genetic recombination** (new gene combination) in crossing-over produces genetic variability in species.

Note:
- Smoking damages cilia. Hence they fail to clear foreign particles from respiratory passages.
- Disorders in lysosomal enzymes leads to lysosomal storage disorders, e.g., Tay-Sachs disease.
- If proteasomes fail to clear abnormal proteins, diseases like Alzheimer's can result.
- Mitochondria is inherited from mother.
- Study of chromosomes and genes, diseases developing due to their alteration is genetics.
- Chromosome is a highly coiled DNA molecule combined with protein molecule.
- Apoptosis—process of programed cell death.
- Necrosis—death of cells in a tissue or organ due to disease, injury or loss of blood supply.
- Largest cell—ovum
- Smallest cell—sperm
- Uncontrolled or abnormal cell division can lead to cancer. Study of this is called oncology.
- Hyperplasia—increase in the number of cells due to cell division.
- Hypertrophy—increase in the size of a cells without cell division.
- Anaplasia—loss of tissue differentiation and function, as seen in cancers.
- Atrophy—decrease in size of cells/tissues (wasting).
- Dysplasia—size, shape and organization of cells is altered 0 due to inflammation or chronic irritation. It can lead to cancer, if the process continues.

3

CHAPTER

Epithelial Tissue

LONG ESSAYS — 10 MARKS

1. Classify epithelial tissue with examples. Explain about simple epithelium in detail.

Ans. **Definition**— epithelium tissue is a basic tissue that covers the body surfaces, lines body cavities, ducts and forms glands.

Epithelial tissue is made of cells resting on a basement membrane. This layer will be supported further by a layer of connective tissue which contains blood vessels, lymphatics and nerves. The cells are interconnected and with the basement membrane by various types of cell junctions.

Classification

Epithelium is broadly classified as simple and compound epithelium.

Epithelium
- Simple epithelium—made of single layer of cells resting on a basement membrane
- Compound/stratified epithelium—consists of multiple layer of cells

Simple epithelium: This type is further classified into various types depending on the type of cells lining.

i. **Simple squamous epithelium (Fig. 3.1)**—made of single layer of flat cells, and on surface view gives pavement-like appearance.
Function—diffusion, filtration and osmosis, e.g., alveolar sacs in lungs, inner lining of blood vessels, etc.

ii. **Simple cuboidal epithelium (Fig. 3.2)**—single layer of cuboidal cells, e.g., tubules of kidney, surface of ovary, lens of eye.

iii. **Simple columnar epithelium (Fig. 3.3)**—single layer of columnar cells. Primarily involved in absorption, secretion, protection and lubrication, e.g., lining of gastrointestinal tract (GIT), gallbladder, glands.

iv. **Pseudostratified epithelium (Fig. 3.4)**—it appears falsely stratified. It consists of tall columnar cells along with short basal cells, hence nuclei are at different levels. It lines the larger excretory ducts of many glands, epididymis, parts of male urethra and auditory tubes. Its functions are: protection and secretion. The lining

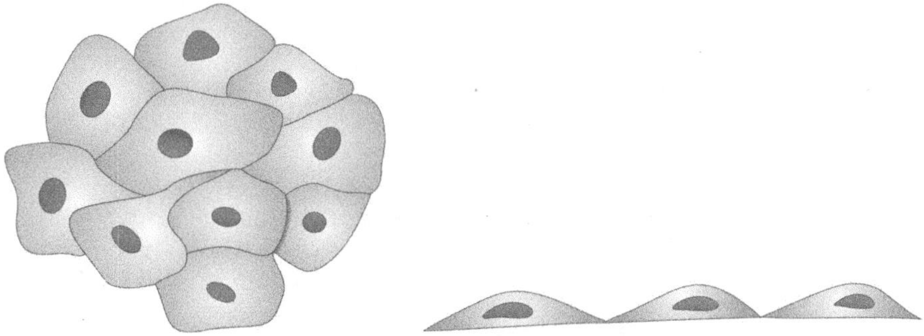

Fig. 3.1: Simple squamous epithelium.

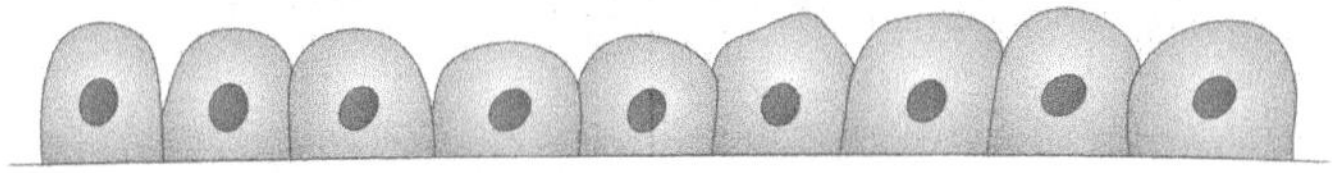

Fig. 3.2: Simple cuboidal epithelium.

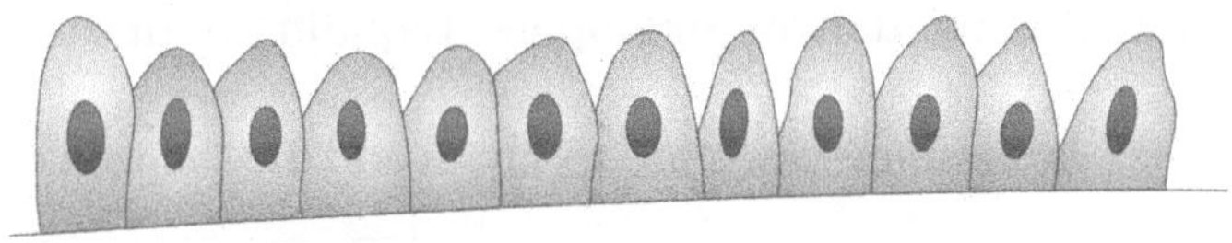

Fig. 3.3: Simple columnar epithelium.

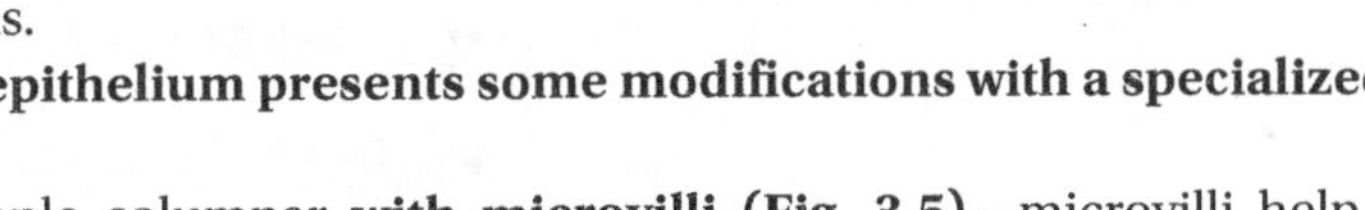

Fig. 3.4: Pseudostratified epithelium.

of trachea and bronchi is by ciliated pseudostratified epithelium with goblet cells.

Simple epithelium presents some modifications with a specialized function. They are:

v. Simple columnar **with microvilli (Fig. 3.5)**—microvilli help to increase the surface area for absorption, e.g., small intestine.
vi. Simple cuboidal with microvilli (called **brush border**)—found in proximal convoluted tubule (PCT) of kidney.
vii. Simple columnar **with cilia and goblet cells (Fig. 3.6)**—cilia are involved in movements, e.g., trachea and bronchi of lungs.
viii. Columnar epithelium **with stereo cilia**—stereo cilia are modified microvilli (followed by comma) and useful in increasing surface area for absorption as in epididymis of the male genital tract.

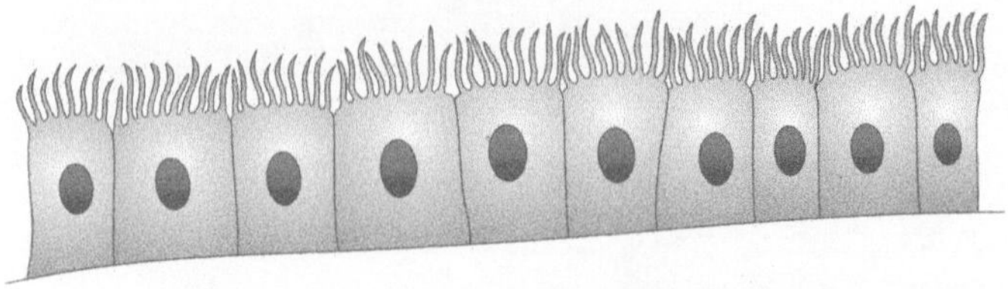

Fig. 3.5: Columnar epithelium with microvilli.

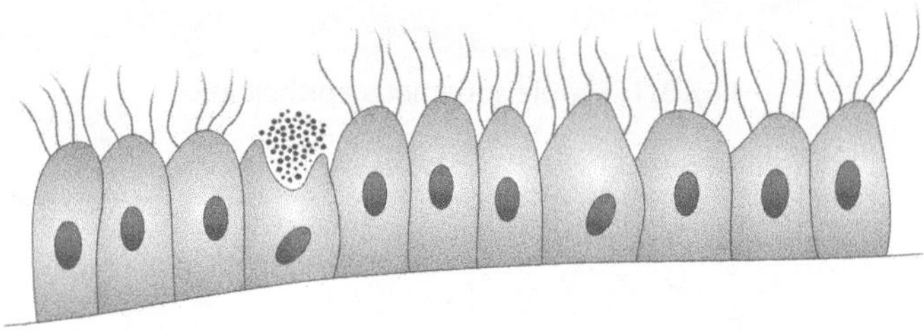

Fig. 3.6: Ciliated columnar with goblet cells.

2. Classify epithelial tissue with examples. Explain about stratified epithelium in detail.

Ans. Epithelial tissue is classified based on cell layers and the shape of cells.

Arrangement of cell layers →
- Simple epithelium
- Pseudostratified epithelium
- Stratified epithelium

Shape of cells

The shape of the cells vary depending on the function →
- Squamous epithelium
- Cuboidal epithelium
- Columnar epithelium
- Transitional epithelium

If these are combined, we get the following broad classification:

Simple epithelium
- Simple squamous
- Simple cuboidal
- Simple columnar—can be with ciliated or nonciliated
- Pseudostratified

Compound epithelium
- Stratified squamous epithelium—keratinized or nonkeratinized
- Stratified cuboidal
- Stratified columnar
- Transitional epithelium

A. **Stratified squamous epithelium (Figs. 3.7 and 3.8).**

It is more durable, protects underlying tissues from external environment as well as from wear and tear.

Stratified squamous epithelium consists of multiple layers of cells (10–12 layers).

- Basal cells are either cuboidal or columnar resting on a basement membrane.
- The next layer of cells become polyhedral, then flat. Superficial most cells are squamous, hence the name.
- The superficial cells are dead; hence the proteins accumulate to form keratin. Later keratin with the dead cells is shed of.
- New cells replace old cells that migrate from the basal cells.

It consist of five layers from deep to superficial. They are:

1. Stratum basale
2. Stratum spinosum
3. Stratum granulosum
4. Stratum lucidum
5. Stratum corneum

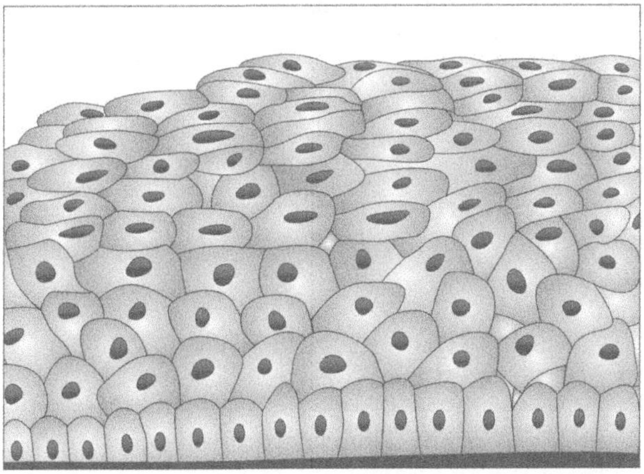

Fig. 3.7: Stratified squamous nonkeratinized epithelium.

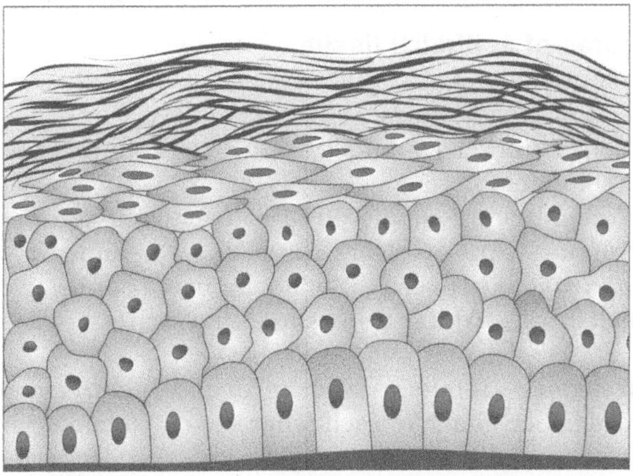

Fig. 3.8: Stratified squamous keratinized epithelium.

Based on the presence or absence of keratin, it is classified into:

i. Nonkeratinized stratified squamous epithelium—without keratin layer on the exposed surface. It is found on moist surfaces and are subjected to considerable wear and tear, e.g., mouth, tongue and vagina.

ii. Keratinized stratified squamous epithelium—here the keratin forms a thick layer adjacent to the superficial squamous cells, e.g., skin. Keratin is a waterproof protein, resists friction and bacterial invasion.

B. **Stratified cuboidal epithelium**—it is made of more than two layer of cuboidal cells. Its main function is secretion, e.g., duct of sweat glands, conjunctiva of eye, pharynx and epiglottis.

C. **Stratified columnar epithelium**—it is made of more than two layer of columnar cells. Functions: protection and provides passage to secretions as in ducts, e.g., milk duct of mammary gland and anal canal.

D. **Transitional epithelium (Fig. 3.9)**—special feature is that the cells of outer layer tend to be large and rounded (called umbrella cells). This feature allows the tissue to stretch when filled with urine, and return to original state after emptying. It also prevents seepage of urine into the underlying tissue layers. It is found in urinary bladder, part of ureters and urethra.

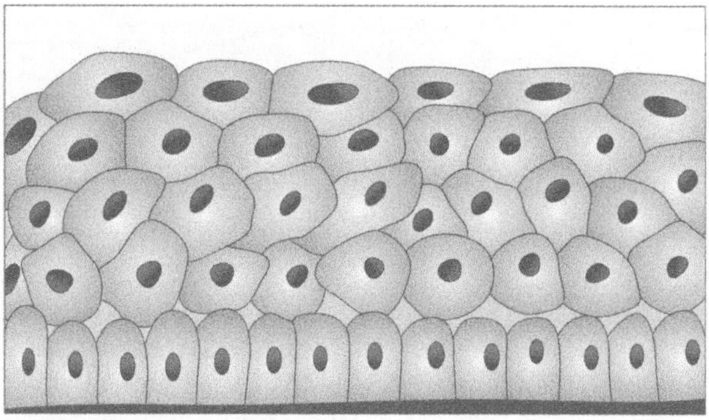

Fig. 3.9: Transitional epithelium.

SHORT ESSAYS — 5 MARKS

3. General features of epithelial tissue.

Ans. Epithelium is a tissue lining the outer surface of the body as well as forms internal lining of the hollow organs, ducts, and blood vessels.

- It chiefly consists of cells arranged as single layer or multiple layers. The cells rest on a basement membrane.
- Basement membrane is made up of connective tissue rich in blood vessels. It provides support to the overlying avascular epithelium.
- Metabolic exchange between the epithelium and connective tissue is by diffusion
- The epithelial cells exhibit three surfaces which differ in function **(Fig. 3.10)**, namely:
  1. **Apical surface**—is free. It is the site for absorption, secretion.
  2. **Lateral surface** attach to each other by cell junctions viz. tight, gap junctions and desmosomes.
  3. **Basal surface**—by which cells attach to the basement membrane.

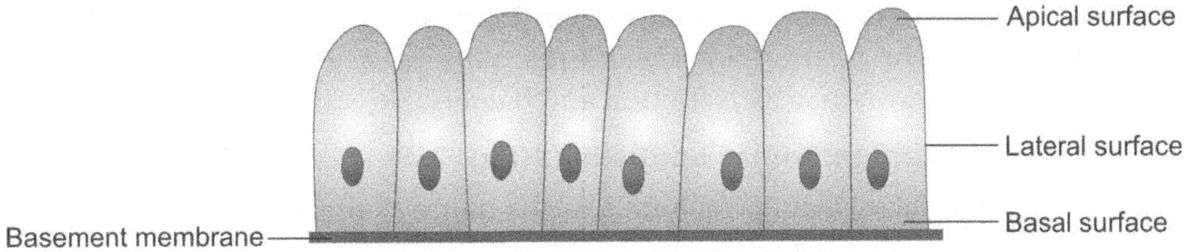

Fig. 3.10: Surfaces of columnar cell.

- It has great capacity for regeneration as it is exposed to wear and tear.
- The functions are:
  - Protection—as in skin.
  - Filtration—as in Bowman's capsule of kidney.
  - Secretion—as in GIT and glands.
  - Absorption—as in GIT.
  - Excretion—as in glomeruli of kidneys.

4. Transitional epithelium (Fig. 3.9).

Ans. Transitional epithelium is a specialized epithelium found lining the urinary passages.
- It is made of 4–5 layers of cells resting on basement membrane.
- Basal cells are low cuboidal.
- The cells of the superficial layer tend to be large and rounded called umbrella cells. This feature allows the epithelial tissue to stretch when filled with urine, and return to original state after emptying.
- It also prevents seepage of urine into the underlying tissue layers.
- When the bladder is full, the epithelium stretches, giving stratified squamous appearance. When the bladder is empty, it appears stratified cuboidal.
- Location—urinary bladder, part of ureters and urethra.

5. Stratified squamous epithelium (Figs. 3.7 and 3.8).

Ans. Stratified squamous epithelium consists of multiple layers of cells. It consists of five layers from deep to superficial. They are:
1. *Stratum basale*—basal cells are either cuboidal or columnar resting on a basement membrane. New cells replace old cells that migrate from the basal cells.
2. *Stratum spinosum*—the next layer of cells become polyhedral with spiny projections.
3. *Stratum granulosum*—it is made of flat cells with keratohyalin granules inside.
4. *Stratum lucidum*—here the cells begin to loose organelles, nuclei disappear.
5. *Stratum corneum*—superficial most cells are squamous, hence the name. They are superficial cells and are dead; hence the proteins accumulate to form keratin. Later keratin with the dead cells are shed off.

Functions—it is more durable, **protects** underlying tissues from external environment as well as from **wear and tear**.

Stratified squamous epithelium is subdivided into two types based on the presence or absence of keratin.

a. **Nonkeratinized stratified squamous epithelium**—without keratin layer on the exposed surface. It is found on moist surfaces and is subjected to considerable wear and tear, e.g., mouth, tongue and vagina.

b. **Keratinized stratified squamous epithelium**—here the keratin forms a thick layer adjacent to the superficial squamous cells. Example: skin. Keratin is a waterproof protein, resists friction and bacterial invasion.

6. Pseudostratified columnar epithelium (Fig. 3.4).

Ans. Pseudo means false. This epithelium gets the name as pseudostratified since:
- All the columnar cell rest on basement membrane.
- But few cells do not reach the superficial surface.
- The nuclei are at different levels as the columnar cells differ in their height.
- Some cells may possess cilia; they help in movement of particles.
- Some have goblet cells dispersed between them which secrete mucus.

Hence there is:

Pseudostratified ciliated columnar epithelium with goblet cells—as in respiratory passages. The mucus traps foreign particles and cilia move it out of the passage.

Pseudostratified nonciliated columnar epithelium—found in larger duct of glands, epididymis and male urethra. Here the epithelium is involved in secretion and absorption.

7. Classify glands.

Ans. A gland may consist of one cell or a group of highly specialized epithelial cell. Their main function is secretion.

Glands can be classified:

A. **According to where they release their secretion:**
   i. **Exocrine**—glands that empty their secretion onto to a surface via ducts/tubes. Their main products are mucous, oil, wax, perspiration and digestive enzyme, e.g., sweat and salivary glands.
   ii. **Endocrine**—glands that empty their secretion directly into bloodstream are endocrine glands, e.g., pituitary, thyroid, etc. Their secretions are called hormones which are chemicals that regulate various physiological activities in the body.

B. **Based on structure:**
   i. Unicellular—it is single celled gland, e.g., goblet cell.
   ii. Multicellular—contain many cells and form majority of the glands.

C. **Based on the shape of the secretory portion (called acini):**
   i. Tubular— the gland is tubular shaped.
   ii. Acinar—flask/spherical shaped secretory portion.
   iii. Tubuloacinar—both tubular and flask shaped acini.

8. Structural classification of exocrine glands.

Ans. Exocrine glands secrete their products through a duct onto a skin surface or lumen of hollow organs.

Majority of them are **multicellular glands**. Second variety is the **unicellular gland** which is a single cell secreting directly onto the surface (e.g., goblet cell).

Multicellular gland—classified based in the branching of ducts and shape of secretory portions of the gland.

Accordingly, the following is the classification:

Classification of exocrine glands

- Simple glands—duct of the gland does not branch
  - Simple tubular
  - Simple branched tubular
  - Simple coiled tubular
  - Simple acinar
  - Simple branched acinar
- Compound glands—duct of the gland branches
  - Compound tubular
  - Compound acinar
  - Compound tubuloacinar

9. Describe about the cell junctions.

Ans. Cell junctions' hold the cells with each other. They attach the plasma membrane of adjacent cells **(Fig. 3.11)**.

a. **Tight junctions**—consists of proteins that seal the space between adjacent cells. They prevent passage of substances into blood or surrounding tissues, e.g., stomach, urinary bladder.

b. **Adherents junctions**—it is made of dense plaque of proteins which surround the cell. It resists separation of cells during movements.

c. **Desmosomes**—here the cells are connected by dense plaque and intermediate filaments. It prevents separation of epidermal cells under tension, and also in cardiac muscle cells.

d. **Hemidesmosomes**—they resemble desmosomes, but connect cells with the basement membrane.

e. **Gap junctions**—the adjacent plasma membranes are separated by narrow intercellular space. Tiny fluid filled tunnels connect the cells that allow small molecules to pass through, e.g., involved in transfer of nutrients or nerve impulses.

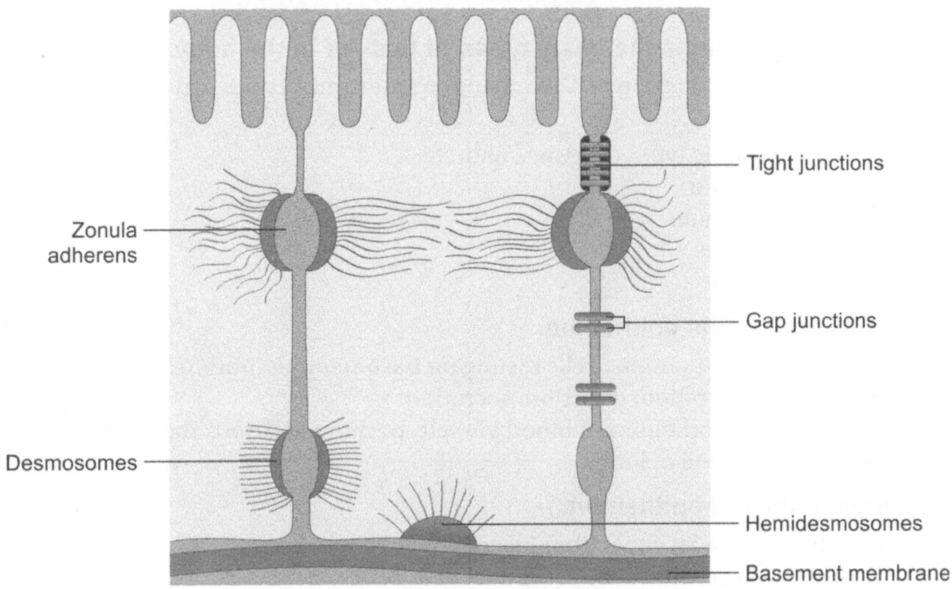

Fig. 3.11: Cell junctions.

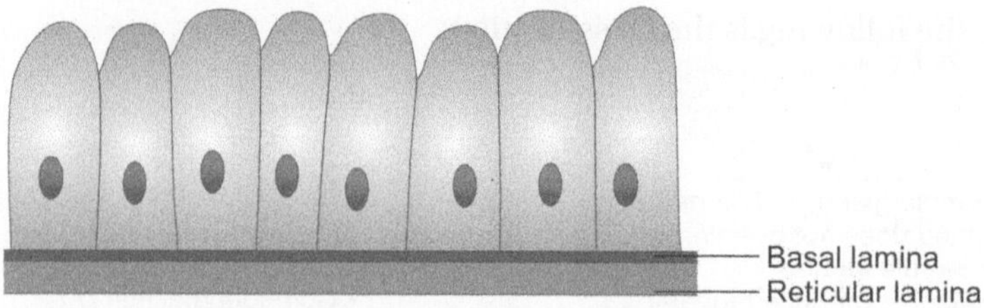

Fig. 3.12: Layers of basement membrane.

10. Explain briefly about basement membrane.

Ans. Basement membrane is a thin extracellular layer which supports the basal surface of the epithelium. It consists of two layers **(Fig. 3.12)**:

i. *Basal lamina*—is closer to the epithelial cell and secreted by them. Laminin molecules in basal lamina attach to hemidesmosomes, thus anchoring the epithelial cells.

ii. *Reticular lamina*—is nothing but the connective tissue containing the collagen fibers and fibroblasts. It supports the epithelium and provides nutrition by diffusion.

Functions of the basement membrane:
- Supports the epithelium.
- Forms surfaces along which epithelial cells migrate during wound healing or growth.
- Prevents large molecules from entering underlying connective tissue.
- Helps to form filtration barrier in kidneys.
- Applied anatomy—basement membrane can get thickened during some pathological conditions like diabetes. It leads to blindness and kidney failure.

SHORT ANSWERS — 2 MARKS

11. Define tissue. Name the basic types of tissues in the body.

Ans. A tissue is defined as group of cells having common embryological origin and performs similar function.

There are four basic types of tissues namely:

a. Epithelial tissue
b. Connective tissue
c. Muscular tissue
d. Nervous tissue

12. Simple squamous epithelium.

Ans. It is made of flat, squamous cells resting on basement membrane.
- Functions— filtration, diffusion, secretion.
- Location—endothelium of blood vessels, peritoneal serous membrane, glomeruli of kidneys, alveoli of lungs.

13. Simple cuboidal epithelium.

Ans. It is made of single layer of cuboidal cells.
- Function—secretion and absorption.
- Location—tubules of kidney, surface of ovary, lens of eye, duct of small glands.

14. Simple columnar epithelium.

Ans. It is made of single layer of columnar cells.

- Function—secretion and absorption.
- Location—stomach, ducts of glands, gallbladder.
- The apical surface of the cell presents some surface modifications which impart additional function like:
  - microvilli (increase surface area for absorption).
  - cilia (for movement of substances).
  - stereo cilia (for absorption).
  - goblet cells (secrete mucus).

15. Write down the functional classification of exocrine glands.

Ans. Exocrine glands are classified into three types based on their mode of secretion.

1. **Merocrine**—most abundant type. Secretory vesicles are expelled by exocytosis, e.g., sweat glands.
2. **Apocrine**—here the apical portion is pinched off along with the secretory vesicles, e.g., mammary gland.
3. **Holocrine**—here the whole cell is ruptured with its plasma membrane, e.g., sebaceous gland of skin.

16. Differentiate exocrine and endocrine glands.

Ans. A gland is defined as a cell or group of cells, that secrete onto a surface, or ducts or directly into bloodstream. All the glands in the body can be exocrine or endocrine.

	Exocrine gland	Endocrine gland (ductless glands)
1.	Need duct for carrying secretions	Release the secretions directly into the bloodstream
2.	Target organs near to the gland	Target organs are far away from the gland that secretes it
3.	For example, sweat gland	For example, thyroid gland

Note:
- Some are mixed glands—pancreas, testis and ovaries
- Contain exocrine and endocrine component.

Notes:

- Epithelium is avascular (no blood supply). It gets nutrition by diffusion from underlying connective tissue.
- Basement membrane can thicken in diseases like diabetes. It will lead to changes in blood vessels of eye, kidneys, etc. This can lead to blindness and kidney failure.
- In cases where epithelial cells can be easily obtained, screening tests can be performed. For example, cervical epithelial cells are scraped (called pap smear) to find out presence or absence of cancerous condition of female genital tract.
- **Metaplasia:** It is the conversion of one type cell to another type, e.g., nonkeratinized squamous epithelium of esophagus converts to columnar type.
- **Dysplasia:** It is the term used to denote replacement of mature epithelial cells with immature cells. It is precursor of cancer/neoplasia.

4

CHAPTER

Connective Tissue

SHORT ESSAYS — 5 MARKS

1. Classify connective tissue in detail.

Ans. Connective tissue binds different tissues of the body together. It consists of an intercellular matrix, fibers and cells.

Classification: *Refer* the flowchart below

- **Embryonic connective tissue**—here the mesenchymal cells are embedded in semifluid connective tissue. It forms the chief connective tissue in embryo and fetus.
- **Connective tissue proper**
  - *Loose connective tissue*—it is a vascular, delicate, flexible tissue where the fibers and the matrix are loosely arranged. It is helpful as packing material between various tissue components, e.g., lamina propria, endomysium.
  - *Adipose tissue*—matrix is filled with adipocytes.
  - *Reticular tissue*—matrix mainly consists of network of reticular fibers. It forms architectural framework for some cellular organs, e.g., lymph node, spleen
  - *Dense connective tissue*—it is located in places where tensile forces is more. The matrix contains densely packed collagen fibers. This gives strength and resistance to traction forces.
    a. Dense regular—the collagen fibers are arranged in an orderly manner, e.g., tendon, ligament, aponeurosis.
    b. Dense irregular—the collagen fibers are oriented in different directions, e.g., dermis of skin.
  - *Elastic tissue*—elastic fibers impart strength and elasticity, e.g., ligamentum nuchae.

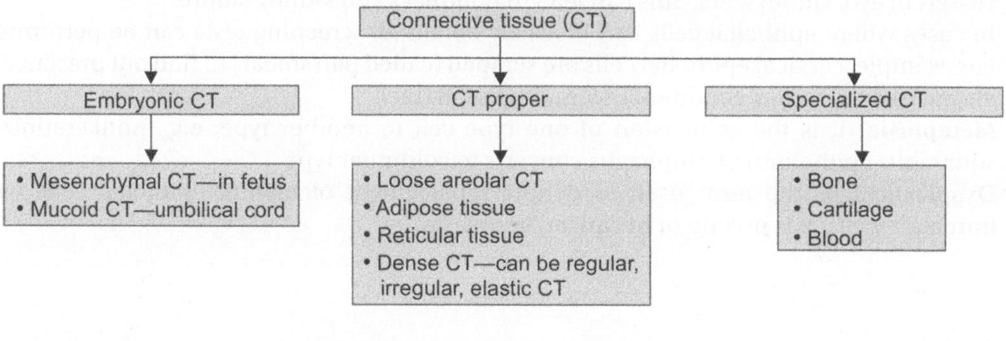

- **Specialized connective tissue**—they have special properties due to their composition. It includes bone, cartilage, blood (dealt in appropriate chapters).

2. General properties of connective tissue.

Ans. Connective tissue is an abundant and widely distributed tissue in the body.

Functions include:

- Support
- Protection and insulation
- Compartmentalization of similar functional structures
- Involved in transport of substances (blood)
- Energy storage (like adipose tissue)
- Source of immune response

Note: It is highly vascular (rich blood supply)

It principally consists of:

- *Extracellular matrix*—is the space between widely separated cells. It consists of ground substance with fibers embedded in it.
- *Connective tissue fibers*
- *Connective tissue cells*

Table 4.1: Components of connective tissue.

Ground substance—may be fluid, gelatinous, semifluid or calcified	• Present between the fibers and CT* cells • Made of water and organic molecules like hyaluronic acid, glucosamine, chondroitin sulfate, etc. • Nature of the matrix determines the function of the CT* • Involved in tissue development, migration and proliferation • Function—supports, binds, acts as a medium for exchange, for metabolic support
CT* fibers	
1. **Collagen** 2. **Elastic** 3. **Reticular**	• Abundant, strong, made of collagen protein • Stretchable, strong, made of elastin protein • Finer fibers, support some glands, lymphoid organs
CT* cells	
1. **Fibroblasts** 2. **Macrophages** 3. **Adipocytes** 4. **Neutrophils, eosinophils** 5. **Plasma cells** 6. **Mast cells**	• Abundant cell type, synthesize ground substance and CT* fibers • Destroy bacteria and other debris by phagocytosis • Store lipids • For defense against any infection • Produce antibodies in response to infection • Produce histamine during inflammation

*Connective tissue

3. Describe about connective tissue fibers.

Ans. The strength and support provided by the connective tissue is due to the presence of fibers. They are of three types—collagen, elastic and reticular fibers. They are all synthesized by the fibroblasts.

Collagen Fibers

- They are tough, predominant type of fiber.
- Resist pulling forces, yet flexible fibers.
- Their association with water around it determines the CT properties. The collagen in cartilage has more water molecules around it compared to bone, hence cartilage has a cushion effect.
- They do not branch, and are arranged in bundles. This provides tensile strength.
- Location: Bone, cartilage, tendon and ligament.

Elastic Fibers

- They are less abundant, have smaller diameter, branch and form a network.
- It is made of a protein called elastin along with a glycoprotein-fibrillin.
- Due to their unique molecular structure, they can be stretched 150% of their length, as well as capable of recoiling once the force is removed termed elasticity.
- Location: Skin, blood vessels, lungs, etc.

Reticular Fibers

- These are fine collagen fibers, and form a branching network.
- Provide strength and support.
- Forms framework for many soft tissue organs, such as spleen, liver and lymph nodes.

4. Describe about adipose tissue (Fig 4.1).

Ans.
- Adipose tissue is made of cells which store triglycerides.
- Cells called adipocytes are derived from fibroblasts.
- The fat is in form of a large single droplet, fills the whole cell.
- The nucleus is pushed to the periphery with scanty cytoplasm.
- Adipose tissue increases with weight gain.
- In adults, the adipose tissue just described is present, whereas in newborns brown adipose tissue is abundant (described below).

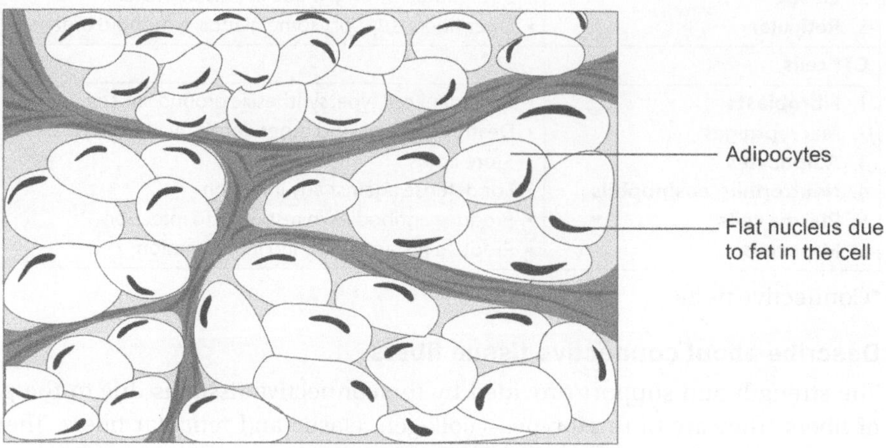

Fig. 4.1: Adipose tissue.

- Location: Around kidney, heart, mesentery, subcutaneous fat over lower abdomen, around eyeball, etc.

Functions—reduces heat loss, energy reserve, supports and protects organs.

- *Brown adipose tissue*—is found in newborn and infants. It is richly vascular. Fat is in form of numerous droplets; cells are rich in mitochondria. It generates heat, beneficial to maintain body temperature.
- *Applied anatomy*—liposuction is a procedure to remove excess fat in locations like thigh, abdomen, breasts, buttocks, arms for improving body contour and proportions.

5. Describe about loose areolar tissue (Fig 4.2).

Ans.
- Loose CT/areolar tissue is widely distributed type of CT.
- Consists of:
  - CT fibers—collagen, elastic, reticular.
  - CT cells—macrophages, fibroblasts, mast cells, plasma cells, adipocytes, WBCs.
  - Semifluid ground substance—hyaluronic acid, chondroitin sulfate, dermatan and keratin sulfate.
- Function—forms packing material throughout the body. It is required for strength, elasticity and support.
- Location—subcutaneous layer of the skin, papillary layer of dermis, lamina propria of mucous membrane.

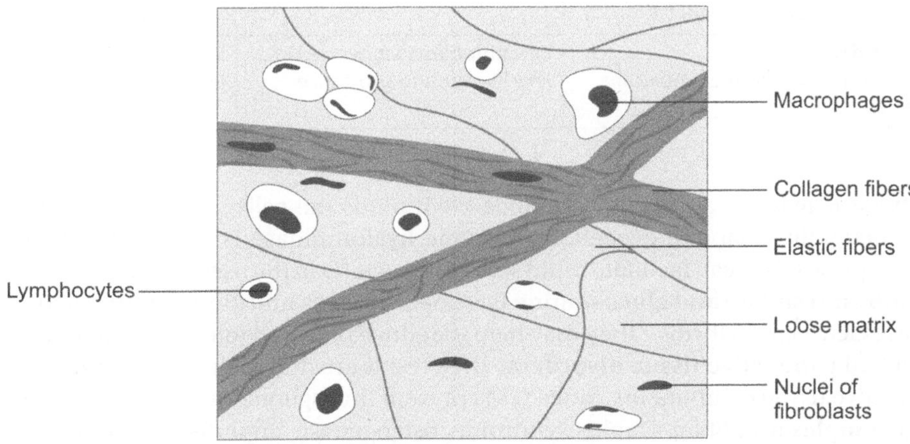

Fig. 4.2: Components of connective tissue.

SHORT ANSWERS 2 MARKS

6. Name the cells of connective tissue.

Ans. The cells of connective tissue can be fixed or free cells.

a. Fixed cells—fibroblasts, adipocyte, macrophages.
b. Free cells—mast cells, plasma cells, leukocytes and free macrophages.

7. Properties of the various CT. (Each type can be asked for two marks question)

Ans. *Refer* **Table 4.2.**

Table 4.2: Description of different connective tissue.

Sl. No.	Type of CT	Properties	Location
1.	**Loose connective tissue** Function—support, elasticity	Widely distributed Fibers are loosely scattered in the semifluid ground substance with few cells	Subcutaneous tissue Dermis of skin Around blood vessels and nerves
2.	**Dense regular CT** Function—helps to attach two structures	Collagen fibers are arranged in a regular fashion	Tendon, ligaments and aponeurosis
3.	**Dense regular CT** Function—provides tensile strength	Collagen fibers are arranged in an irregular fashion with few fibroblasts.	Fasciae, periosteum, capsules of glands, joint capsules
4.	**Adipose tissue** Function—packing material, energy source, support and protection	Adipocytes store triglycerides Adults—white adipose tissue Newborn and children—brown adipose tissue	Around the heart, kidney, eyeball
5.	**Elastic CT** Function—allows expansion and recoil	Elastic fibers with fibroblasts	Lung tissue, elastic arteries, vocal cords
6.	**Embryonic CT** Function—CT basis in fetal life, also gives rise to all other adult CT	Mesenchymal cells embedded in semifluid connective tissue	Forms the chief CT in embryo and fetus
7.	**Mucoid CT** Function—support the umbilical vessels	Few fibroblasts embedded in jelly like ground substance	In umbilical cord as Wharton's jelly

Note:

- **Hyaluronic acid**—is a viscous substance and it binds the cells involved in lubrication of joint, maintains shape of eyeball. An enzyme hyaluronidase is synthesized by bacteria, WBCs, sperms. This can facilitate rapid spread of bacteria in the tissue, as in some infections.
- **Chondroitin sulfate and glucosamine** have been used as nutritional supplements in joint diseases like osteoarthritis. They may help to reduce pain and joint inflammation.
- **Inherited connective tissue disorders:** They result are due to defective genes coding for connective tissue components. Since CT is present throughout, many organs are affected. **Few examples are:** Ehler-Danlos syndrome, osteogenesis imperfecta, Marfan syndrome, epidermolysis bullosa.
- **Autoimmune disorders affecting CT**—polymyositis-dermatomyositis, rheumatoid arthritis, scleroderma, systemic lupus erythematosus (SLE).

5

CHAPTER

Bone and Cartilage

LONG ESSAYS — 10 MARKS

1. Classify the bones with examples. Describe the parts and blood supply of a typical long bone.

Ans. Bones can be classified in various ways:

1. **Regional**
   - Axial skeleton—skull, vertebrae, ribs and sternum
   - Appendicular skeleton—upper and lower limb bones.
2. **Mode of ossification**
   - Membranous—like parietal and frontal bones
   - Cartilaginous—all long bones.
3. **Structure**
   - Spongy—inner part of the bone
   - Compact—outer cortical portion of the bone.
4. **Shape, size and consistency**
   a. Long bones—have two expanded ends connected by a narrow shaft. Shaft consists of outer compact bone and inner spongy bone (medullary cavity). They ossify in cartilage, e.g., humerus, femur.
   b. Short bones—small and polyhedral, e.g., tarsal and carpals.
   c. Flat bones—two plates of compact bone with spongy bone in between. Ossifies from membrane, e.g., parietal, frontal bones.
   d. Irregular bone—irregular in shape and mainly consists of spongy bone, e.g.,vertebrae and hip bone.
   e. Sesamoid bones—they are small bones developing in a tendon. Periosteum is absent, e.g., patella.
   f. Accessory bones—they appear with center of ossification and fail to fuse with the main mass of bone, e.g., sutural bones.
   g. Pneumatic bones—bones contain spaces within them. So, bones are lighter. They add resonance to the sound. Act as air conditioning chamber by adding humidity and temperature to the inspired air, e.g., maxilla, and frontal bone.

Parts of a Long Bone

Long bone has an *outer compact* bone and *inner spongy* bone (medullary/marrow cavity).

Its outermost covering is called ***Periosteum***. Periosteum is a tough, connective tissue sheath. It is helps in growth, nutrition to the bone as well provides attachment to the tendons.

Long bone consists of a shaft and two expanded ends **(Fig. 5.1)**.

- **Diaphysis**—is the long, cylindrical and central portion of the bone. It ossifies from primary center.
- **Epiphysis**—expanded terminal end of the bone. It ossifies from secondary center. They form joints with the adjacent bones.
- **Metaphysis**—portion of the diaphysis in contact with epiphyseal cartilage. It contributes to increase in length of the bone. It is the most actively growing area of the bone and has rich blood supply. Hence, it is common site for infection.

Epiphyseal cartilage: Plate of hyaline cartilage in between epiphysis and diaphysis of growing bone.

Medullary or the marrow cavity: It is a hollow internal cavity, filled with yellow bone marrow in adults. In fetal life and young children, it contains red bone marrow and involved in hemopoiesis.

Blood supply to the long bone—following are the sources of nutrition to the bone **(Fig. 5.2)**:

- Nutrient artery—enters the bone through nutrient foramen and supplies cortex and medullary cavity of the bone.
- Metaphyseal artery—it is branch from muscles attached to the bone.
- Epiphyseal artery—usually derived from anastomoses around joints.
- Periosteal arteries—they are derived from adjacent muscles and supply the periosteum.

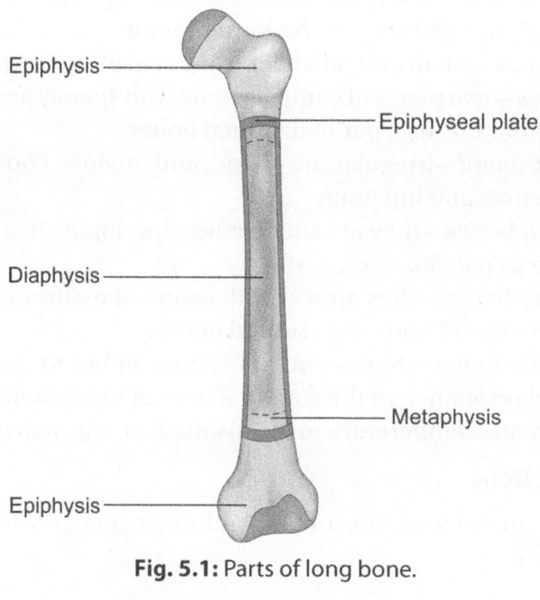

Fig. 5.1: Parts of long bone.

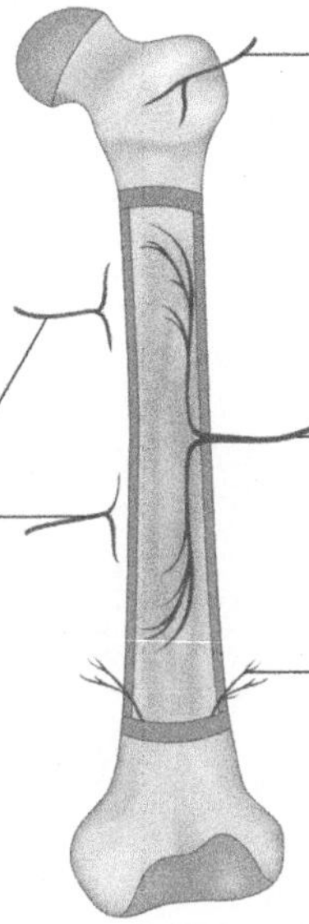

Fig. 5.2: Blood supply of long bone.

SHORT ESSAYS 5 MARKS

2. Classify the bones based on their shape (Fig. 5.3).

Ans. The bones form the main skeletal framework for the body. They are classified as follows:

a. **Long bones**—have two expanded (termed epiphysis) ends connected by a narrow shaft (the diaphysis). The shaft consists of outer compact bone and inner spongy bone (medullary cavity). They ossify in cartilage, e.g., humerus, femur.
b. **Short bones**— they are small and polyhedral, e.g., tarsal and carpals
c. **Flat bones**— consist of two plates of compact bone with spongy bone in between. Ossifies from membrane, e.g., bones of skull, scapula.
d. **Irregular bone**—irregular in shape and mainly consists of spongy bone, e.g., vertebrae and hip bone.
e. **Sesamoid bones**—they are small bones developing in a tendon. Periosteum is absent, e.g., patella.
f. **Accessory bones**—they appear with center of ossification and fail to fuse with the main mass of bone, e.g., sutural bones.
g. **Pneumatic bones**—they contain air spaces with epithelial mucosal lining. So bones are lighter. They add resonance to the voice. Act as air conditioning chamber by adding humidity and temperature to the inspired air, e.g., maxilla and frontal bone.

3. Enumerate the functions of skeletal system.

Ans. **Skeletal system performs the following functions (Table 5.1):**

a. Structural framework of the body is by bone and cartilage
b. For protection of underlying organs, e.g., brain, heart, liver, etc.
c. Required for movements—this function is brought about by formation of joints.

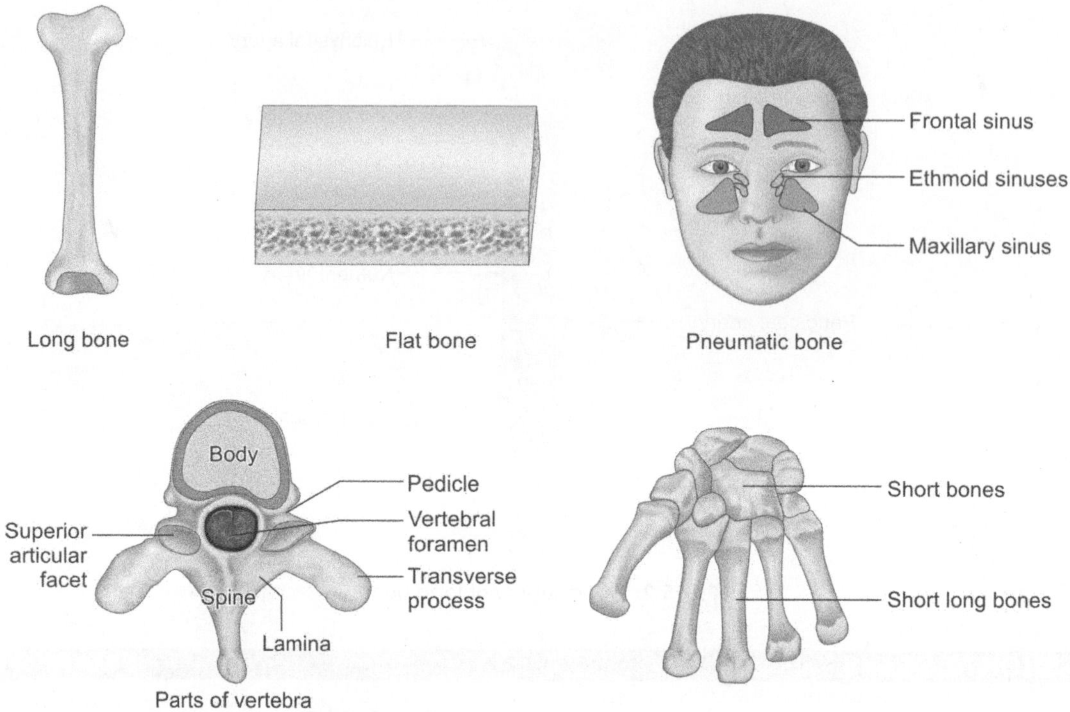

Fig. 5.3: Classification bones based on shape.

d. Involved in homeostasis of calcium and other minerals.
e. Hematopoiesis—this is one of the location both in fetal and adult life, where production of blood components take place.
f. Attachment to skeletal muscles—thereby movements are possible across joints.

Table 5.1: Disorders of skeletal system due to imbalance of hormones and vitamins.

Sl. No.	Name	Clinical syndrome
1.	Growth hormone increase	• During childhood—gigantism • Adults—acromegaly
2.	Growth hormone decrease	Dwarfism (called pituitary dwarfism)
3.	Vitamin D deficiency—leads to inadequate calcification of extracellular matrix	• Rickets—in children • Osteomalacia—in adults
4.	Calcium deficiency	Rickets, osteopenia and osteoporosis

4. Describe the structure of different parts of long bone.

Ans. The following are the parts of a long bone **(Figs. 5.1 and 5.4)**:

a. **Periosteum**—is the outermost covering. It consists of collagen fibers and osteocytes. Periosteum is involved in growth, nutrition to the bone as well gives attachment to tendons.
b. **Cortex—**it is the outer layer made of compact bone. It gives strength to the bone.
c. **Marrow cavity**—is hollow space within the diaphysis. In adults it is filled with yellow bone marrow and blood vessels.

d. **Diaphysis**—central cylindrical part of the long bone. It ossifies from primary center.
e. **Epiphysis**—expanded terminal end of the bone, proximal and distal. They ossify from secondary centers. It has cancellous bone surrounded by thin layer of compact bone.
f. **Metaphysis**—portion of the diaphysis in contact with epiphyseal cartilage. It is the most actively growing area of the bone. It has rich blood supply. Hence, it is common site for infection.
g. **Epiphyseal cartilage**—after growth is completed, it unites with epiphysis and diaphysis called fusion of the bone (synostosis). It is a plate of hyaline cartilage and helps in increase in the length of long bone.

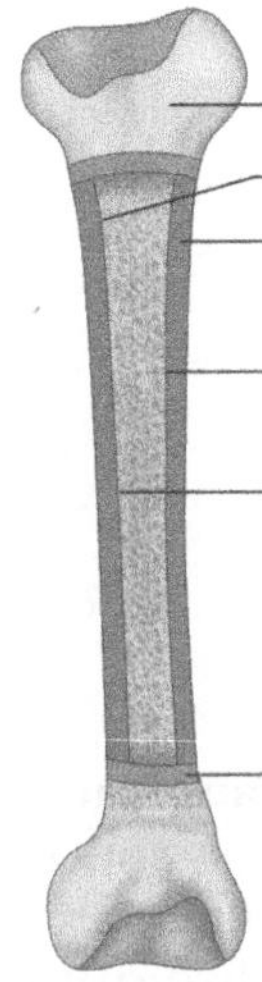

Fig. 5.4: Gross features of long bone.

5. Structure of a compact bone (or histological features of a long bone) (Fig. 5.5).

Ans. Compact bone is a hard bony tissue beneath the periosteum. It is present in all the bones. Function—protection, support, resists weight.

On histological sections, the compact bone presents the following features:

- Periosteum
- Haversian system
- Circumferential lamellae
- Interstitial lamellae

Periosteum—is the tough, connective tissue covering of the bone. It is made of outer fibrous and inner cellular layer. The inner cellular layer is lined by osteoblasts, hence involved in growth and repair.

Haversian system (osteon)—is the structural unit of the compact bone. It has a central Haversian canal surrounded by 6-12 **concentric lamellae**. Haversian canal provides passage for blood vessels, nerves and lymphatics.

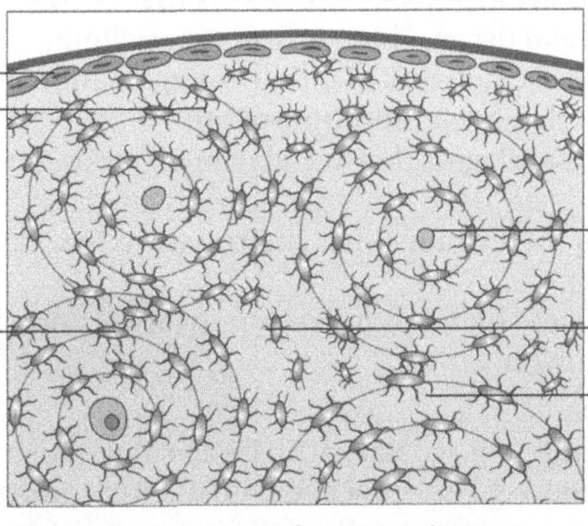

Fig. 5.5: Histology of compact bone.

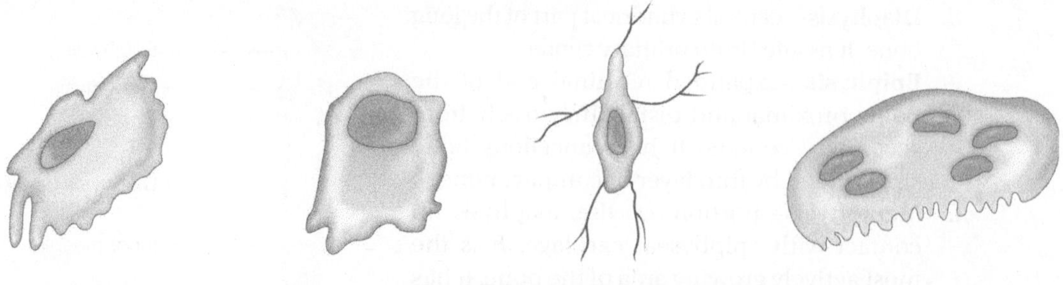

Fig. 5.6: Cells of the bone.

Concentric lamellae—are parallel layers of extracellular osteoid matrix. These lamellae contain both organic and inorganic materials. Organic material is the matrix with collagen fibers embedded in it. Inorganic minerals like calcium will be deposited in the form of hydroxyapatite crystals.

- Collagen is responsible for the mechanical strength of the bone.
- Calcium provides hardness and rigidity to the bone.
- In between the lamellae, are the **lacunae** containing **osteocytes. Canaliculi** radiate from these lacunae containing processes of osteocytes. Canaliculi help to intercommunicate between the lacunae and with the Haversian canal. This arrangement is essential for providing nutrition, oxygen, etc.
- **Circumferential lamellae** are present just beneath the periosteum as well as outside the endosteum.
- **Interstitial lamellae**—are present in between the osteons.

Following are the cells present in a bone (Fig. 5.6):

- **Osteoprogenitor cells**—they give rise to osteoblasts.
- **Osteocyte**—involved in normal maintenance of the bone.
- **Osteoblasts**—give rise to osteocytes. They synthesize organic matrix and fibers. They also help in deposition of bone in the lamellae.
- **Osteoclasts**—helps in resorption of bone. They are important in bone removal and remodeling.
- **Bone lining cells**—are found lining the endosteum.

6. Classify cartilages. Describe the histology of hyaline cartilage.

Ans. Cartilage is a skeletal tissue which is firm yet resilient.

- It consists of dense network of either collagen and/or elastic fibers embedded in a gel-like matrix rich in chondroitin sulfate.
- Strength of the cartilage is due to collagen fibers, and resiliency is due to chondroitin sulfate.
- Large amount of extracellular matrix with few cartilage cells (chondrocytes) embedded in it.
- It does not possess blood or nerve supply. It gets nutrition from perichondrium by process of diffusion.

It is of three types:

1. Hyaline cartilage, e.g., costal cartilage, cartilages of trachea.
2. Elastic cartilage, e.g., external acoustic meatus, pinna, Eustachian tube.
3. Fibrocartilage, e.g., intervertebral disc, menisci of knee joint.

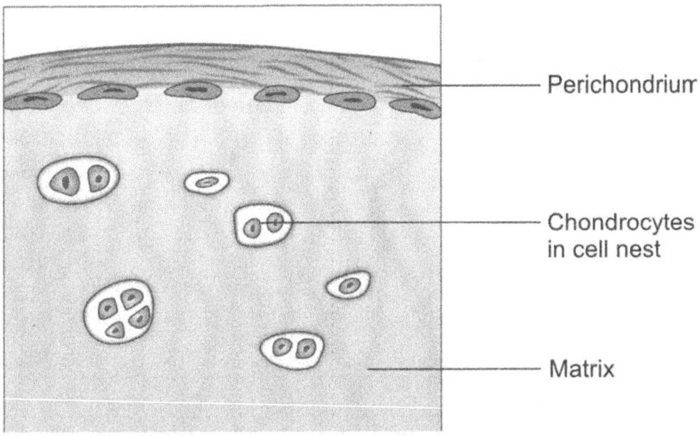

Fig. 5.7: Structure of hyaline cartilage.

Structure of Hyaline Cartilage (Fig. 5.7):

- Outer layer of perichondrium—which is made of outer fibrous and inner cellular layer. It has blood vessels and nerves, and is the source of new cartilage cells. (perichondrium is absent in articular cartilage and epiphyseal plate).
- Matrix is bluish-white, translucent and homogenous (collagen fibers not made out by regular staining, hence homogenous).
- Type II collagen fibers are embedded in it.
- The chondrocytes are arranged singular or in groups in **lacunae** within the extracellular matrix.
- **Functions:** Provides smooth articular surface at joints, major type of skeletal tissue in fetus, helps in increase in the length of long bone.
- Can undergo calcification, hence prone for fracture.
- *Example*—at the end of long bones, anterior ends of ribs (costal cartilage), nose, parts of larynx, trachea, bronchi, fetal skeleton.

7. Enumerate the bones forming the axial and appendicular skeleton.

Ans. Axial skeleton consists of the bones along the longitudinal axis of the body. Appendicular skeleton consists of bones of the upper and lower limb. The bones are enlisted in **Table 5.2**.

Table 5.2: Components of skeleton.

Axial skeleton		Appendicular skeleton	
Skull	Cranium—08 Face—14 Auditory ossicles—6 Hyoid—1	**Upper limb**	***Pectoral girdle*** a. Clavicle—2 b. Scapula—2
Vertebral column- 26	Cervical—7 Thoracic—12 Lumbar—5 Sacrum—01 Coccyx—1 to 3		***Free upper limb*** Humerus—2 Radius—2 Ulna—2 Carpals—16 Metacarpals—10 Phalanges—28

Contd...

Contd...

Axial skeleton		Appendicular skeleton	
Thorax	Sternum—1 Ribs—24	**Lower limb**	***Pelvic girdle*** Hip bone— 2
			Free lower limb Femur—2 Tibia—2 Fibula—2 Tarsal—14 Metatarsals—10 Phalanges—28
Total	80		126
Total bones in the human adult skeleton—206			

8. Enumerate the bones of skull and face.

Ans. The skull or the cranium is made of 22 bones and supported on the upper end of vertebral column.

These are again classified as:

- Cranial bones—protect the brain.
- Facial bones—form part of the skeleton of face.

They are listed in **Table 5.3**.

Table 5.3: Bones of skull and face.

Cranial bones	Facial bones
Frontal—1 Parietal—2 Temporal—2 Occipital—1 Sphenoid—1 Ethmoid—1 Inferior nasal concha—2 Vomer—1	Nasal—2 Lacrimal—2 Maxilla—2 Mandible—1 Zygomatic—1 Palatine—2

9. Mandible.

Ans. Mandible is the only movable bone of the skull. It gives attachment to the muscles of mastication. It is involved in the formation of temporomandibular joint.

Parts: Body, pair of rami on either side and two processes—coronoid and condyloid process **(Fig. 5.8)**.

- Lateral surface of ramus—masseter muscle.
- Medial surface—mandibular foramen for inferior alveolar nerves and vessels. Medial pterygoid muscle insertion.
- Symphysis menti—unites two halves of the body.
- Inner surface of the body—related to submandibular and sublingual salivary glands.
- Outer surface of the body—few muscles of face attach.
- Mandible ossifies in membrane.
- Alveolar/upper border has sockets for teeth.
- The condyloid process forms temporomandibular joint (TMJ) with temporal bone.

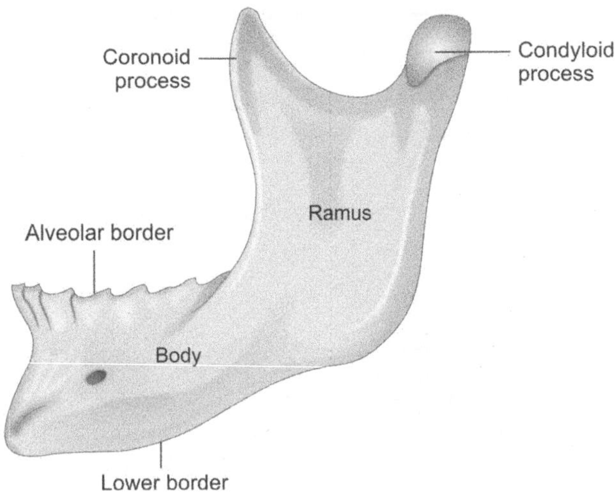

Fig. 5.8: Parts of mandible.

Muscle attachments:
- Temporalis—coronoid process.
- Lateral pterygoid—neck of mandible (condyloid process).
- Masseter—lateral surface of ramus.
- Medial pterygoid—medial surface of ramus.
- Lower border of body—platysma.
- Mandible also provides attachment to few muscles of face, tongue, pharynx.

10. Different regions and curvatures of vertebral column.

Ans. Vertebral column is made of vertebrae, intervertebral discs, ligaments and joints. During fetal life, 33 vertebrae make up the vertebral column. Later, vertebrae in sacrum and coccygeal region fuse, resulting in 26 vertebrae in adults.

The different **regions** are **(Fig. 5.9)**:

a. Cervical region—7 cervical vertebrae.
b. Thoracic region—12 thoracic vertebrae.
c. Lumbar region—5 lumbar vertebrae.
d. Sacral region—1 (5 fused sacral vertebrae).
e. Coccyx—1 (made of 4 fused coccygeal vertebrae).

The adult vertebral column is straight when viewed from front. When viewed from side, it presents **curves (Fig. 5.10)**:
- Cervical and lumbar curvature—convex anteriorly.
- Thoracic and sacral curvature—concave anteriorly.

In the fetus, a single curve is present.
- Around 3rd month—due to development of erect head, cervical curve is formed.
- As the child stands up and walks, lumbar curve develops.

Hence, curves can be **(Fig. 5.10)**:
- **Primary curves**—thoracic and sacral. They are present at birth.
- **Secondary curves**—cervical and lumbar. They develop due to secondary factors.

These curvatures are helpful for the following:
- Increases the strength of vertebral column
- For balance in upright posture

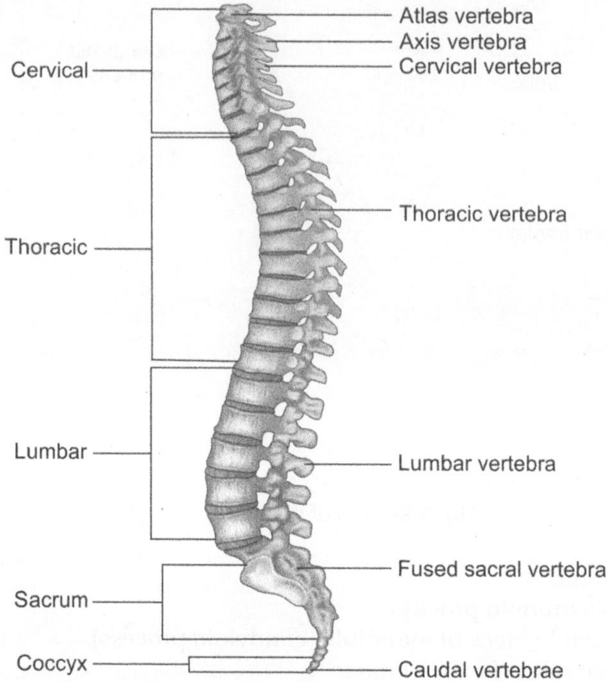

Fig. 5.9: Regions of vertebral column.

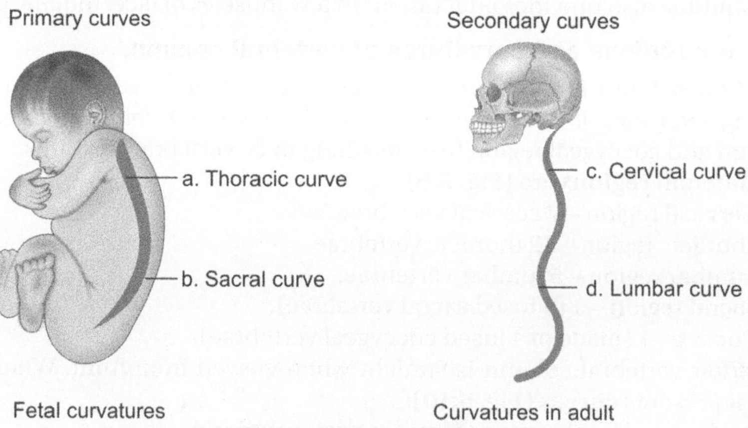

Fig. 5.10: Curves of the vertebral column.

- Shock absorber
- Protection from fracture.

11. Bones forming thoracic cage (Fig. 5.11).

Ans. Thorax is a bony cage formed by sternum (breast bone), costal cartilage, ribs and bodies of the thoracic vertebra. It protects the vital organs—the heart and lungs.

***Sternum*—**is a long, flat bone in the anterior midline of bony thorax. It consists of three parts- manubrium, body and xiphoid process. Junction between body and

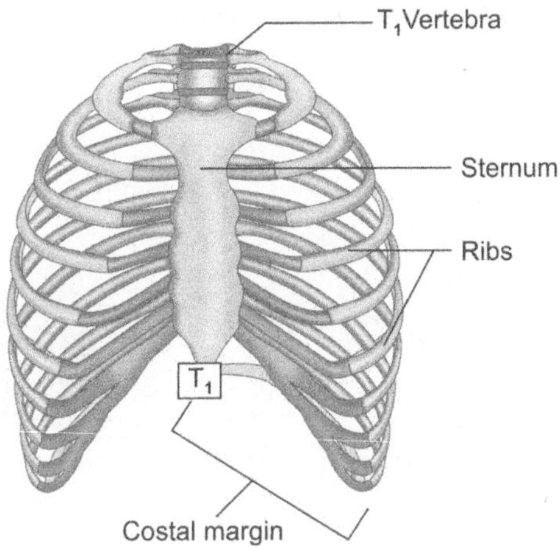

Fig. 5.11: Bones of thoracic cage.

manubrium forms the sternal angle. Second rib and costal cartilage lies at the level of sternal angle. Manubrium has a notch in its center called jugular/suprasternal notch. On each side, lateral to the notch is the clavicular notch.

Ribs—lateral to sternum are 12 pairs of ribs connected to sternum via costal cartilage. 1st and 2nd ribs are attached to manubrium. 3rd to 7th is attached to body of the sternum. 8th to 12th ribs are not attached to sternum. 11th and 12th ribs are called floating ribs, as they are attached only to the body of T11 and T12 vertebra.

Thoracic vertebrae—are 12 in number. They are located on the posterior aspect of the thorax.

12. Describe about fontanelles.

Ans. Fontanelles are mesenchyme filled spaces in between the bones of newborn. They are the soft spots in the skull, and the mesenchyme is not ossified. They are gradually ossified by intramembranous ossification and finally replaced by sutures.

Functions

- Since fontanelles are not ossified, they make the newborn skull flexible.
- This enables the newborn easy passage through birth canal.
- Allows for rapid growth of brain during infancy.

Named fontanels **(Fig. 5.12)**

- Unpaired **anterior fontanelle**—is located in the midline between the frontal and parietal bones.
- Unpaired **posterior fontanelle**—is located in the midline between the two parietal and occipital bones. It closes around 2 months after birth.
- Paired **anterolateral fontanelle**—located between frontal, parietal, temporal and sphenoid bones. They close around 3 months.
- Paired **posterolateral fontanelle**—located between parietal, temporal, occipital bones. They close around 12 months.

Note: Anterior fontanelle is the largest one. It is placed at the junction between coronal, sagittal and frontal sutures. It is diamond shaped. It measures 4 × 2.5 cm. It allows easy passage of fetal skull through the birth canal. It closes around 18–24 months.

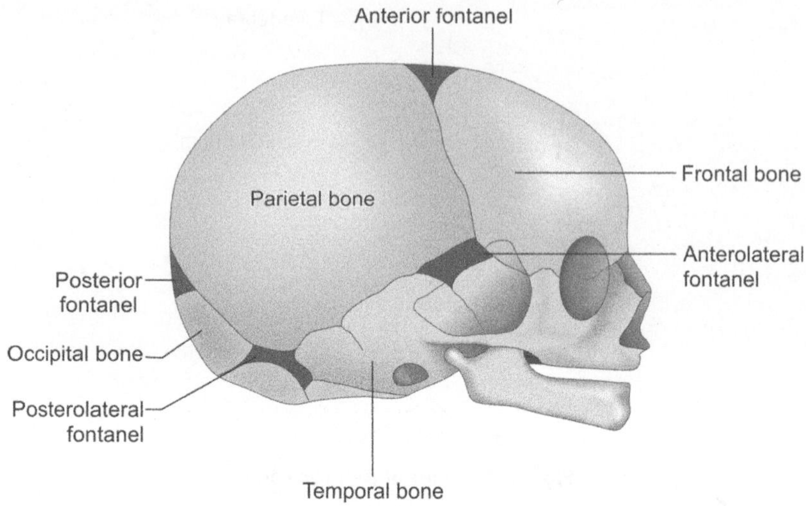

Fig. 5.12: Fetal skull with fontanels.

Clinically, it has many applications:

- During examination of an infant, anterior fontanelle is palpated.
- Sunken fontanelle—indicates dehydration.
- Bulging fontanelle—indicates increased intracranial pressure.
- It is also beneficial for taking blood from the superior sagittal sinus in newborns.

13. Name the parts of a vertebra.

Ans. Vertebral column consists of 26 vertebrae. The vertebral body forms the central column in the midline and is weight-bearing.

Each vertebra varies region wise. But a typical vertebra is made of **(Fig. 5.13)**:

- Body—thick, anterior portion. It bears weight.
- Vertebral arch—consists of pedicle and laminae.
- Vertebral arches enclose vertebral foramen along with the vertebral body.
- Processes—superior and inferior articular facets, transverse processes, spine.
- Spinal canal—vertebral foramina of all vertebrae is the spinal canal. It contains spinal cord and meninges, internal vertebral plexus, spinal arteries.

14. Blood and nerve supply of long bone.

Ans. The bone has a rich blood supply. Following are the sources of blood supply to a long bone **(Fig. 5.2)**:

a. Periosteal arteries—are branches of adjacent muscular arteries. They enter through Volkmann's canal to supply periosteum and outer compact bone.

b. Nutrient artery—enters through nutrient foramen. It divides into ascending and descending branches. It supplies inner compact bone, spongy bone, red bone marrow of the shaft.

c. Epiphyseal arteries—supply the ends (epiphysis).

d. Metaphyseal arteries—supply the metaphysis. They are branches from arteries supplying joints and are in shape of hair pin loop. This predisposes metaphysis to infection.

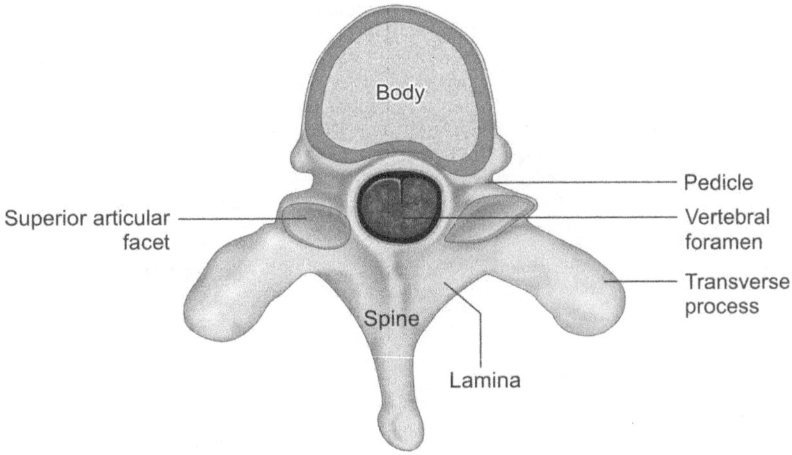

Fig. 5.13: Parts of vertebra.

Nerve supply—nerves accompany the blood vessels. Nerves supplying periosteum are pain fibers. Hence in case of fracture, bone tumor or during biopsy, there is pain.

15. Different type of fractures.

Ans. Fracture is a break in the bone. The various types are:

1. Stress fracture—microscopic fracture without any evidence of injury. It results due to repeated strenuous activity. Tibia and metatarsals are commonly involved.
2. Simple (closed) fracture—bone is fractured without skin damage/any wound. Bone is broken without displacement of the bony fragments.
3. Compound/open fracture—the broken ends of bones protrude through the skin.
4. Comminuted fracture—bone is broken into smaller fragments.
5. Greenstick fracture—is seen in children. One side of the bone breaks, other side bends. This is because the bone is not ossified fully.

16. Parts of scapula and the joints forms by it.

Ans. Scapula consists of **(Fig. 5.14)**:

- Body—triangular. It has medial, lateral and superior borders.
- Processes—triangular spine, coracoid and acromion process (acromion forms the highest point on the shoulder).
- Angles—superior, lateral and inferior.
- Fossae—supraspinous, infraspinous, subscapular fossae.
- Has an articular glenoid cavity at its lateral angle.

Joints formed by scapula:

a. Acromioclavicular joint.
b. Shoulder joint with the head of humerus.

17. Humerus.

Ans. Humerus is the bone of the arm, longest and strongest bone of upper limb. It consists of the following parts **(Fig. 5.15A)**:

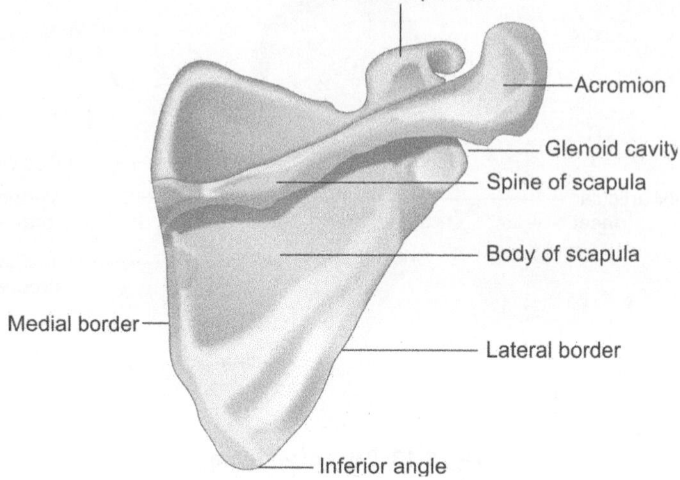

Fig. 5.14: Parts of scapula.

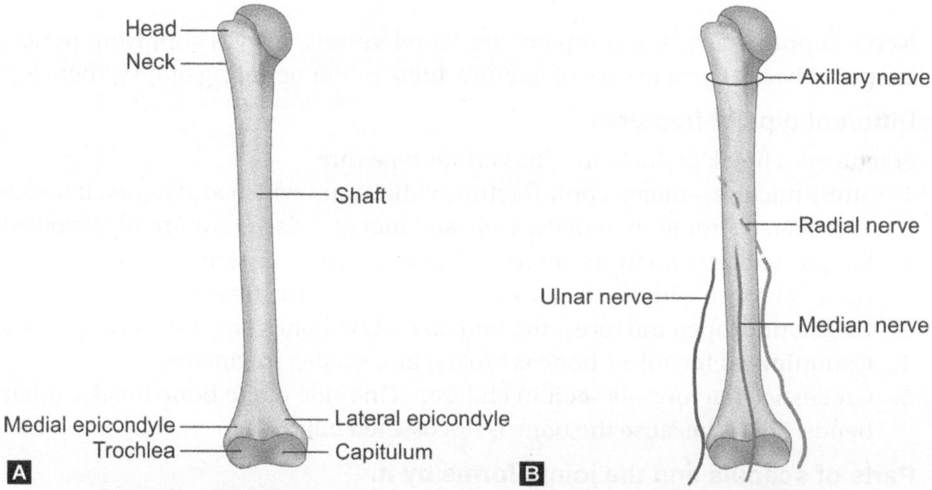

Figs. 5.15A and B: (A) Parts of humerus; (B) Nerves related to humerus.

a. Upper end—has head which forms shoulder joint. Also has greater and lesser tubercles for muscle attachments (greater tubercle is the lateral most point on the shoulder).
b. Shaft—is cylindrical. It has a deltoid tuberosity for deltoid insertion. Spiral groove is on posterior surface and related to radial nerve.
c. Lower end—presents medial and lateral epicondyles, capitulum, trochlea, radial and coronoid fossa.
d. Two necks—anatomical neck is distal to the head. Surgical neck is junction between upper end and the shaft.
e. *Surgical neck* is more prone for fractures. It is also related to axillary nerve. Dislocation of head of humerus (shoulder dislocation) can compress axillary nerve.

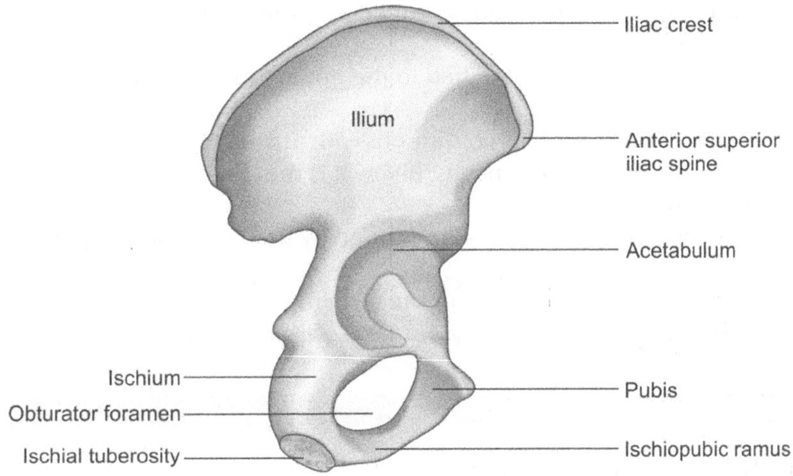

Fig. 5.16: Parts of hip bone.

Joints formed:
- Shoulder joint with scapula
- Elbow joint

Nerves related **(Fig. 5.15B)**:
- Axillary nerve to the surgical neck.
- Musculocutaneous neve to the shaft, anteriorly.
- Radial nerve in the spiral groove.
- Ulnar nerve to the medial epicondyle.

18. Hip bone.

Ans. Hip bone belongs to the pelvic girdle. It consists of three components—ilium, ischium and pubis **(Fig. 5.16)**.

A. Ilium:
- Upper expanded portion.
- Iliac crest is prominent bony landmark at its upper border.
- It ends in anterior and posterior superior iliac spines.
- Presents *greater sciatic notch* behind—forms a foramen through which structures from pelvis enter the gluteal region: Most significant being the *sciatic nerve.*
- Lesser sciatic foramen—internal pudendal vessels and nerves enter pelvis.
- Iliac fossa—presents arcuate line. It demarcates false pelvis above, true pelvis below.

B. Ischium:
- Lower smaller portion.
- Has rough area—ischial tuberosity for attachment to hamstring muscles of back of thigh.
- Remaining portion is subcutaneous, the area over which we sit. Since it is just below the skin, it hurts if sat on bony surface.
- *Ischial spine* is related to *pudendal nerve* used to *give pudendal block.*

C. Pubis:
- Is the anterior portion.
- Forms pubic symphysis with the opposite pubic bone.

- Presents pubic crest, pubic tubercle; provide attachment to ligaments and muscles.
- Inguinal ligament is attached to the pubic tubercle and anterior superior iliac spine.
- Pectineal line becomes continuous with arcuate line to form *pelvic brim*. Above the pelvic brim is false pelvis, below it is the true pelvis.

D. Acetabulum:
- It is a cup shaped depression formed by point of union of pubis, ischium and ilium.
- Articulates with head of femur to form hip joint.
- The three bones also enclose *obturator foramen*, closed by obturator membrane.

SHORT ANSWERS — 2 MARKS

19. Name the parts of a long bone.

Ans. The long bone consists of two ends connected by a shaft **(Fig. 5.1)**.
- The ends are called epiphysis, and the shaft is the diaphysis.
- In between the epiphysis and diaphysis, zone of growing bone is present in children called metaphysis.
- Periosteum—is the outer protective layer of the bone.
- Medullary cavity—it is a hollow cylindrical space within the diaphysis. It is filled with yellow bone marrow and blood vessels in adult bone.

20. Periosteum.

Ans.
- It is a tough connective tissue sheath around the bones.
- Consists of—(a) an outer fibrous layer and (b) inner cellular layer.
- Functions—carries blood supply, helps in fracture repair, and is the site for attachment of muscles and ligaments.

21. Flat bone with example.

Ans. Flat bones are called so since they are flat in appearance. They consist of outer- and inner tables with spongy bone inside. They are united with adjacent bones by a type joint called suture. Most bones of the skull are flat bones, e.g., temporal, frontal, parietal bones.

22. Name the bone cells.

Ans. The bone cells are involved in synthesis and maintenance of bone tissue.
They are as follows **(Fig. 5.6)**:
- Osteocytes—involved in normal maintenance of the bone
- Osteoblasts—give rise to osteocytes. They synthesize matrix and fibers
- Osteoclasts—resorption of bone. They are important in bone removal and remodeling.
- Osteoprogenitor cells—they are the stem cells giving rise to osteoblasts.

23. Name the skull sutures.

Ans. A suture is a fibrous joint made of dense irregular connective tissue. They are present only in skull. Some of the important sutures are as follows **(Fig. 5.17)**:

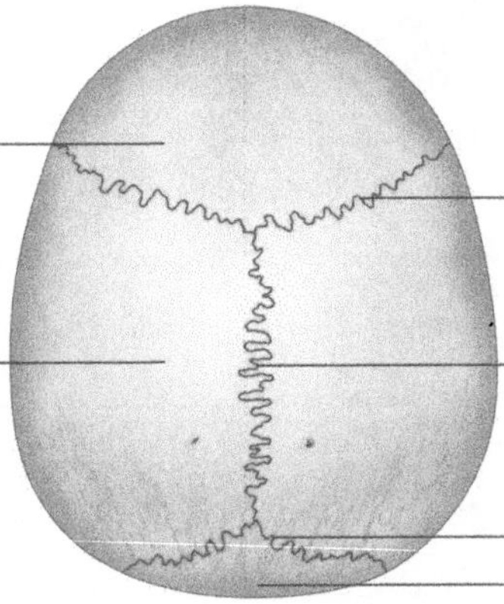

Fig. 5.17: Skull sutures.

- Sagittal suture—present in the midline uniting the parietal bones.
- Coronal suture—present perpendicular to the sagittal suture in between frontal and parietal sutures.
- Lambdoid suture—it is present between parietal and occipital bones.
- Metopic suture—in between the two halves of the frontal bone.

24. Sesamoid bones.

Ans. Sesamoid bones resemble a seed, hence the name. They are small bones developing in a tendon. The periosteum is absent. They are located at places where tendons change their direction. Haversian system is absent, e.g., patella, fabella.

25. Paranasal air sinuses.

Ans. Paranasal air sinuses are the cavities present inside the skull bones. They have an inner lining of mucous membrane that is continuous with that of the nasal cavities. The secretions of the paranasal sinus drain into the nasal cavity.

Functions:

- Makes the skull bones lighter.
- Adds resonance to the voice and increases its quality.

The air sinuses are as follows **(Fig. 5.18):**

- Frontal air sinus
- Maxillary air sinus
- Ethmoidal air sinuses
- Sphenoidal air sinus

26. Name the cranial fossae in the skull and their relations.

Ans. Cranial fossae are bony depressions in the floor of the cranial cavity which are related to brain convolutions, blood vessels and contain various foramina. They adapt to the shape of the developing brain.

- Anterior cranial fossa—related to the frontal lobe of cerebrum.
- Middle cranial fossa—related to the temporal lobe of cerebrum.
- Posterior cranial fossa—related to the cerebellum.

27. Elastic cartilage.

Ans. Elastic cartilage is a basic type of cartilage forming skeletal framework for organs of sound production (larynx) and hearing. It presents the following features **(Fig. 5.19):**

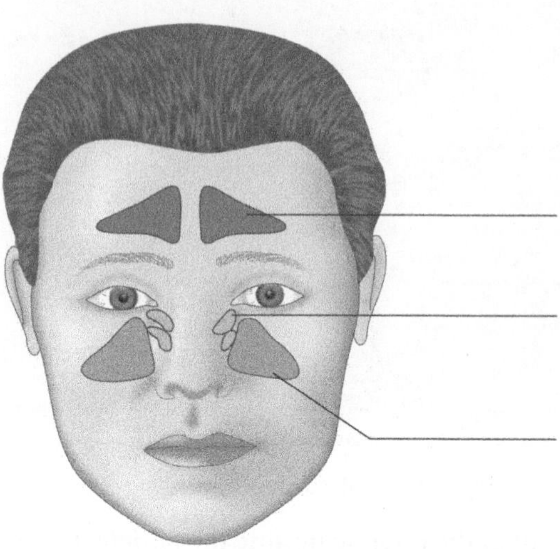

Fig. 5.18: Paranasal sinuses.

a. Outer covering by a layer of perichondrium.
b. Cartilage cells in single or in groups.
c. Ground substance contain yellow elastic fibers ground substance contains elastic fibers which are arranged in form of network, e.g., cartilages of larynx, pinna, Eustachian tube.

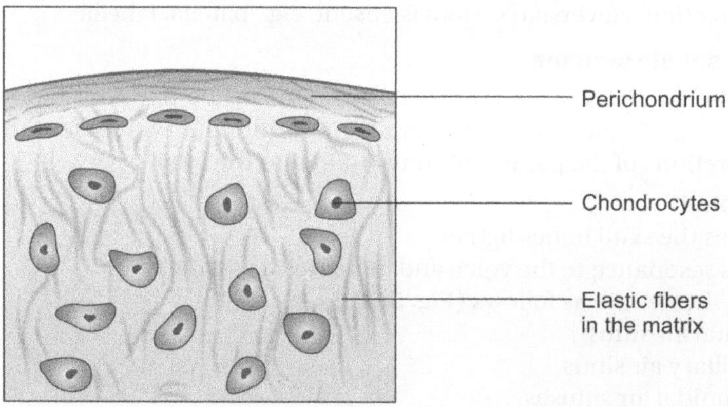

Fig. 5.19: Structure of elastic cartilage.

28. Hyaline cartilage.

Ans. Hyaline cartilage is very important since it is the main skeletal framework during fetal life. In adults, this is replaced by bone. It exhibits the following features **(Fig. 5.7)**:

a. Covered by perichondrium.
b. Homogeneous, glass like basophilic ground substance.
c. Contains network of type II collagen fibers.
d. Fibers have same refractive index as ground substance.
e. Chondroblasts arranged in group of 2, 3 or 4 cells in cell nest, e.g., costal cartilages, nasal cartilage, etc.

29. Name the different types of epiphysis.

Ans. Epiphysis is the part of bone ossified from secondary center **(Fig. 5.20)**.

a. Pressure epiphysis—transmits body weight, e.g., head of femur and humerus.
b. Traction epiphysis—it is produced due to the pull of muscles, e.g., trochanters of femur.
c. Atavistic epiphysis—phylogenetically independent bone, and attached to another bone for nutrition, e.g., coracoid process of scapula.

30. Name the bones forming orbit.

Ans. Bony orbit contains the eyeball and associated nerves, blood vessels, fat. It is in the form of a pyramid, apex behind and base towards the face. It is said to consist of four walls:

- Roof—frontal and sphenoid bones.
- Lateral wall—zygomatic and sphenoid bones.
- Medial wall—ethmoid, maxilla, lacrimal, sphenoid bones.
- Floor—maxilla, zygomatic and palatine bones.

31. Nasal septum.

Ans. Nasal septum is a vertical partition that divides the nasal cavity into two halves. It is made of three components:

1. Vomer
2. Perpendicular plate of ethmoid bone
3. Septal cartilage.

DNS—refers to deviated nasal septum (not in the midline of nose).
Septoplasty—refers to any surgery done to correct deformities of the septum.
Broken nose—refers to injury to the septal cartilage as a result of trauma.

32. Hyoid bone.

Ans. Hyoid bone is unique, as it does not articulate with any other skull bone. It is suspended by muscles and ligaments from the styloid process of skull.
Location—anterior region of neck, below the mandible.

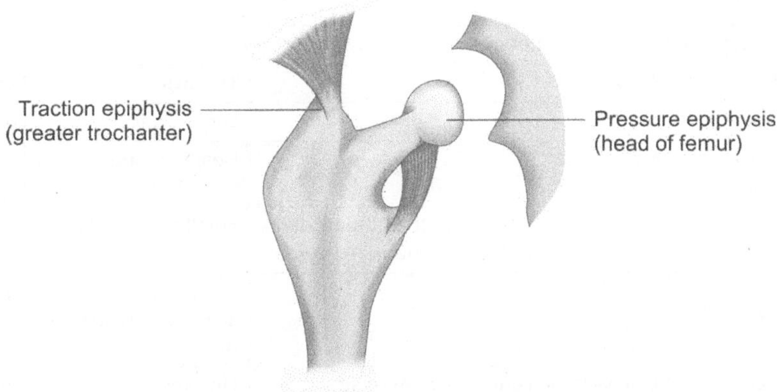

Fig. 5.20: Types of epiphysis.

Functions—supports tongue, gives attachment to the muscles of the tongue, neck and pharynx. It can be fractured during strangulation along with the laryngeal cartilages and trachea.

33. Name the contents of vertebral canal.

Ans. Vertebral canal is formed by vertebral foramen of all the vertebrae. It contains spinal cord, meninges covering, spinal arteries, internal vertebral venous plexus.

34. What are the functions of vertebral column?

Ans. Vertebral column forms a part of axial skeleton. It is made of vertebrae joined by intervertebral joints and intervertebral disc.

- Movement of the trunk
- Transmission of body weight
- Encloses and protects spinal cord
- Attachment to pelvic and pectoral girdle
- Attachment to muscles.

35. Name the bones of lower limb.

Ans. The skeleton of the lower limb consists of 30 bones in each free limb.

The hip bone (consisting of pubis, ilium, and ischium) attaches it to the vertebral column.

The bones include—femur (thigh bone), patella, tibia and fibula (leg bones). The tarsal bones are—talus, calcaneum, navicular, cuboid, medial, intermediate and lateral cuneiforms. The foot is made of 5 metatarsals and 14 phalanges.

36. Name the different vertebrae of vertebral column.

Ans. The vertebral column (backbone) is made up of 33 vertebrae **(Table 5.4)**.

They include:

- Cervical—7
- Thoracic—12
- Lumbar—5
- Sacral—5 (fused to form sacrum)
- Coccyx—4.

Table 5.4: Comparison between the different vertebrae.

Features	Cervical	Thoracic	Lumbar
Size	Small	Large	Largest
Vertebral body	Small, oval	Heart shaped	Largest, kidney shaped
Vertebral foramen	Triangular, slightly large. It accommodates cervical enlargement of the spinal cord.	Small and circular	Slightly oval
Transverse process	Small	Present. It articulates with the ribs	Large and blunt
Foramina	One vertebral and two transverse foramina. Vertebral artery passes through the transverse foramen	One vertebral foramen	One vertebral foramen

37. Name the cartilages with examples.

Ans. Cartilage is skeletal tissue which is firm yet resilient. It is of three types:

a. Hyaline cartilage, e.g., costal cartilage, cartilages of trachea
b. Elastic cartilage, e.g., external acoustic meatus, pinna, Eustachian tube
c. Fibrocartilage, e.g., intervertebral disc, menisci of knee joint.

38. Name the parts of manubrium sternum.

Ans. Manubrium sternum (breastbone) is anterior most bone of the thoracic cage. It is made of three parts namely **(Fig. 5.21)**:

- Manubrium
- Body
- Xiphoid process.

It articulates with the anterior end of the ribs via costal cartilages.

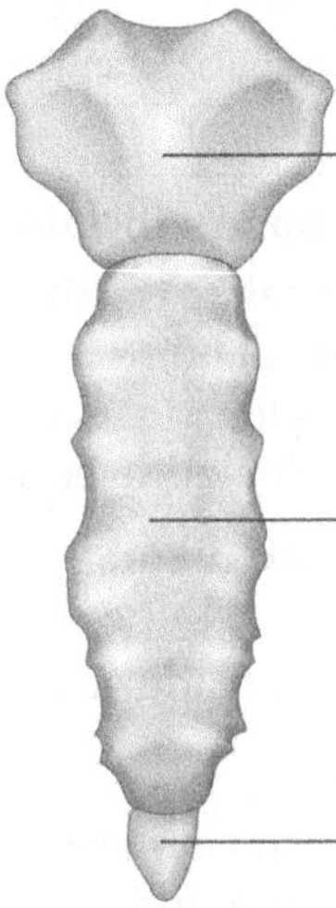

Fig. 5.21: Parts of sternum.

39. Name the parts of the mandible.

Ans. Mandible forms the skeleton of lower jaw, is the only movable bone in the skull. It provides attachment to the muscles of mastication, face, oral cavity. It is involved in the formation of temporomandibular joint. It provides support to the lower set of teeth (16 in number in adults).

It consists of **(Fig. 5.8)**:

- Curved body in the center.
- Two rami attached perpendicular to the mandible.
- Two processes—coronoid and condyloid process.

40. What is a foramen? Give any two examples.

Ans. The foramen means a whole in the bone through which blood vessels, nerves, etc., pass. Skull has numerous foramina (pleural of foramen). Other bones have minute foramina for blood vessels and nerves. The prominent one is called nutrient foramen, e.g., foramen ovale, optic foramen **(Table 5.5)**.

Table 5.5: Important foramina of the skull.

Sl. No.	Name of the foramen	Structures passing through it
1.	Foramen magnum	• Medulla oblongata • Meninges • Spinal accessory nerve • Vertebral and spinal vessels
2.	Carotid canal	• Internal carotid artery • Sympathetic nerves
3.	Foramen ovale	Mandibular nerve
4.	Foramen spinosum	Middle meningeal artery
5.	Foramen rotundum	Maxillary nerve

Contd...

Contd...

Sl. No.	Name of the foramen	Structures passing through it
6.	Jugular foramen	Internal jugular vein 9th,10th and 11th cranial nerves
7.	Stylomastoid foramen	Facial nerve
8.	Olfactory foramina	Olfactory nerve rootlets
9.	Mandibular foramen	Inferior alveolar nerve and vessels
10.	Optic canal	Optic nerve and ophthalmic artery

41. Name the bones forming hard palate (Fig. 5.22).

Ans.
- The hard palate is a thin horizontal plate that forms the roof of the oral cavity.
- It consists of bone covered with mucoperiosteum.
- The bones forming hard palate are—the palatine process of maxilla and horizontal process of palatine bone.

42. Intervertebral disc.

Ans. Intervertebral disc (IVD) is a fibrocartilaginous plate in between the bodies of the vertebrae. It is made of an *outer annulus fibrosus and an inner nucleus pulposus.*

Functions:
- Forms strong joints with the vertebra and helpful in movements of the column.
- Absorb shock and compressive forces
- Bears weight and transmission of weight

Clinical anatomy: *Prolapsed disc* is a common cause for back pain as the age advances. It can compress on the nerve roots of the spinal cord.

43. Classify ribs.

Ans. The thoracic cage consists of 12 pair of ribs.
- The first 7 ribs connect sternum and called vertebrosternal (true ribs)
- The 8, 9, 10th ribs are attached to the sternum via costal cartilages- vertebra-chondral ribs

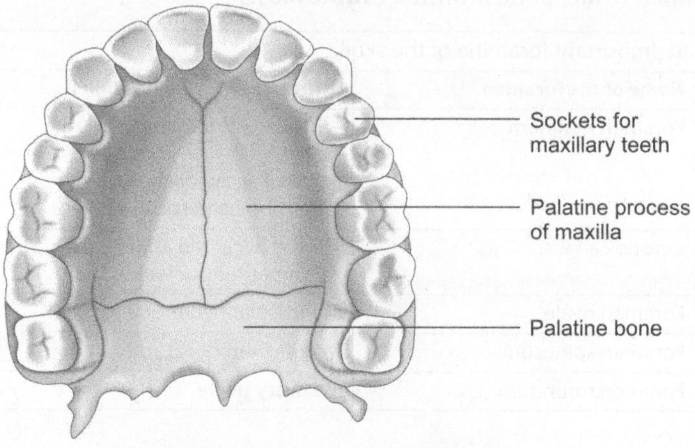

Fig. 5.22: Bones forming hard palate.

- The 9th and 12th ribs attach to the vertebra—floating ribs
- 3rd to 9th ribs have similar features, hence called **typical ribs.**

Remaining ribs are the **atypical ribs**, i.e., 1, 2, 10, 11 and 12th ribs

44. Xiphoid process.

Ans.
- Xiphoid process is the lowest part of the sternum (breastbone).
- It gives attachment to some abdominal muscles. It is made of hyaline cartilage, and does not ossify till 40 years of age.
- During cardiopulmonary resuscitation, xiphoid process may be drawn inside the abdomen leading to damage to internal organs like liver.

45. Name the situations when bone formation (ossification) occurs.

Ans.
- Bone formation in embryo and fetus.
- Growth of bones—childhood and adolescence.
- Remodeling of bone (replacement of old with new bone).
- After fracture.

46. Define endochondral and membranous ossification.

Ans. **Membranous ossification**—involves development of bone in sheets of mesenchyme, e.g., skull bones, mandible, clavicle, etc.

Endochondral ossification—bone develops from a cartilaginous model, e.g., all the long bones.

47. Enumerate the factors that affect bone growth and remodeling.

Ans.
- **Minerals**—Calcium and phosphorous are essential. Others are magnesium, fluoride and manganese.
- **Vitamins**—Vitamin A stimulates osteoblasts. Vitamin C required for collagen synthesis. Vitamin D helps in absorption of calcium from digestive tract. Vitamin B_{12} and K are required for synthesis of bone proteins.
- **Hormones**—during childhood growth and thyroid hormones, insulin-like growth factor are essential. During adolescence, estrogen and androgens are responsible for growth spurt. They cause increase in length of the bone, and later bone growth ceases. Calcitriol and parathormone are required for bone remodeling.

48. Bone remodeling.

Ans. It is the process of replacement of old bone with new bone. Old bone is resorbed; new bone is deposited. It is influenced by exercise, diet, lifestyle. Remodeling varies across the bones. Lower end of femur is replaced every 4 months, some part of femur is never replaced. If newly formed bone is subjected to stress, it is stronger and thicker than the old bone.

49. Atlas vertebra.

Ans.
- First cervical vertebra.
- Body and spine are absent.
- Has anterior and posterior arches, two lateral masses.
- Superior articular facet forms atlanto-occipital joint (permits 'yes' movement).

50. Axis vertebra.

Ans.
- Second cervical vertebra.
- Has a body, bifid spine.

- Body has a dens (odontoid process) which forms atlanto-axial joint with atlas (permits 'no' movement).
- Fracture of dens can injure the medulla oblongata.

51. Features of thoracic vertebra.

Ans.
- Small, heart shaped body in front. Body articulates with head of the ribs. Two facets are present on either side of the body for this.
- Circular vertebral foramen.
- Spine is prominent and directed downwards.
- Transverse process articulates with tubercle of corresponding rib.

52. Joints formed by sacrum.

Ans.
- Two sacroiliac joints on either side—auricular surface with ilium.
- Lumbosacral joint—body of sacrum with L5 vertebra.
- Above two joints are important in weight transmission to the hip bone, lower down to the lower limb.
- Sacrococcygeal joint.

53. Sacral hiatus.

Ans.
- Sacral hiatus is formed due to the failure of fusion of L5 and sometimes L4 laminae.
- This gap is continuous above with vertebral canal.
- The sacral canal contains sacral and coccygeal nerves.
- Caudal anesthesia can be given through sacral hiatus.

54. Sternum.

Ans.
- It is the anterior most bone in the midline of the thoracic cage.
- It has three parts—manubrium, body and xiphoid process.
- Joints—sternoclavicular, with first 7 ribs, manubriosternal joint.
- Manubriosternal joint (sternal angle) marks the level of 2nd costal cartilage—useful to count the ribs, and in surface anatomy.
- Sternum is split in cardiothoracic surgeries.

55. Pelvic (hip) girdle.

Ans. Pelvic or hip girdle (bony pelvis) is made of two hip bones on either side, posteriorly completed by sacrum.

Joints:
- Pubic symphysis in the middle
- Right and left sacroiliac joints behind.

Functions:
- Connects lower limb to the trunk.
- Provides support to the vertebral column.
- Pelvic organs are located inside—bladder, prostate (males), uterus and fallopian tube (females), rectum and anal canal.
- Transmission of weight.

56. Boundaries of pelvic brim.

Ans. Anterior to posterior it consists of:
- Pubic symphysis
- Pubic crest

- Pectineal line
- Arcuate line
- Ala of sacrum
- Sacral promontory

The pelvic brim demarcates true and false pelvis.

57. False or greater pelvis.

Ans.
- This part of bony pelvis is superior to pelvic brim.
- Boundaries—lumbar vertebrae behind, iliac fossae on either side, anterior abdominal wall in front.
- Contents—urinary bladder (when full), lower intestines (in both genders), uterus, ovaries, uterine tube (females).

58. True (lesser) pelvis.

Ans.
- This part of bony pelvis is inferior to the pelvic brim.
- The pelvic outlet—is formed by pubic arch, ischial tuberosities, sacrotuberous ligament and coccyx.
  - *Inlet*—is the pelvic brim.
  - *Outlet*—muscles of pelvic floor.
- *Cavity*—is bounded by pubic symphysis in front, sacrum and coccyx behind, ilium and ischium laterally.
- *Contents*—rectum and anal canal, prostate in males, cervix and vagina in females.

59. Pelvic axis.

Ans.
- Pelvic axis is an imaginary line in the true pelvis.
- It joins center point of pelvic inlet to the center point of pelvic outlet.
- It is the axis followed by the fetus during childbirth.
- *Pelvimetry*—is a clinical examination technique to assess the pelvis. It is done manually or by ultrasound. This helps to know whether the child can pass through the birth canal normally or not.
- If pelvic canal is too small, cesarean section is planned.

60. Femur (*refer* Figure 5.23).

Ans.
- Longest, strongest, heaviest bone.
- The upper end has—head, neck, greater- and lesser trochanters. Head forms *hip-joint* with acetabulum.
- Fracture neck of femur, commonly referred to as broken hip; is common in elderly females.
- Shaft presents linea aspera. It gives attachment to muscles.
- Lower end has medial and lateral femoral condyles and forms *knee joint*. Adductor tubercle is an important bony landmark.

Notes:
- Healing of the cartilage is poor as it does not have blood supply.
- Spine of C7 vertebra is long, and prominent projection hence called *vertebra prominence*. It is useful in counting the spine below it.
- Humerus—called funny bone. Because, medial epicondyle is related to the ulnar nerve on its posterior surface. When we hit our elbow, it leads to severe pain due to the nerve here.

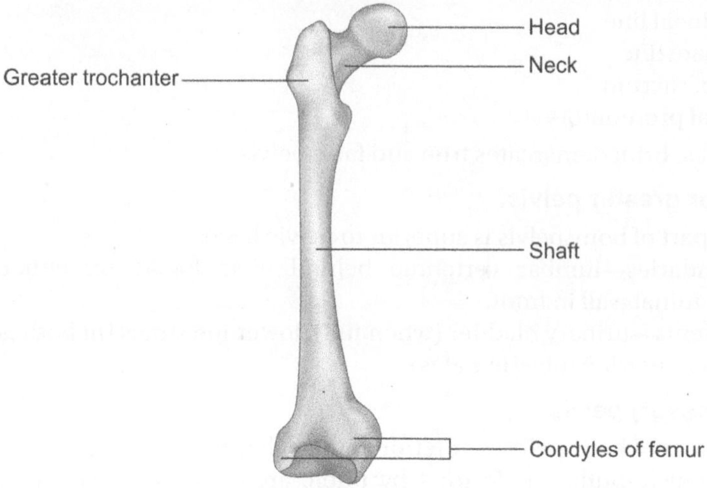

Fig. 5.23: Parts of femur.

- Cleft palate—when bones forming hard palate fail to fuse, cleft palate results. It leads to difficulty in breathing and swallowing. It may be associated with cleft lip. These can be corrected by surgery.
- Scoliosis—lateral bending of the vertebral column.
- Kyphosis (hunch back)—forward bending of the thoracic spine.
- Lordosis—exaggerated lumbar curvature.
- Spina bifida—this results due to failure of laminae of a vertebra to fuse in the midline. It can be of various degrees. Meninges can herniate with or without spinal cord (meningocele, meningomyelocele, respectively).
- Osteoporosis—the rate of bone resorption exceeds that of bone deposition. Bones are porous, can fracture easily.
- Osteomyelitis—infection of bone, by bacteria. It leads to fever, pain, pus formation.
- Osteosarcoma—tumor of the bone affecting osteoblasts.
- *Fibula*—is commonly used in *bone grafting*. A piece of bone along with nutrient artery is grafted to the site of repair. Walking and running can be performed normally even after fibula is removed.
- Tibia bears the body weight and transmits to ankle and foot.

6

CHAPTER

Joints

LONG ESSAYS — 10 MARKS

1. Classify the joints with examples. Describe the structure of synovial joint.

Ans. Joints are places where two bones or cartilages meet. Based on the structure joints can be classified as follows:

Based on function—it relates to the degree of movement permitted by the joint. The joints are classified as follows:

a. **Synarthrosis**—is an immovable joint, e.g., fibrous joints.
b. **Amphiarthrosis**—these are slightly movable joint, e.g., cartilaginous joints.
c. **Diarthrosis**—these are freely movable joints, e.g., synovial joints.

Based on structure—three types which are as follows **(Fig. 6.1)**:

a. **Fibrous joints**—here fibrous tissue (dense irregular connective tissue) unites the articulating bones. Joint cavity is absent; hence they are immovable joints. They are of three types:
   i. Sutures—found between the skull bones.
   ii. Syndesmosis—holds bones together, e.g., interosseous membrane between radius and ulna.
   iii. Gomphosis—a peg fitting in a socket, e.g., thin periodontal membrane unites root of tooth with its socket.
b. **Cartilaginous joints**—the articulating bones lack synovial cavity and are joined by hyaline or fibrocartilage. These are slightly movable joints. They are of two types:
   i. Primary cartilaginous/synchondrosis—a plate of hyaline cartilage unites the bones, e.g., epiphyseal plate (made of hyaline cartilage) connecting epiphysis and diaphysis of long bones, first manubriosternal joint.
   ii. Secondary cartilaginous/symphysis—the bony surfaces are covered by hyaline cartilage and a plate of fibrocartilage connects the two bones, e.g., symphysis pubis, manubriosternal joints, intervertebral joints.
c. **Synovial joints**—they are freely movable joints. It consists of a joint cavity, capsule and articular cartilage covering the bone surfaces, e.g., shoulder and hip joint.

Structure of a synovial joint:

i. Presence of **a joint cavity**—which allows considerable movement.
ii. Articular ends are covered with hyaline cartilage called **articular cartilage**—they reduce friction between the bones and act as shock absorber.

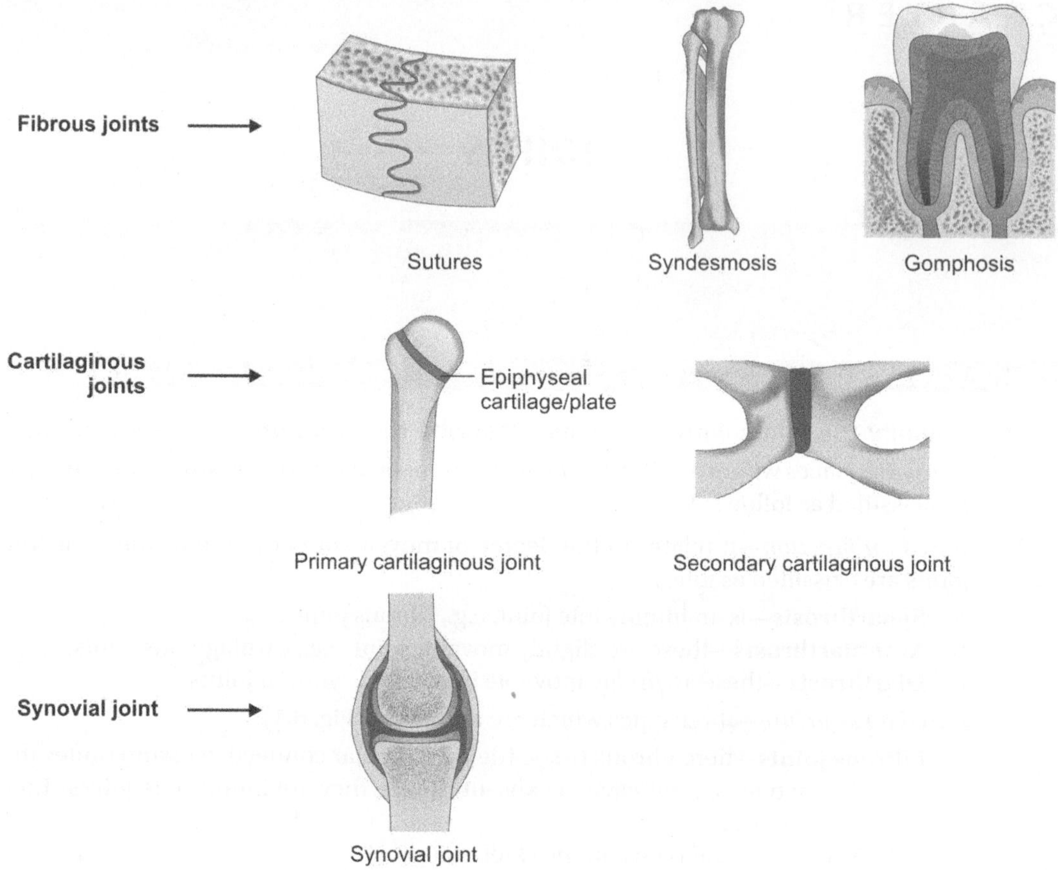

Fig. 6.1: Structural classification of joints.

iii. Bones are held together by **joint (articular) capsule**—the capsule is made of two layers—outer fibrous layer and inner synovial membrane.

iv. **Synovial membrane**—it consists of areolar tissue with elastic fibers. It has rich blood supply. It synthesizes synovial fluid.

v. Joint cavity is filled with **synovial fluid**—the synovial fluid is viscous, pale/clear fluid secreted by the synovial membrane. It performs the following functions:
   - Nutrition to the cartilage—supplies nutrients and oxygen, removes metabolic wastes and carbon.
   - Lubrication.
   - Shock absorber.
   - Removes microbes by phagocytic action.
   - Removes debris within the joint.

vi. **Ligaments**—they are made of regularly arranged dense regular connective tissue. They strengthen the joint and resist strain.

vii. **Accessory ligaments, articular discs and labra:**
   - **Accessory ligaments**—can be extracapsular (outside the joint) and intracapsular ligaments (are inside the joint).

- **Articular discs or Menisci**—they are crescent shaped plates of fibrocartilage. They are attached to the capsule and divide the joint into compartments. This allows separate movements to occur in each space. They help in—shock absorption, distribute weight, better fit between the bones, e.g., knee joint and temporomandibular joint (TMJ).
- **Labrum**—is a plate of fibrocartilage attached to the margins of articular bone. It deepens the cavity, e.g., shoulder and hip joints.

2. Describe the structure of a synovial joint with help of neat labeled diagram. Classify synovial joint with examples.

Ans. Synovial joint is a freely movable joint, with a synovial cavity and fibrous capsule.

Structure of a synovial joint (Fig. 6.2):

i. Presence of **a joint cavity**—which allows considerable movement.
ii. Articular ends are covered with hyaline cartilage called **articular cartilage**—they reduce friction between the bones and act as shock absorber.
iii. Bones are held together by **joint (articular) capsule**—the capsule is made of two layers—outer fibrous layer and inner synovial membrane.
iv. **Synovial membrane**—it consists of areolar tissue with elastic fibers. It has rich blood supply. It synthesizes synovial fluid.
v. Joint cavity is filled with **synovial fluid**—the synovial fluid is viscous, pale/clear fluid secreted by the synovial membrane. It performs the following functions:
   - Nutrition to the cartilage—supplies nutrients and oxygen, removes metabolic wastes and carbon dioxide.
   - Lubrication
   - Shock absorber
   - Removes microbes by phagocytic action
   - Removes debris within the joint.
vi. **Ligaments**—they are made of regularly arranged dense regular connective tissue. They strengthen the joint and resist strain.
vii. **Accessory ligaments, articular discs and labra:**
   - **Accessory ligaments**—can be extracapsular (outside the joint) and intracapsular ligaments (are inside the joint).
   - **Articular discs or Menisci**—they are crescent shaped plates of fibrocartilage. They are attached to the capsule and divide the joint into compartments. This allows separate movements to occur in each space. They help in—shock absorption, distribute weight, better fit between the bones, e.g., knee joint and temporomandibular joint (TMJ).

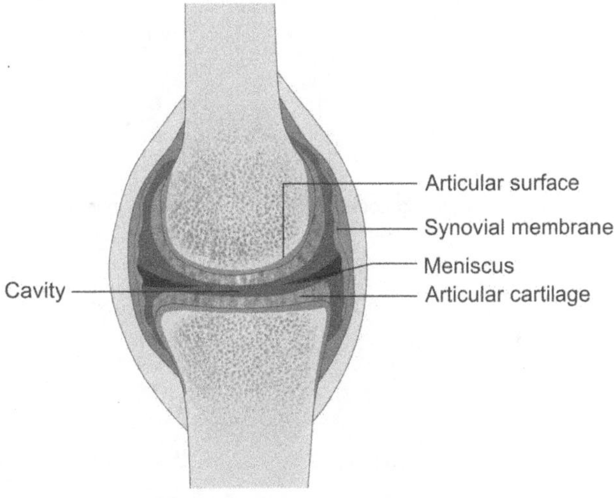

Fig. 6.2: Structure of synovial joint.

- **Labrum**—is a plate of fibrocartilage attached to the margins of articular bone. It deepens the cavity, e.g., shoulder and hip joints.

Classification of synovial joints: Based on the *shape of the articular surface* they are of following types **(Fig. 6.3):**

1. Plane joint—surfaces are flat, e.g., intertarsal joints.
2. Hinge joint—convex surface of one fits into concave surface of other bone. Flexion and extension possible, e.g., elbow, interphalangeal joints.
3. Pivot joint—central pivot surrounded by bony ring or ligament, e.g., proximal radioulnar and atlantoaxial joints. Movements—rotation, supination.
4. Condyloid joint—ellipsoid articular surface, e.g., metacarpophalangeal joints. Movements—flexion, extension, adduction, abduction.
5. Saddle joint—articular surfaces have both convex and concave surfaces, e.g., carpometacarpal joint of the thumb. Movements—flexion, extension, adduction, abduction, circumduction.
6. Ellipsoid joint—surfaces are ellipse in shape, e.g., wrist joint.
7. Ball and socket joint—globe like end of one bone fits in cavity of other bone. Freely movable joint, e.g., shoulder and hip joints. Movements—flexion, extension, adduction, abduction, circumduction, medial and lateral rotation.

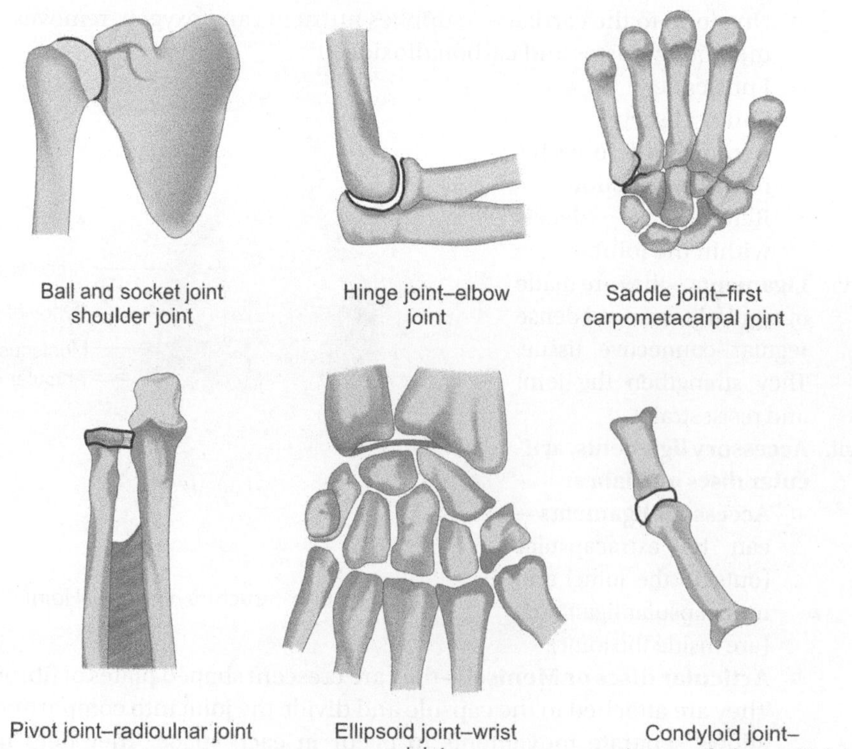

Fig. 6.3: Classification of synovial joint.

Based on the degree of movement (axis along which it occurs), they are:

a. Uniaxial—joint moves in a single plane, e.g., elbow joint (flexion and extension)
b. Biaxial—the joint moves in two planes, e.g., wrist joint (flexion, extension, abduction and adduction).
c. Multiaxial—the joint moves in any plane, e.g., shoulder joint (along with above movements, rotation possible).

Based on the number of bones involved, they are classified as:

a. Simple—two bones are involved, e.g., shoulder and knee joints.
b. Compound joints—three or more bones form a joint, e.g., radiocarpal joint.
c. Complex joint—three or more bones with an intra-articular structure like menisci, e.g., knee joint.

3. Hip joint.

Ans. Hip joint is an important joint which connects trunk with the lower limb.

Type—ball and socket variety of synovial joint.

Articular surfaces (Fig. 6.4):

a. Head and neck of femur
b. Acetabular cavity of the hip bone.

Since the head of femur is smaller than acetabular cavity, the entire head is inside acetabular cavity. Hence the joint is more stable, but movements are restricted.

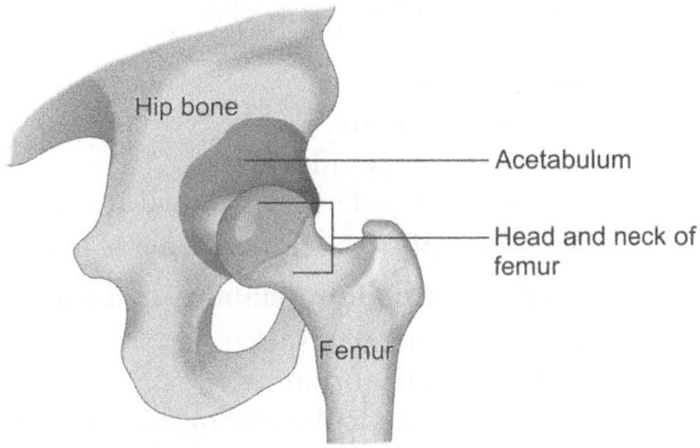

Fig. 6.4: Bones forming hip joint.

Ligaments of the joint (Fig. 6.5):

- Articular cartilage covers both head of femur and acetabulum.
- Capsule—is very strong, attached to the margins of acetabulum and onto the neck of femur.
- Iliofemoral ligament—strongest ligament in the body. It extends from anterior superior iliac spine to intertrochanteric line of femur. It prevents hyperextension.
- Ischiofemoral ligament—extends from ischium to femur. It tenses during abduction and strengthens the capsule.
- Pubofemoral ligament—prevents over-abduction. It extends from anterior inferior iliac spine to femur.
- Transverse acetabular ligament.

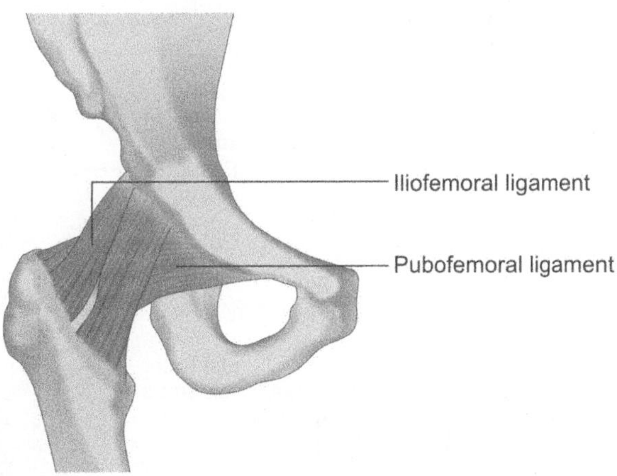

Fig. 6.5: Ligaments of hip joint.

- Acetabular labrum—is a ring of fibrocartilage, increases the depth of acetabular cup. It prevents dislocation of head of femur.
- Ligament of head of femur—from the acetabular fossa to the head of femur. It carries blood vessels to the head of femur.

Movements occurring at the joint—hip joint is very strong, since the capsule and accessory ligaments are strong, head fits well in the acetabular cup, and the muscles around it. But the movements are of limited range compared to the shoulder joint.

1. Flexion and extension
2. Medial and lateral rotation
3. Adduction and abduction
4. Circumduction

Relations (Fig. 6.6):

Anterior—iliopsoas, rectus femoris, pectineus, femoral vessels and nerve.

Posterior—gluteal muscle, piriformis, obturator internus, sciatic nerve.

Inferior—adductor muscles.

Arterial supply

1. Obturator artery
2. Medial circumflex artery
3. Superior and inferior gluteal arteries

Nerve supply—sciatic nerve, nerve to rectus femoris and obturator nerve.

Factors maintaining stability of the joint:

- Deep acetabular socket
- Acetabular labrum
- Strength of the Iliofemoral and ischiofemoral ligament
- Surrounding muscles.

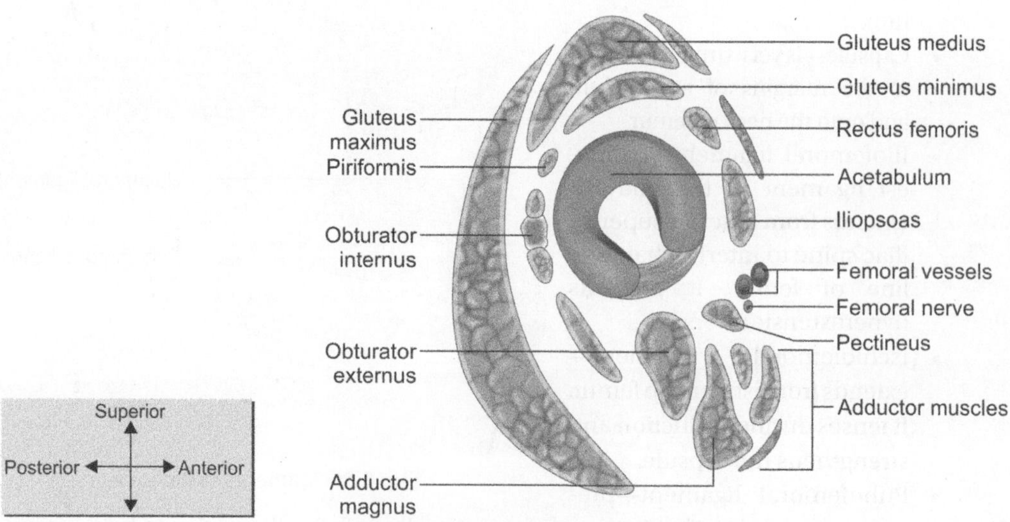

Fig. 6.6: Relations of hip joint.

Applied anatomy:

- Congenital dislocation of hip joint is common.
- Tuberculosis can affect the joint.
- Coxa vara—neck-shaft angle is decreased.
- Coxa valga—neck-shaft angle is increased.
- Arthroscopy—interior of the joint can be visualized using an endoscope for any pathology.
- Arthroplasty—severely damaged joints can be replaced with artificial one by surgery called arthroplasty. It can be partial (only femur) or total hip replacement (both femur and acetabulum).

4. Knee joint.

Ans. **Type of joint**—compound, modified hinge variety synovial joint.

Bones involved (Fig. 6.7)—condyles of femur above, condyles of tibia below, and patella.

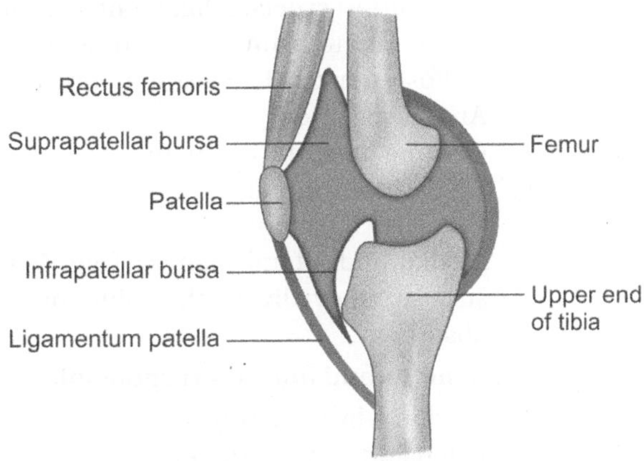

Fig. 6.7: Bones forming knee joint.

Ligaments of the joint are as follows (Fig. 6.8):

a. Capsular ligament—it is attached to the area above the medial and lateral condyle of femur. Below it is attached to area below the tibial condyles.
b. Ligamentum patella—extends from tip of patella to tibial tuberosity.
c. Tibial and fibular collateral ligaments attach the bones on either side of the joint—they connect condyles of femur with tibial condyles. Tibial collateral ligament is attached to medial meniscus.

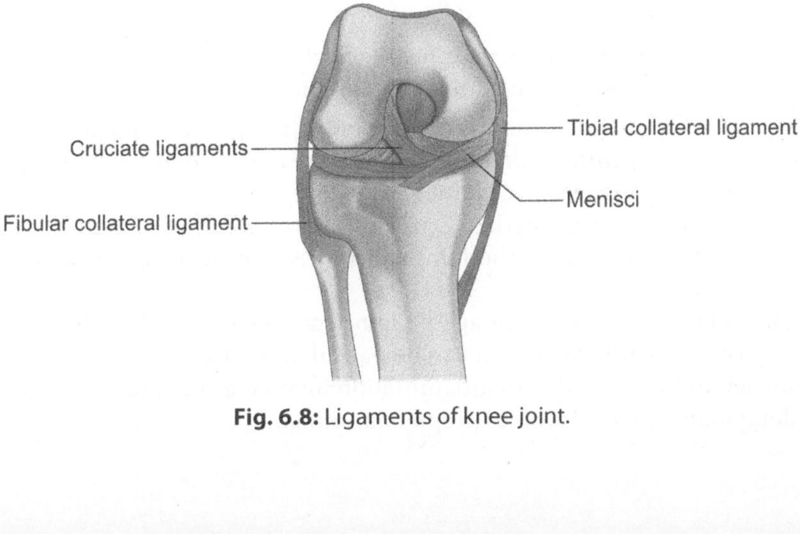

Fig. 6.8: Ligaments of knee joint.

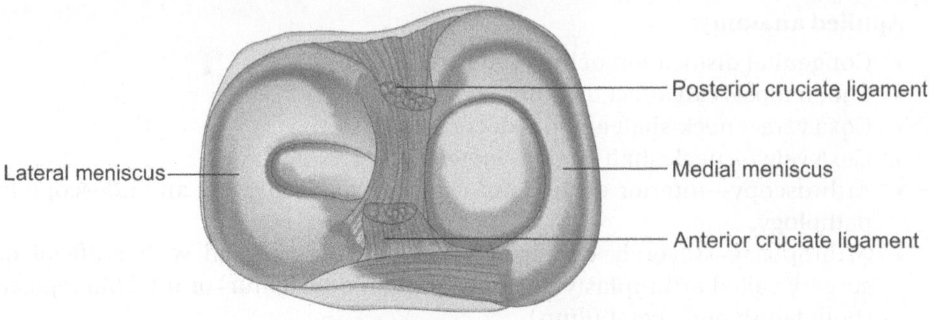

Fig. 6.9: Menisci in knee joint.

d. Anterior and posterior cruciate ligaments:
   - Anterior cruciate ligament prevents hyperextension, prevents tibia sliding anterior to femur. It is commonly damaged in knee injuries.
   - Posterior cruciate ligament prevents tibia sliding posterior to femur.

e. Arcuate ligament
f. Oblique popliteal ligament
g. Transverse ligament
h. Coronary ligament
i. Medial and lateral menisci **(Fig. 6.9)**—plates of fibrocartilage resting on tibial surface. They divide the joint into two compartments. Menisci act as shock absorbers.

Movements and muscles responsible:

a. Flexion—by hamstrings
b. Extension—by quadriceps femoris
c. Medial rotation—semimembranosus, semitendinosus, popliteus
d. Lateral rotation—biceps femoris.

Blood supply—genicular branches of popliteal artery form genicular anastomosis which supplies the joint.

Nerve supply—femoral, tibial, common peroneal and obturator nerve.

Bursae around the joint—suprapatellar, prepatellar, infrapatellar, etc.

Applied anatomy

Knee joint is prone to injury, as it bears weight and is a mobile joint. Its stability is maintained by the menisci, collateral and cruciate ligaments muscles.

- Rupture of medial meniscus is common during sports. Damage *to tibial collateral ligament is associated with damage to medial meniscus* as they are firmly attached.
- Osteoarthritis involves knee joint early.
- The joint can get dislocated.
- Arthroscopy—interior of the joint can be visualized using an endoscope for any pathology.
- Arthroplasty—severely damaged joints can be replaced with artificial one by surgery called arthroplasty. It can be partial or total knee replacement.
- Housemaid's knee—due to inflammation involving subcutaneous bursa.
- Clergyman's knee—involves prepatellar bursa.

- Knee replacement—involves replacement of damaged tibial and femoral articular surfaces with prosthesis.

SHORT ESSAYS 5 MARKS

5. Movements of the synovial joints.

Ans. Synovial joints are structurally suited for various movements. It occurs in different axis—uniaxial, biaxial or polyaxial.

The joint movements can be classified into four major categories **(Table 6.1)**:

Table 6.1: Classification of movements of synovial joints.

Categories of movement	Name	Description
Angular: Here there is increase or decrease in the angle between the two bones.	Flexion	Decrease in angle between the bones
	Extension	Increase in angle between the bones
	Abduction	Movement of the limb away from the midline
	Adduction	Movement of the limb towards the midline.
	Circumduction	• Flexion, abduction, extension, adduction, rotation occur in succession • Distal part of the limb moves in a circle
Gliding: It is the gliding of two bones without change in angle		Occurs in intercarpal joints
Rotation: Here a long bone moves in a longitudinal axis		In limbs, they can rotate medially or laterally
Special types: These occur at specific joints in the body	Elevation and depression	Temporomandibular (TM) joint
	Protraction and retraction	Temporomandibular (TM) joint
	Inversion and eversion	Subtalar joint
	Dorsiflexion and plantar flexion	Ankle
	Supination and pronation	Radioulnar joints
	Opposition	Metacarpophalangeal joint of thumb

6. Shoulder joint.

Ans. Shoulder joint is an important joint which connects the upper limb with the trunk.

Type—ball and socket variety of synovial joint, multiaxial joint.

Bones involved (Fig. 6.10)—
a. glenoid cavity of scapula
b. head of humerus. The head of humerus is large, can dislocate inferiorly.

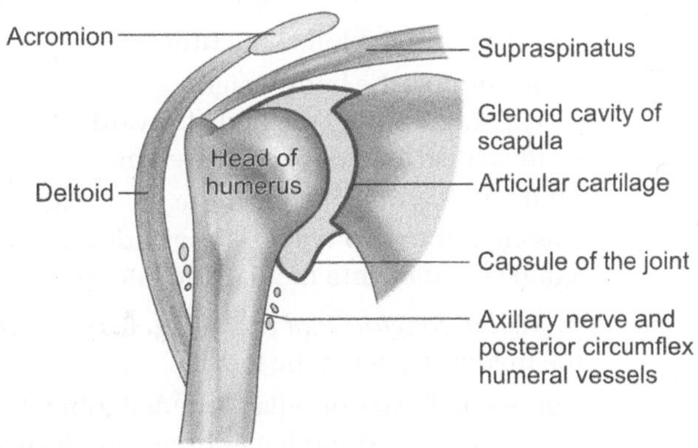

Fig. 6.10: Shoulder joint.

Ligaments

- Capsule—extends from the margins of the glenoid cavity to neck of humerus. Inferomedial aspect it is lax.
- Coracohumeral ligament.
- Glenohumeral ligament.
- Glenoid labrum—made of fibrocartilage. It makes the shallow glenoid cavity more deep.
- Transverse humeral ligament.

Musculotendinous/rotator cuff—four muscles form a covering over the capsule of the joint and strengthen it. They anchor humerus to the scapula.

- Anterior—subscapularis
- Posterior—infraspinatus
- Superior—supraspinatus
- Inferior—teres minor

Important relations—the joint is mainly supported by muscles around it. It is covered with deltoid. *Inferiorly the capsule is lax, and related to axillary nerve.*

Movements at the shoulder joint: Shoulder joint is highly mobile due to lax capsule and shallow glenoid cavity.

a. Flexion—biceps, pectoralis major, deltoid (anterior fibers).
b. Extension—deltoid (posterior fibers), latissimus dorsi.
c. Abduction—supraspinatus, middle fibers of deltoid, trapezius, serratus anterior.
d. Adduction—pectoralis major, latissimus dorsi, teres major.
e. Medial rotation—pectoralis major, latissimus dorsi, teres major.
f. Lateral rotation—infraspinatus, teres minor.
g. Circumduction—all the above muscles.

Applied anatomy

a. Dislocation of the head of humerus can occur, especially inferiorly where the capsule is lax.
b. Axillary nerve is in danger in inferior dislocation of the head of humerus.

7. Describe the arches of foot.

Ans. The foot in humans is not flat. The bones of the foot are arranged to form arches.

They perform the following **functions**:

- To support the body weight.
- Walking—propel the body forward.
- Ideal distribution of body weight.

All the bones of foot contribute to formation of arches **(Fig. 6.11)**. Foot arches can be classified into **two types—longitudinal and transverse arches**. Longitudinal arch is again classified into medial and lateral.

A. Medial longitudinal arch **(Fig. 6.12)**: It is the highest and very important arch on the medial aspect of the foot.

Bones—i. Posterior pillar—medial tubercle of calcaneum, talus, navicular.
ii. Anterior pillar—three cuneiforms, first three metatarsals.

Summit—talus.

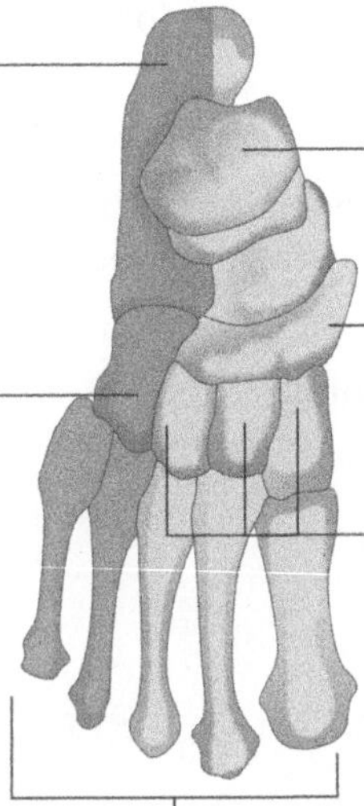

Fig. 6.11: Bones forming arches of foot.

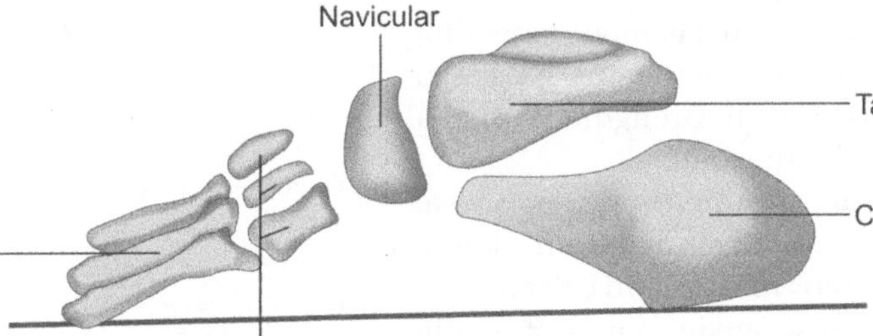

Fig. 6.12: Medial longitudinal arch.

B. Lateral longitudinal arch **(Fig. 6.13)**: It is located over the lateral aspect of the foot.

Bones— i. Posterior pillar—lateral tubercle of calcaneum.

ii. Anterior pillar—cuboid, 4th and 5th metatarsals.

Summit—**talocalcaneal** joint.

C. Transverse arches: These are formed by head of metatarsals, navicular and cuboid.

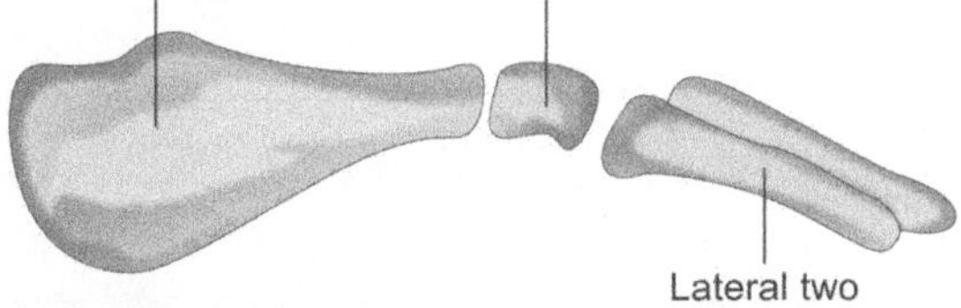

Fig. 6.13: Lateral longitudinal arch.

Factors that maintain the arch of foot:

a. Bones—shape of the bones of foot.
b. Ligaments—long and short plantar ligaments, spring ligament, transverse ligament of heads of metatarsals.

c. Muscles of leg—peroneus longus, tibialis posterior, flexor digitorum longus, flexor hallucis longus.

Applied anatomy

- Flat foot/ Pes planus—concavity of medial longitudinal arch is lost.
- High arched foot—medial arch is excessively curved.

8. Describe the ankle joint.

Ans. **Type of joint**—hinge variety of synovial joint.

Articular surfaces (Fig. 6.14):

a. Superior—by lower end of tibia with medial malleolus, laterally by fibula and lateral malleolus.
b. Inferior—talus.

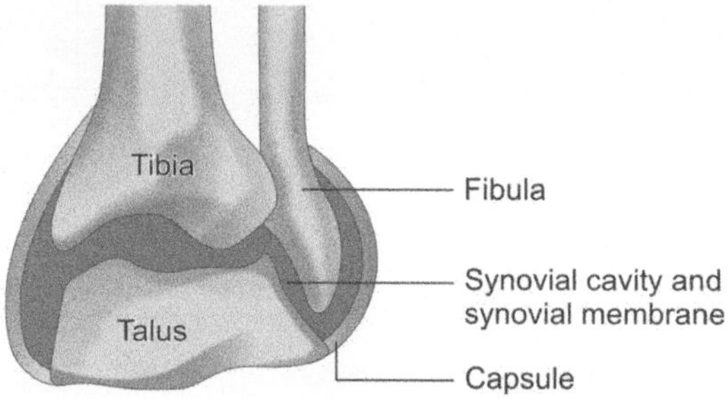

Fig. 6.14: Bones forming ankle joint.

Ligaments (Figs. 6.15A and B):

- Articular capsule—it is weak in front and behind. This permits plantar and dorsiflexion.
- Deltoid ligament—it is a strong, flat, triangular ligament extending from lower tibia to talus, navicular, calcaneum. It strengthens medial aspect of the joint.
- Lateral ligament—it is weak ligament. Extends from lateral malleolus to talus and calcaneum.

Movements—ankle joint is quite a stable joint due to its articular surfaces, ligaments and the tendons around it. Dorsiflexion and plantar flexion are possible.

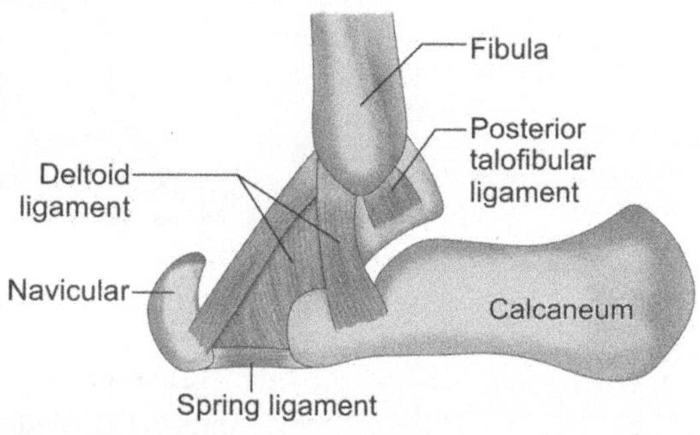

Fig. 6.15A: Ligaments of ankle joint.

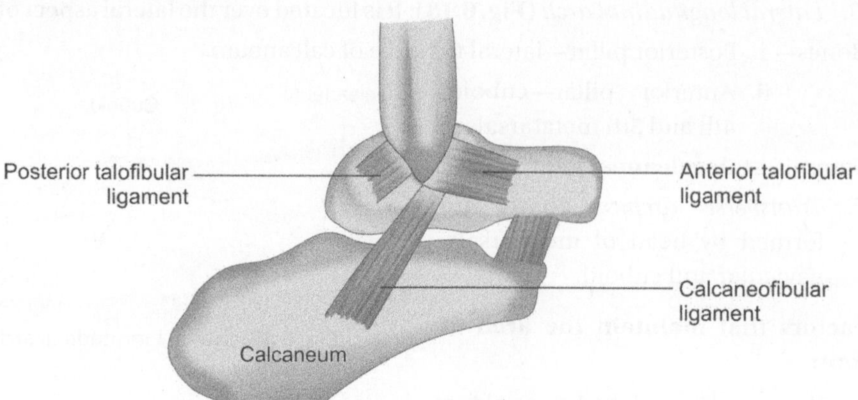

Fig. 6.15B: Ligaments of ankle joint.

Applied anatomy—ankle joint is a frequently injured joint in the body.

- Excessive inversion leads to **sprain**. Sprain is treated by rest, ice, compression and elevation. Severe ones require immobilization, or surgery.
- **Pott's fracture**—both medial and lateral malleoli are fractured.

9. Enumerate the components in synovial joint.

Ans. Synovial joint is formed between two bones, connected by a capsule and lined by synovial membrane. It is a freely movable joint. The various components and their function is **(Table 6.2)**.

Table 6.2: Components of synovial joint and their function.

Synovial joint component	Function
Articular cartilage— it covers the articular surfaces of the bones and made of hyaline cartilage	• Reduces friction between the joint surfaces • Shock absorber
Synovial membrane—this lines the inner surface of the articular capsule. It is made of areolar tissue with elastic fibers	Synthesizes synovial fluid
Synovial fluid—it is viscous, pale, yellow clear fluid, produced by synovial membrane	• For lubrication • For nutrition to the articular cartilage
Articular disc—it is a plate of fibrocartilage which divide the joint into compartments	• Helps to stabilize the joints • Acts as shock absorber • Reduces frictional wear and tear
Menisci—they are incomplete articular discs. Made of fibrocartilage	• Improves fit of articular surfaces • Aids in lubrication • Divides the joint into compartments, so that different movements are possible • Weight distribution
Ligaments—they connect any two bones together. They are made of dense irregular connective tissue	Binds the bones/cartilage
Capsule—encloses the synovial joint and unites the articular bones. It has an outer fibrous and inner synovial layer	• Allows movement at the joint as it is flexible • Prevents dislocation

10. Describe the elbow joint.

Ans. Elbow joint is a hinge variety of synovial joint.

Articular surfaces (bones forming the joint) (Fig. 6.17):

- Superior—trochlea and capitulum at the lower end of humerus.
- Inferior—trochlear notch of ulna and head of radius respectively.

Ligaments

1. Capsular ligament.
2. Ulnar collateral ligament—medial epicondyle to ulna.
3. Radial collateral ligament—lateral epicondyle to radius.

Movements—since it is a hinge joint, only flexion and extension are possible.

Applied anatomy

a. Dislocation of head of radius is common in children.
b. Tennis elbow—pain over the lateral epicondyle.

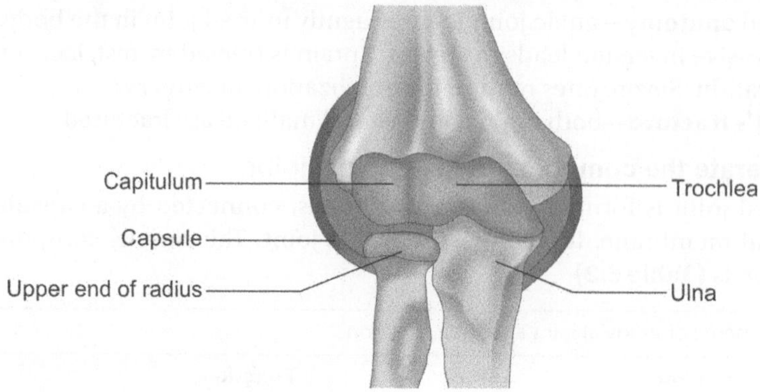

Fig. 6.16: Bones of elbow joint.

11. Wrist joint.

Ans. Wrist joint is a biaxial, ellipsoid variety of synovial joint.

Articular surfaces (Fig. 6.17):

a. Lower end of radius with articular disc of ulna.
b. Scaphoid, lunate and triquetral.

Ligaments:

a. Fibrous capsule
b. Radial collateral ligament laterally
c. Ulnar collateral ligament medially
d. Palmar radiocarpal ligament
e. Dorsal radiocarpal ligament.

Blood supply: By branches of radial and ulnar arteries.

Nerve supply—radial, median and ulnar nerves.

Movements possible—flexion, extension, adduction, abduction, circumduction.

Applied anatomy:

- Fall on the wrist—can lead to scaphoid bone fracture.
- Colles' fracture—leads to fracture of distal end of radius.

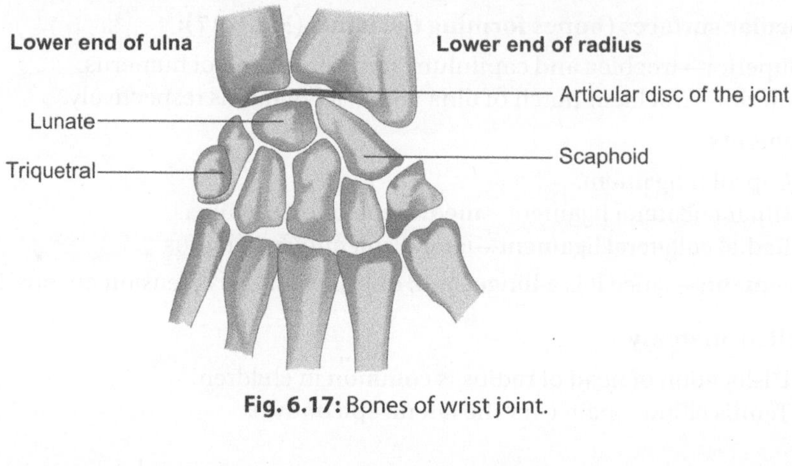

Fig. 6.17: Bones of wrist joint.

12. Temporomandibular joint (TMJ).

Ans. Temporomandibular joint is the only movable joint in the skull.

Bones forming

a. Above—mandibular fossa and articular tubercle of temporal bone.
b. Below—head and neck of the mandible.

Peculiarity—the bones never come in contact during movements. They are separated by articular disc.

Ligaments (Fig. 6.18):

- Articular capsule—covers the articular bones and forms lateral ligament of the joint. The articular surfaces are covered by fibrocartilage.
- Lateral ligament—strengthens the joint form the lateral aspect.
- Articular disc—is made of fibrocartilage. It separates the joint cavity into upper- and lower compartments.
- Sphenomandibular ligament—from the spine of sphenoid to the mandible.
- Stylomandibular ligament—from styloid process to angle of mandible.

Movements: The movements possible include:

- Elevation—depression of the mandible as in opening and closing the mouth.
- Protraction (forward protrusion of mandible)—retraction. They are required for chewing (side to side movements).

Muscles causing the movements:

- Elevation—masseter, temporalis and medial pterygoid.
- Depression—lateral pterygoid.
- Protraction—medial and lateral pterygoid.
- Retraction—posterior fibers of temporalis.

Applied anatomy

- TMJ can dislocate in anterior direction.
- Trismus—difficulty in opening the mouth.
- Arthritis—can involve the joint.

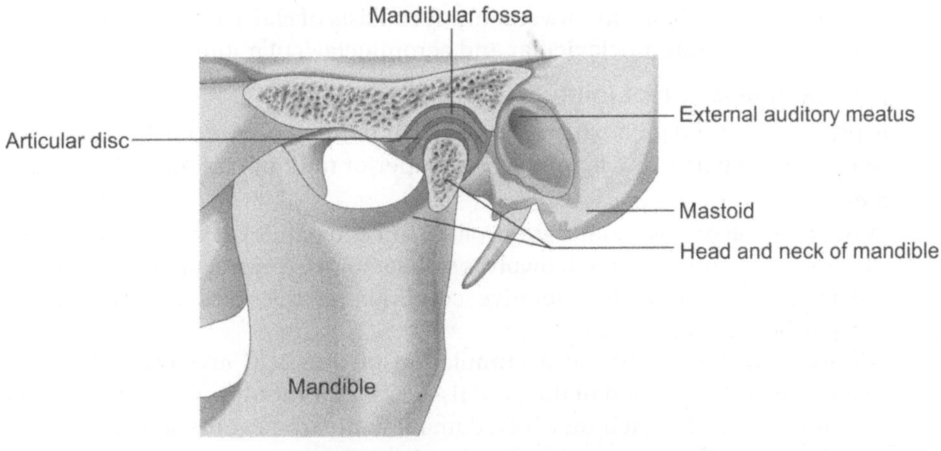

Fig. 6.18: Temporomandibular joint.

SHORT ANSWERS 2 MARKS

13. Name the four ligaments of knee joint.

Ans. a. Tibial and fibular collateral ligaments attach the bones on either side of the joint.
b. Anterior and posterior cruciate ligaments.
c. Arcuate ligament.
d. Oblique popliteal ligament.

14. Bursae of joints.

Ans. Bursae are sac-like structures that are present in relation to the joints. They prevent friction between two adjacent structures like bone-bone, bone-ligament, bone-muscle. It is made of outer fibrous layer and inner synovial lining.

Example: Suprapatellar bursa in relation to knee joint. It helps to prevent friction between quadriceps femoris and lower end of femur.

Applied anatomy: Inflammation of bursa is called bursitis.

15. Synovial (tendon) sheaths.

Ans. Tendon sheaths are similar to bursa, but found around a tendon which is prone for constant friction. They are made of outer fibrous layer and inner synovial lining.

Location: Tendons passing through osseofibrous tunnel as in the long flexor tendons through the carpal tunnel.

16. Give two examples of hinge joint.

Ans. Hinge or Ginglymus joint, here convex surface of one bone fits into concave surface of another bone. They produce an angular, opening-closing type of movements. It occurs at a single axis, i.e., uniaxial, e.g., interphalangeal joints, elbow joint.

17. Give two examples of ball and socket joint.

Ans. Shoulder and hip joint are the examples of ball and socket joint. It consists of ball-like surface of one bone fitting into socket like surface of another bone. They are multiaxial joints—flexion, extension, adduction, abduction and rotation are possible.

18. Name the bones forming pectoral girdle.

Ans. The pectoral girdle connects upper limb with the trunk. It also provides attachment to various muscles, helps in movements. It consists of clavicle and scapula. The joints connecting are the sternoclavicular and acromioclavicular joints.

19. Give example for pivot joint.

Ans. The pivot or trochoid joint consists rounded or pointed part of one bone with a ring of other bone and partly by a ligament, e.g., superior radioulnar joint, atlantoaxial joint.

Notes:

- **Rheumatic arthritis**—joints are swollen, stiff and painful. It is due to auto-immunity against body's own tissues. It involves smaller joints. It can lead to physical disability.
- **Osteoarthritis**—is a degenerative condition of the joint cartilage. It involves weight-bearing larger joints.
- **Gouty arthritis**—is due to accumulation of uric acid crystals within the joint, leading to inflammation of the joint tissues. It commonly involves joints of foot.
- **Sprain**—forceful stretching which damages or tears a ligament of a joint.
- **Strain**—partially torn muscle or tendon. It results due to sudden pull on the muscle.

7
CHAPTER

Muscle Tissue

SHORT ESSAYS — 5 MARKS

1. Enumerate the differences between the three types of muscle tissue.

Ans. Muscle tissue is responsible for movement. The three types of muscle tissue based on structure and location are skeletal, cardiac and smooth muscles. Following are the differences exhibited by them **(Table 7.1)**.

Table 7.1: Comparison of different types of muscle.

Skeletal muscle (striated muscle)	Smooth muscle	Cardiac muscle
Attached to skeleton	It is related to viscera, e.g., gastrointestinal (GIT), excretory system	It is present exclusively in the myocardium of the heart
Long and cylindrical fibers	Spindle shaped cells	Cylindrical fibers which branch and communicate
Nucleus is oval, placed peripherally, and multinucleated	Single oval nucleus in the center of the cell	Single oval nucleus in the center of the cell
Voluntary	Involuntary	Involuntary
Shows prominent longitudinal and transverse striations, i.e., striated	Nonstriated/smooth	Striated
Supplied by spinal/somatic nerve	Innervation is by autonomic nervous system	Innervation is by autonomic nervous system
Absence of intercalated disc	Absence of intercalated disc	Presence of intercalated disc
Absence of branching and anastomosis of fibers	Absence of branching and anastomosis of fibers	Presence of branching and anastomosis of fibers

2. Describe thoracoabdominal diaphragm with its openings.

Ans.
- Diaphragm is the musculoskeletal partition between the abdominal and thoracic cavities.
- Superior surface presents two dome shaped bulging into the thorax with central tendon in between the two domes/cupola.

Origin

a. *Sternal fibers*—from xiphoid process.
b. *Costal fibers*—lower six ribs.
c. *Vertebral origin*—right and left crus which are attached to lumbar vertebrae.

Insertion—into the central tendon of the diaphragm.

Nerve supply—phrenic nerve.

Action—it is the *principal muscle for inspiration*. It also increases the intra-abdominal pressure which is required in activities like micturition, defecation and during child-birth.

Diaphragm has *openings* meant to allow passage of structures from thorax to abdomen and vice-versa.

Major openings are **(Fig. 7.1):**

At T8 vertebral level—inferior venacava passes from abdomen to thorax

At T10 vertebral level—esophagus and vagus nerve, from thorax to abdomen

At T12 vertebral level—aorta, thoracic duct, pass from thorax to abdomen.

Through *minor openings,* the following structures pass—superior epigastric and musculophrenic vessels, intercostal nerve, sympathetic chain, greater and lesser splanchnic nerves.

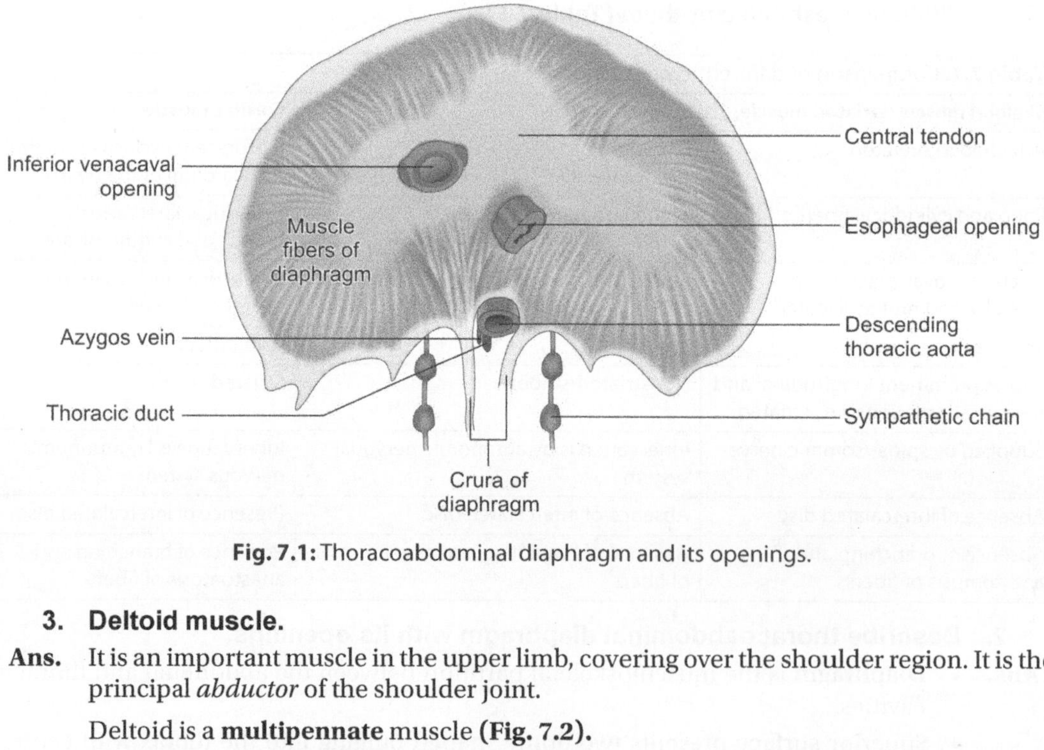

Fig. 7.1: Thoracoabdominal diaphragm and its openings.

3. Deltoid muscle.

Ans. It is an important muscle in the upper limb, covering over the shoulder region. It is the principal *abductor* of the shoulder joint.

Deltoid is a **multipennate** muscle **(Fig. 7.2).**

Origin—anterior fibers from clavicle, middle fibers from acromion process of scapula, posterior fibers from spine of scapula.

Insertion—into the deltoid tuberosity of humerus.

Nerve supply—axillary nerve.

Action—abduction at the shoulder joint. It is also involved in flexion and extension at this joint.

Applied anatomy

a. It is an important site for intra-muscular injection, since the area offered by it is wide. Injections are given hand breadth below the tip of acromion. One should be cautious as the axillary nerve passes close to site of injection.
b. The muscle can get paralyzed due to injury to the axillary nerve. This results in loss of contour over the shoulder, inability to abduct the shoulder joint.

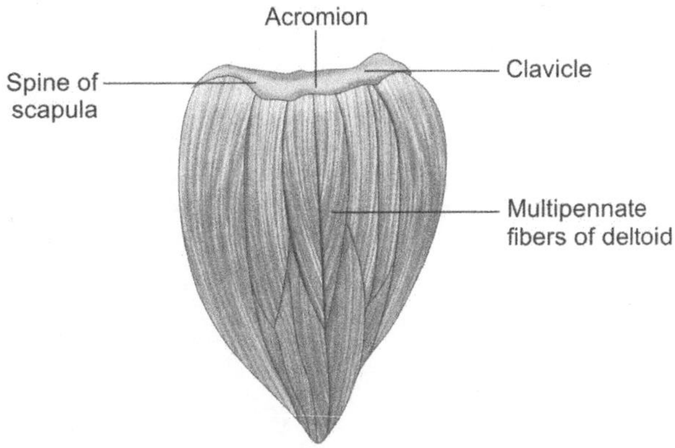

Fig. 7.2: Deltoid muscle.

4. Gluteus maximus muscle.

Ans. It is a prominent muscle over the buttocks. It is clinically important *since intramuscular injections are given over it.*

- **Origin (Figs. 7.3 A and B)**
  - From the gluteal surface of the ilium behind the posterior gluteal line.
  - Dorsal surface of sacrum and coccyx.
  - Sacrotuberous ligament.
  - Thoracolumbar fascia.
- **Insertion**
  - One-fourth of the muscle into gluteal tuberosity of femur.
  - Three-fourth of the muscle into iliotibial tract.
- **Nerve supply**—inferior gluteal nerve.
- **Action**—it is a powerful extensor of hip joint. It also rotates the hip laterally.

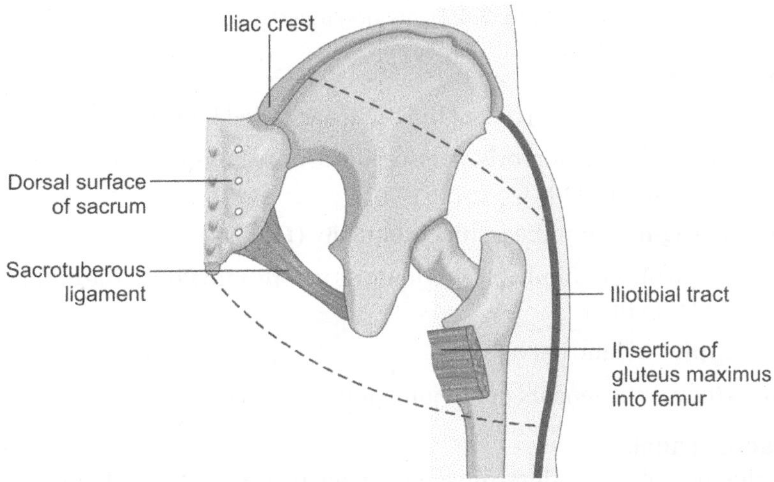

Fig. 7.3A: Gluteus maximus.

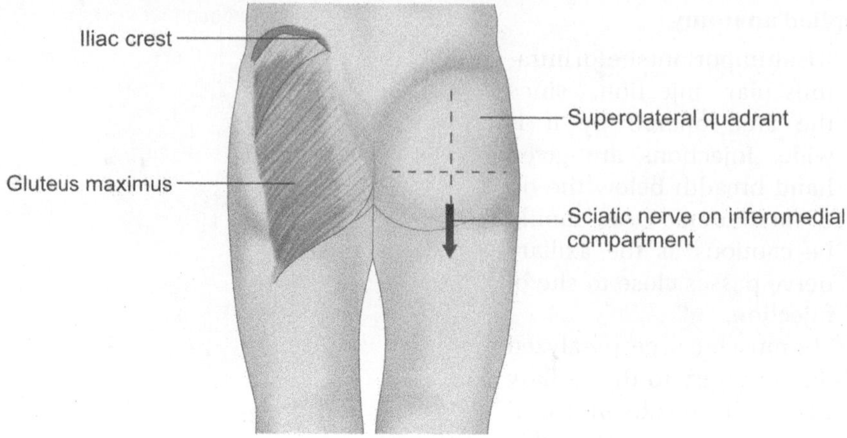

Fig. 7.3B: Gluteus maximus and site of injection.

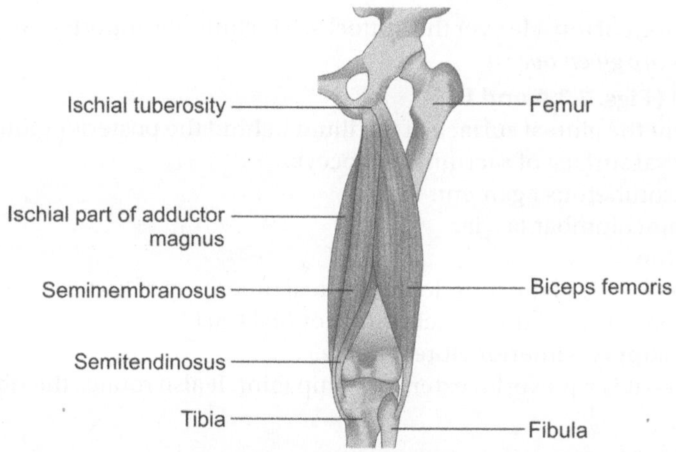

Fig. 7.4: Hamstring muscles.

5. Hamstring muscles.

Ans. The muscles present over back of the thigh are called hamstring muscles.

They include—biceps femoris, semitendinosus, semimembranosus and ischial part of adductor magnus muscle.

Common origin—from the ischial tuberosity **(Fig. 7.4)**.

Insertion—to tibia or fibula. Biceps femoris inserts into fibula, the other three muscles are inserted into tibia.

Nerve supply—sciatic nerve.

Action—they are extensors of hip joint and cause flexion at knee joint.

6. Adductor canal.

Ans.
- Adductor canal is an intermuscular space over middle third, medial aspect of the thigh.

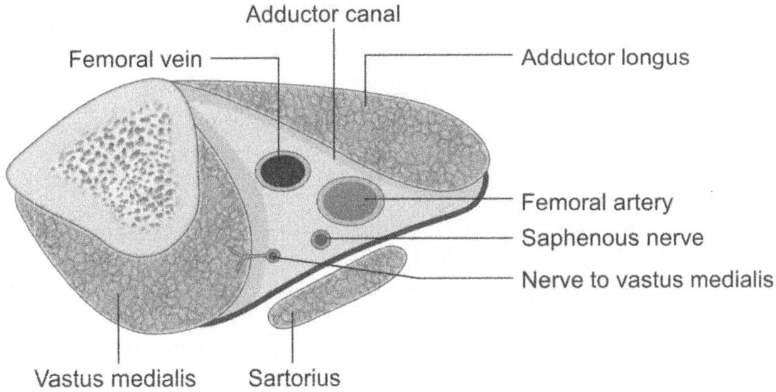

Fig. 7.5: Adductor canal.

- Also called as subsartorial or Hunter's canal.
- It extends from the apex of femoral triangle to the opening in adductor magnus muscle.
- The femoral artery and vein pass through the adductor canal.

It has the following **boundaries (Fig. 7.5):**

A. Anteromedially—vastus medialis.
B. Anterolaterally—sartorius.
C. Posterior wall—adductor longus above and adductor magnus below.

- **Contents**—saphenous nerve, nerve to vastus medialis, femoral artery and vein.
- **Applied anatomy**—any blunt injury here leads to injury to both the femoral vessels.

7. Sternocleidomastoid muscle.

Ans. Sternocleidomastoid muscle is an important landmark in the neck, as it crosses from lateral side of neck to midline.

- **Origin**: sternal head: Upper part of manubrium sterni.
- **Clavicular head:** Medial 1/3rd of superior surface of clavicle **(Fig. 7.6)**.
- **Insertion:** Lateral surface of mastoid process of temporal bone.
- **Nerve supply**: Spinal accessory nerve (eleventh cranial nerve).
- **Action**: Flex the head and neck on trunk. It also rotates the chin to the opposite side.

Applied anatomy—*wry neck*: the muscle is involved due to any pathological lesion or due to injury. The neck is rotated to one side.

8. Trapezius muscle.

Ans. Trapezius is important, prominent muscle over nape (back) of the neck.

- **Origin**—external occipital protuberance, ligamentum nuchae, superior nuchal line, C7 spine.
  - T1-T12 spines **(Fig. 7.7)**
- **Insertion**—lateral 1/3rd of the clavicle, medial margin of acromion, upper lip of spine of scapula.
- **Nerve supply**—spinal accessory nerve (eleventh cranial nerve).
- **Action**—elevates, rotates, and retracts the scapula along with various other muscles.

Applied anatomy: Paralysis of muscle leads to drooping of the shoulder, winged scapula.

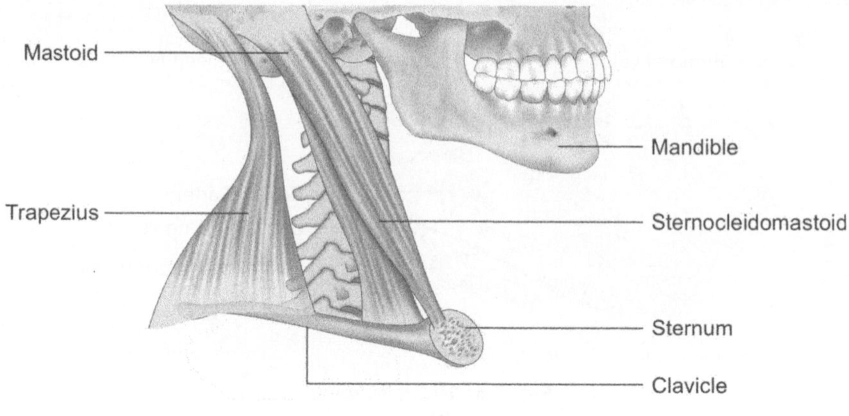

Fig. 7.6: Sternocleidomastoid.

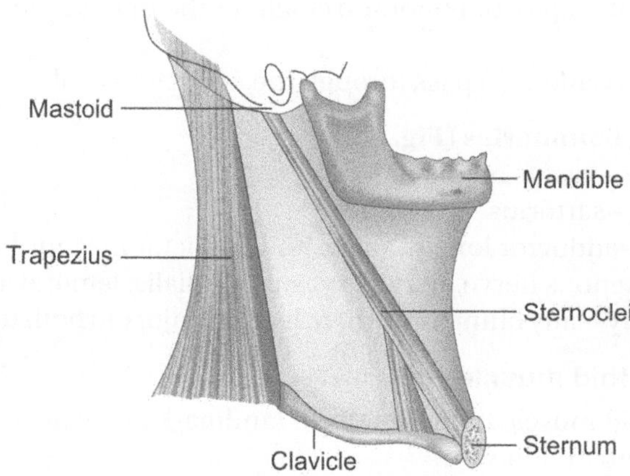

Fig. 7.7: Trapezius.

9. Muscles of the calf.

Ans.
- The calf muscles comprise of **medial and lateral head of gastrocnemius, and soleus (together called *triceps surae*) (Fig. 7.8)**
- **Origin**—medial and lateral head of gastrocnemius arise from medial and lateral femoral condyles respectively. The soleus arises from—upper 1/4th of posterior surface of fibula, soleal line of tibia.
- **Insertion**—these muscles unite to form a long and

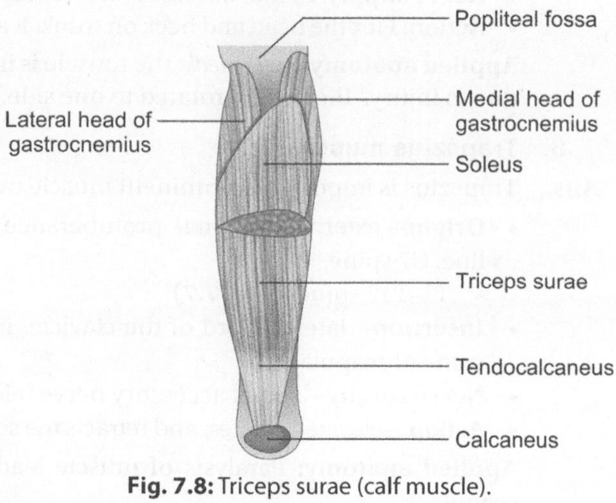

Fig. 7.8: Triceps surae (calf muscle).

strongest tendon in the body called *tendocalcaneus*. It is attached to posterior surface of calcaneum.

- **Nerve supply**—tibial nerve.
- **Action**—brings about plantar flexion of foot at ankle joint. They also flex knee joint.

Note: The soleus muscle has perforating veins which connect superficial and deep veins of leg. The veins do not possess valves. The contraction of the muscle squeezes the venous blood against gravity. Hence **soleus is called "the peripheral heart".**

10. Quadriceps femoris muscle.

Ans.
- The quadriceps femoris comprises group of muscles which are powerful extensors of knee joint.
- It consists of **four parts —vastus lateralis, vastusmedialis, vastus intermedius and rectus femoris (Fig. 7.9)**
- It is a big and bulky muscle group in front of thigh.
- **Origin**—from femur. Rectus femoris has origin from ilium of hip bone.

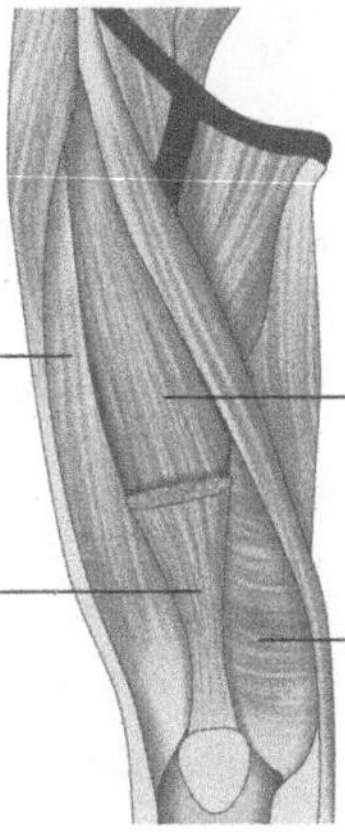

Fig. 7.9: Quadriceps femoris.

- They have a common **insertion into ligamentum patella** which is attached to **tibial tuberosity. Patella** develops as a **sesamoid bone** in this tendon.
- **Nerve supply**—femoral nerve.
- **Action**—rectus femoris flexes hip joint. Quadriceps as whole is a **powerful extensor of knee joint.**

11. Cubital fossa.

Ans. Cubital fossa is a triangular space situated in front of elbow.

Its **boundaries** are **(Fig. 7.10):**

a. Baseline joining medial and lateral epicondyles
b. Lateral—brachioradialis
c. Medial—pronator teres
d. Floor—supinator, brachialis
e. Roof—bicipital aponeurosis, cutaneous nerves of forearm, cubital vein.

Contents (lateral to medial side) radial nerve, biceps tendon, brachial artery with its terminal branches and the median nerve.

12. Popliteal fossa.

Ans. Popliteal fossa is a diamond-shaped space behind the knee.

Boundaries (Fig. 7.11)

A. Above and lateral—tendon of biceps femoris.
   Above and medial—semimembranosus and semitendinosus.
B. Below and lateral—plantaris, lateral head of gastrocnemius.
   Below and medial—medial head of gastrocnemius.

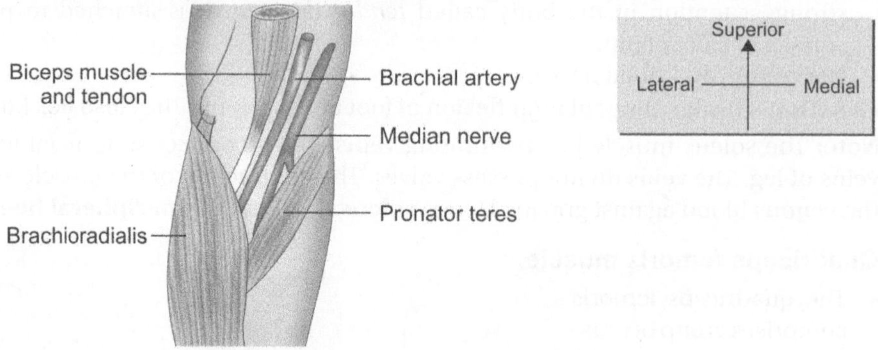

Fig. 7.10: Cubital fossa.

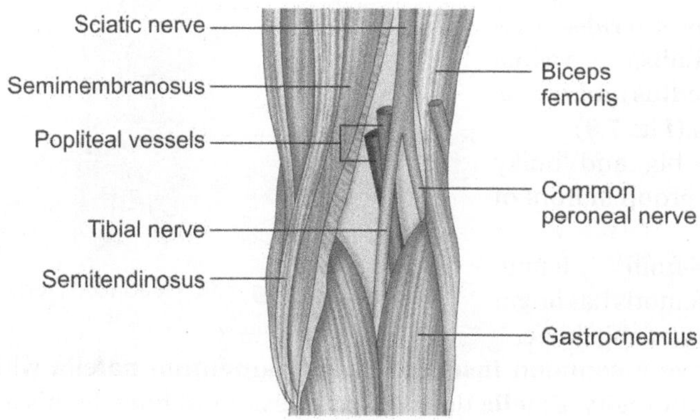

Fig. 7.11: Popliteal fossa.

C. **Roof**—Skin, subcutaneous vessels and nerves, popliteal fascia.
Floor—lower end of femur, oblique popliteal ligament.

Contents—tibial and common peroneal nerves, popliteal artery and vein, lymph nodes, fat, genicular nerves and vessels.

13. Boundaries and contents of axilla.

Ans. Axilla is a pyramidal space between the medial surface of upper arm and lateral chest wall.

Boundaries (Fig. 7.12)

- Anterior—pectoralis major and minor, clavipectoral fascia and subclavius.
- Posterior wall—subscapularis, teres major and latissimus dorsi.
- Medial wall—upper four ribs, intercostal muscles.

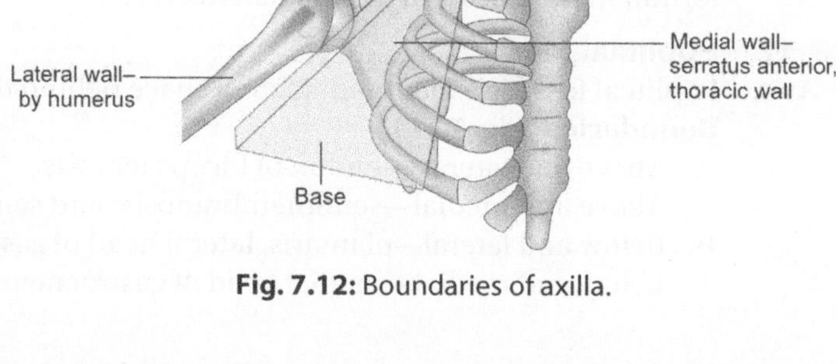

Fig. 7.12: Boundaries of axilla.

- Lateral wall—upper end of humerus.
- Apex—bound by first rib, clavicle and superior border of scapula.
- Base—skin and superficial fascia.

Contents (Fig. 7.13)—axillary artery and vein, axillary group of lymph nodes, infra-clavicular part of brachial plexus.

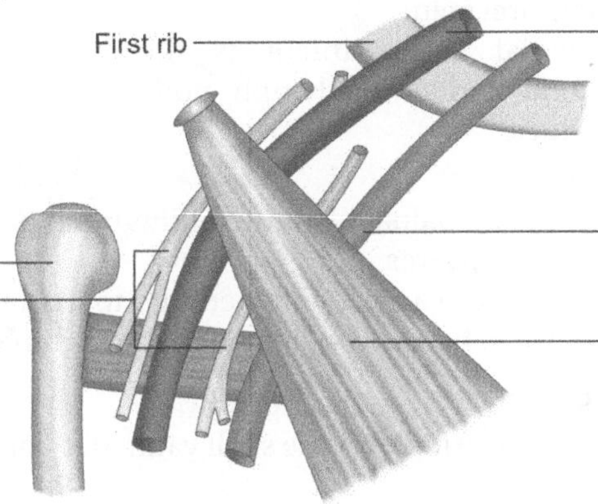

Fig. 7.13: Contents of axilla.

14. Femoral triangle.

Ans. It is a triangular space located in upper part of front of thigh.

Boundaries (Fig. 7.14):

- **Medial**—adductor longus
- **Lateral**—sartorius
- **Apex**—where lateral and medial borders meet
- **Base**—inguinal ligament
- **Roof**—fascia lata
- **Floor**—adductor longus, pectineus, psoas major and iliacus.

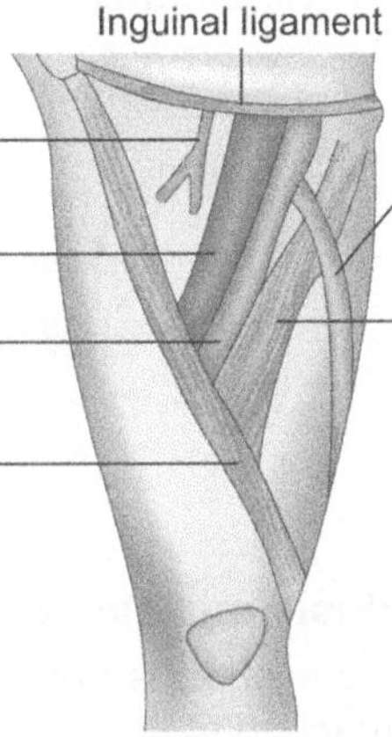

Fig. 7.14: Femoral triangle.

Contents of the femoral triangle—(Fig. 7.14) from medial to lateral side:

- **Femoral vein**—continues as external iliac vein. The great saphenous vein drains into it in the triangle.
- **Femoral artery**—it begins as continuation of external iliac artery.
  It gives various branches in the triangle and continues as popliteal artery at opening in adductor magnus.
- **Femoral nerve**—after a short course, it divides into branches supplying the muscles in front of thigh as well as skin over the thigh. The nerve also supplies hip- and knee joints.
- **Inguinal lymph nodes**—is in the roof of triangle. They are arranged in T-shaped manner, and are superficial and deep groups. They drain the lower limb, anterior abdominal wall below the umbilicus, back of trunk and buttocks.

Femoral sheath (Fig. 7.15):

- Upper parts of femoral vessels are enclosed by femoral sheath.
- It has **three compartments.**
  - **Lateral**—femoral artery and femoral branch of genitofemoral nerve.
  - **Middle**—femoral vein.
  - **Medial**—medial compartment is the femoral canal containing lymph node and lymphatics.

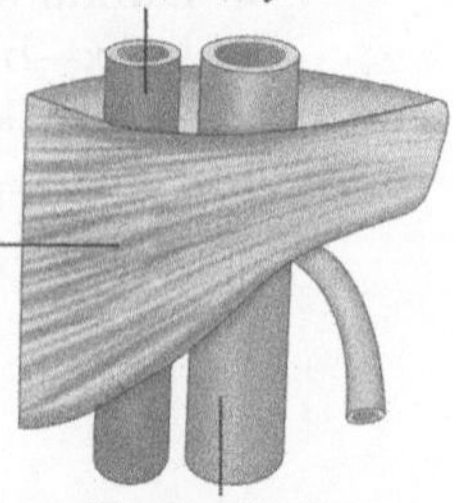

Fig 7.15: Femoral sheath with contents.

Applied anatomy

- Femoral pulse can be palpated at the midinguinal point. It is also used for various catheterization procedures.
- Inguinal lymph nodes can get enlarged due to infection and inflammation of the lower limb. They can be easily palpated in the inguinal region.

15. Layers of scalp.

Ans. Scalp is a soft tissue covering over the skull vault. It is consists of five layers **(Fig. 7.16)**.

i. Skin.
ii. Connective tissue—is dense. Contains blood vessels and nerves. These blood vessels are firmly adherent to the surrounding connective tissue.
iii. Aponeurosis—contributed by epicranial aponeurosis in the central portion. Frontalis and occipital belly are attached to it.
iv. Loose areolar tissue.
v. Pericranium.

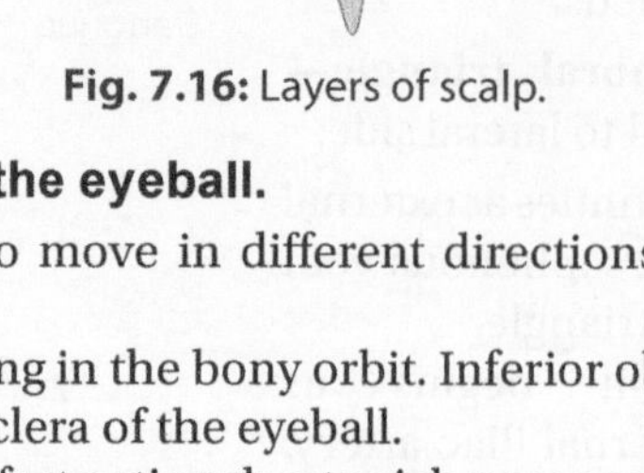

Fig. 7.16: Layers of scalp.

16. Extrinsic muscles of the eyeball.

Ans.

- The eyeball is able to move in different directions due to the extrinsic muscles attached to it.
- Origin—tendinous ring in the bony orbit. Inferior oblique from floor of maxilla.
- Insertion—into the sclera of the eyeball.
- They are precise and fast acting due to rich nerve supply.

There are three group of extraocular muscles as described in the **Table 7.2**. They include **(Fig 7.17):**

a. Superior and inferior rectus.
b. Medial and lateral rectus.
c. Superior and inferior oblique.

Levator palpebrae superioris is closely related, and brings about elevation of upper eyelid.

Table 7.2: Action and nerve supply of extraocular muscles.		
Eyeball muscles	**Action**	**Nerve supply**
Superior and inferior rectii	Move the eyeball superiorly and inferiorly respectively	All the muscles are supplied by 3rd cranial nerve, i.e., the oculomotor except: Superior oblique—by trochlear (4th) nerve Lateral rectus—abducent (6th) nerve
Medial and lateral rectus	Cause adduction and abduction respectively	
Superior oblique	Depression and abduction (moves the eyeball inferiorly and laterally)	
Inferior oblique	Elevation and abduction (moves the eyeball superiorly and laterally)	
Levator palpebrae superioris	Elevates the upper eyelid (does not act on the eyeball)	

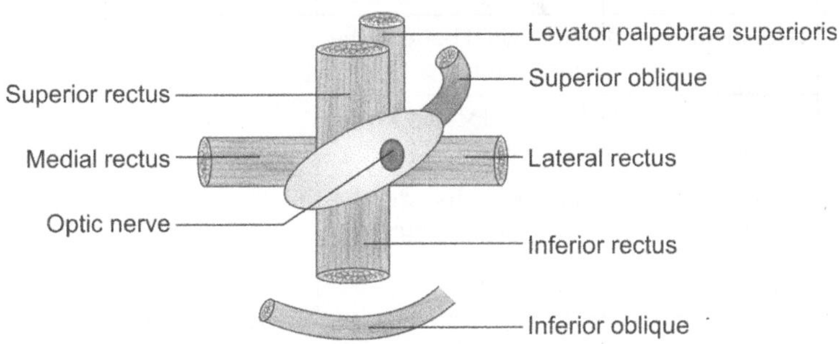

Fig. 7.17: Extraocular muscles of eyeball.

Applied anatomy: Strabismus is a condition in which the right and left eyeballs are aligned in different axis.

External strabismus—due to involvement of oculomotor nerve. Eyeball cannot be moved inferiorly and medially.

Internal strabismus—due to involvement of abducent nerve. The eyeball cannot move laterally.

The action and nerve supply of extraocular muscles are given in **Table 7.2**.

17. Describe the muscles of tongue.

Ans. The muscles of tongue are grouped into intrinsic and extrinsic muscles **(Fig. 7.18 and Table 7.3)**.

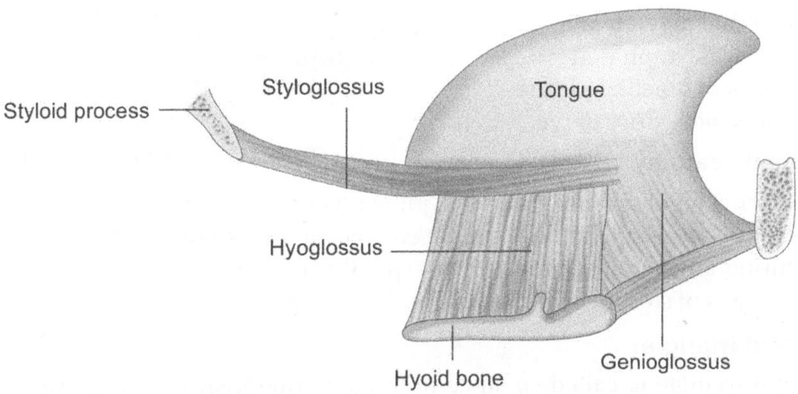

Fig. 7.18: Muscles of tongue.

Table 7.3: Description of muscles of tongue.

Tongue muscles	Names	Attachments	Additional features	Nerve supply
Extrinsic muscles	Genioglossus	From mandible to the tongue. Forms main bulk of the tongue	Genioglossus is called safety muscle of the tongue. It pulls the tongue anteriorly. • Styloglossus and palatoglossus pull the tongue up • Genioglossus and hyoglossus depress the tongue	Hypoglossal nerve except palatoglossus (by pharyngeal plexus)
	Styloglossus	From the styloid process to side of tongue		
	Palatoglossus	From soft palate to the side of tongue		
	Hyoglossus	From hyoid bone to the sides of tongue		
Intrinsic muscles	Transverse linguae	They are located within the tongue		Hypoglossal nerve
	Verticalis linguae. Superior and inferior longitudinal muscles	Action—change the shape of the tongue		

18. Posterior triangle.

Ans. The neck is divided by the sternocleidomastoid anterior and posterior triangles. The posterior triangle is behind the sternocleidomastoid.

The triangle has the following **boundaries (Fig. 7.19):**

Anterior—posterior border of sternocleidomastoid.

Posterior—anterior border of trapezius.

Base—middle 1/3rd of clavicle.

Contents

a. Subclavian artery
b. External jugular vein
c. Cervical lymph nodes
d. Trunk of brachial plexus
e. Spinal accessory nerve.

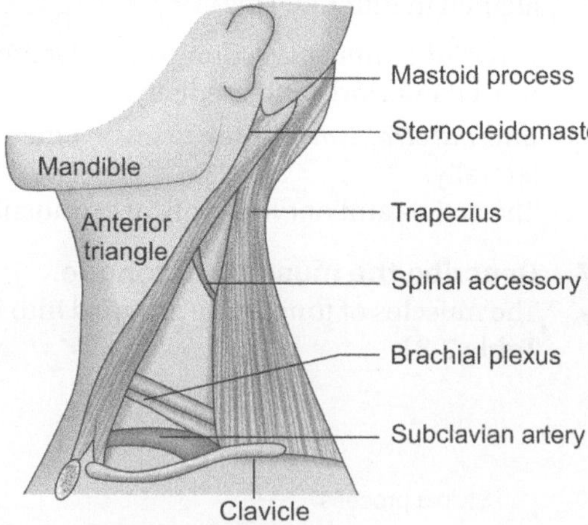

Fig. 7.19: Posterior triangle of neck.

Applied anatomy

- External jugular vein—is used as jugular venous manometer.
- Deep cervical lymph nodes can get enlarged in various diseases.
- During any surgical procedures—spinal accessory nerve is in danger. It leads to paralysis of sternocleidomastoid and trapezius.

19. Carotid triangle.

Ans. Carotid triangle is called so since it contains the great vessels (carotid vessels and internal jugular vein) of the neck.

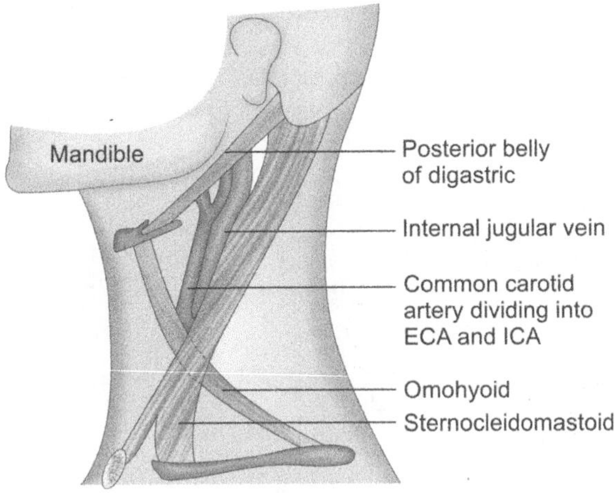

Fig. 7.20: Carotid triangle.
(ECA: external carotid artery; ICA: internal carotid artery)

Its boundaries are (Fig. 7.20):

a. Anterior—superior belly of omohyoid.
b. Posterior—sternocleidomastoid.
c. Superior—anterior belly of digastric.

Contents:

a. Arteries—**common carotid, internal carotid, external carotid** and its branches viz. superior thyroid, facial, lingual, occipital, ascending pharyngeal.
b. Veins—**internal jugular vein** and its tributaries.
c. Nerves—vagus, spinal accessory, hypoglossal, sympathetic chain.
d. Deep cervical lymph nodes.

Applied anatomy: Carotid artery pulsations can be felt in this triangle at the level of upper border of thyroid cartilage.

20. Anterior abdominal wall muscles.

Ans. The anterior abdominal wall comprises of three layer of flat muscles and a vertical rectus abdominis. The flat muscles are **external- and internal oblique abdominis, transversus abdominis** (superficial to deep) **(Figs. 7.21 and 7.22)**.

Origin—they are attached to the costal margin and from the iliac crest.

Insertion—they form broad aponeurosis which unite in the midline to form the linea alba. The aponeurotic layers of the flat muscles enclose the rectus abdominis resulting in formation of rectus sheath.

The **rectus abdominis** takes origin from pubic symphysis, and inserted into the xiphoid process. It has three transverse tendinous intersections (made of fibrous connective tissue) which increase the strength of the muscle. The levels of intersections are—one at umbilicus, at xiphoid process, third in between these two.

Nerve supply—lower 5 intercostal and subcostal nerves.

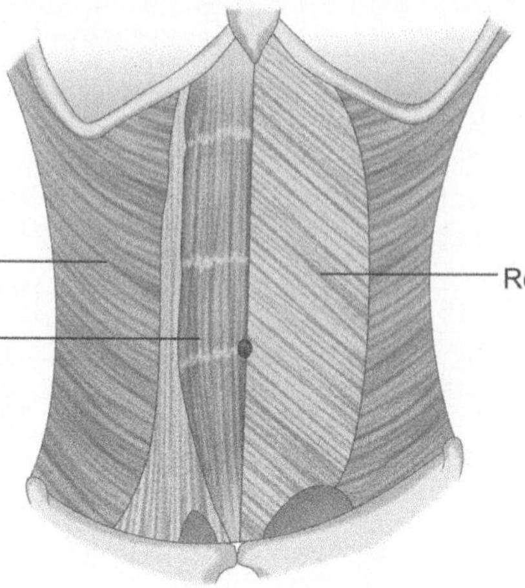

Fig. 7.21: Muscles of the anterior abdominal wall.

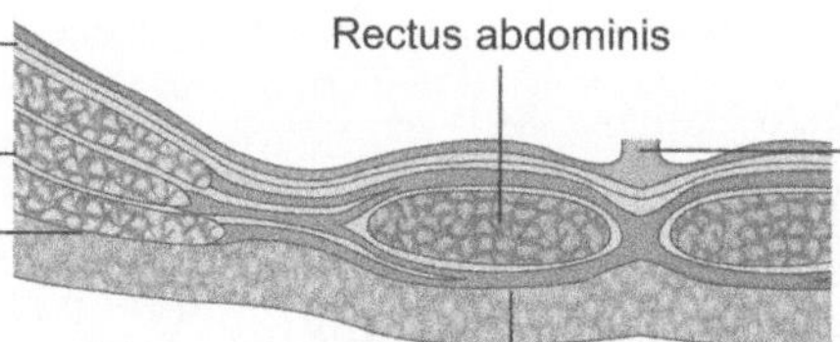

Fig. 7.22: Abdominal wall muscles with rectus sheath.

Actions:

- Support and protect the abdominal organs.
- Lateral flexion, anterior flexion, rotation of the vertebral column.
- Compress the abdominal viscera.
- Required for defecation, urination and child birth.

Applied anatomy—weakness of the muscles can lead to inguinal hernia.

21. Microscopic anatomy of skeletal muscle.

Ans. *Refer* **Figure 7.23.**

- The skeletal muscle cells are called **myocytes**. The myocytes fuse to form an elongated muscle fiber.
- The muscle fibers are cylindrical and arranged parallel to each other.
- Each fiber measures about 10-100 microns in diameter and length can vary from 10 to 40 cm.
- The plasma membrane is called **sarcolemma.**
- The fiber shows striations in form of **dark and light bands**. They are result of regular arrangement of actin and myosin myofibrils. The actin and myosin filaments are the contractile proteins.
- The myofibrils are numerous and push the nuclei to the periphery. Hence the skeletal muscles have characteristic **peripherally placed multiple nuclei**.
- Each fiber has an outer covering of connective tissue called endomysium.

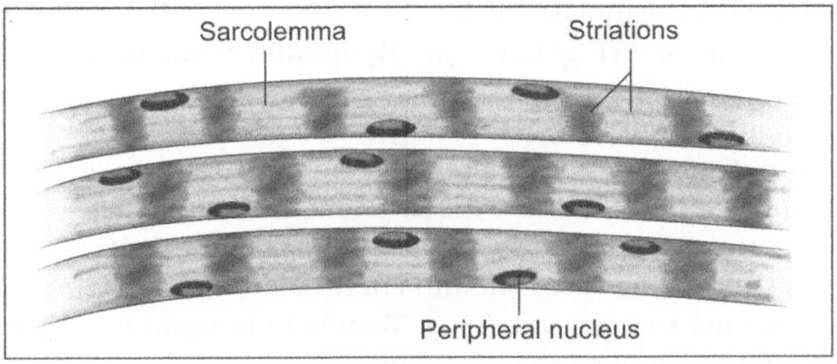

Fig. 7.23: Histology of skeletal muscle.

The skeletal muscle has all the other organelles present in a cell. They can be visualized under electron microscope. They include—**sarcoplasmic reticulum (SR)**, mitochondria (also called **sarcosome**), glycogen, Golgi apparatus, etc. The sarcoplasmic reticulum and T-tubules from sarcolemma form **triads**. The SR is involved in storing calcium ions required for muscle contraction. The red color of skeletal muscle is due to **myoglobin** pigment. Myoglobin binds oxygen and releases it by diffusion.

In transverse section—the connective tissue covers the muscle and muscle bundles/ fascicles. It supports and protects the skeletal muscle. They also carry blood vessels, nerves, and lymphatics. They are from outside to inside as follows:

- **Epimysium:** Covers the whole muscle.
- **Perimysium:** Covers the muscle bundles/fascicles. Muscle fascicles are group of muscle fibers.
- **Endomysium:** Covers the individual muscle fibers.

The individual muscle fibers are irregular with polygonal outline. Nucleus is peripheral.

22. Microscopic anatomy of cardiac muscle.

Ans. *Refer* **Figure 7.24**

- Cardiac muscle fibers (they are nothing but elongated cells) are cylindrical, and the fibers branch and communicate with each other.
- The outer plasma membrane is called **sarcolemma.**
- Invaginations of sarcolemma form **transverse t-tubules**. They help in rapid conduction of action potential.
- Nucleus is in the center.

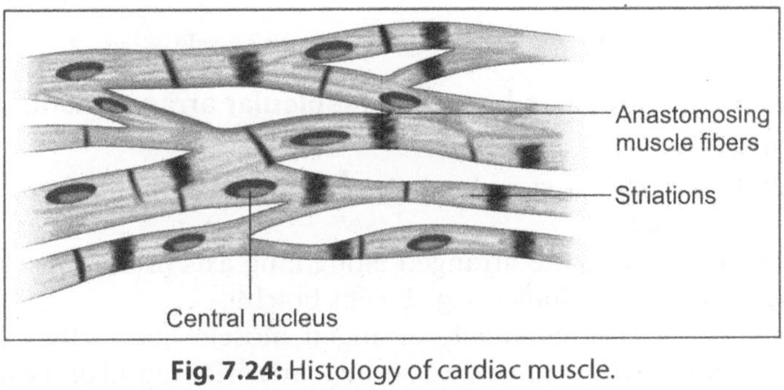

Fig. 7.24: Histology of cardiac muscle.

- **Sarcoplasm** is the cytoplasm of the muscle fiber. It is rich in myoglobin and glycogen.
- Glycogen helps in ATP generation. **Myoglobin** binds oxygen and releases when required.
- Plenty of mitochondria, help in ATP generation.
- Presence of **striations as in skeletal muscle**—which are result of regular arrangement of actin and myosin myofibrils. The striations are in form of **dark and light bands**.
- Prominent feature is the presence of **intercalated disc**—these are irregular transverse thickening of sarcolemma between two cardiac muscle cells. It is made of desmosomes and gap junctions. They help in rapid transmission of impulses, hence forms a *physiological syncytium*.
- Smooth endoplasmic reticulum forms membranous sacs around the myofibrils. Its dilated end abuts transverse T-tubules to form *diads*. It stores calcium ions and released when required.

23. Microscopic anatomy of smooth muscle.

Ans. *Refer* **Figure 7.25.**

- Smooth muscle—it should be smooth muscle is involuntary muscle, without striations.
- Cells are spindle shaped. Nucleus is central and oval.
- Length varies from 30–200 µm, diameter in the middle is 3–8 µm.
- Sarcoplasm contains actin and myosin filaments. But the density is less, not orderly arranged like in a striated muscle.
- Lack transverse tubules.
- Caveolae—are pocket like invaginations of plasma membrane containing extracellular calcium.
- Dense bodies are present near the plasma membrane to which thin filaments are attached. They correspond to Z-discs of striated muscle.

Location: Blood vessels, wall of hollow organs like GIT, trachea and airway passages, genitourinary tract, skin, etc.

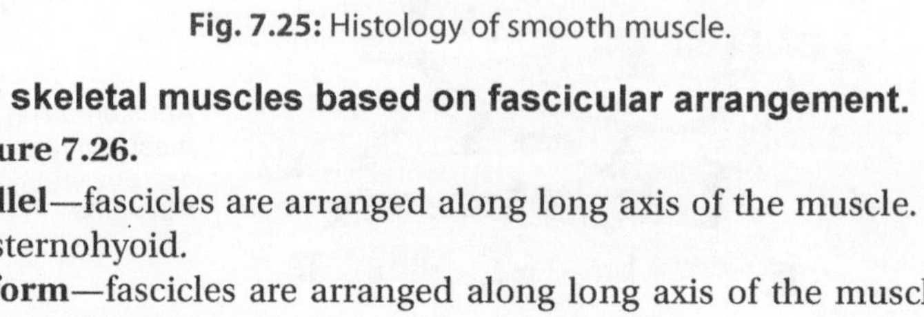

Fig. 7.25: Histology of smooth muscle.

24. Classify skeletal muscles based on fascicular arrangement.

Ans. *Refer* **Figure 7.26.**

1. **Parallel**—fascicles are arranged along long axis of the muscle. Tendons are flat, e.g., sternohyoid.
2. **Fusiform**—fascicles are arranged along long axis of the muscle, tendon tapers giving fusiform appearance, e.g., biceps brachii.
3. **Concentric**—circumferentially arranged muscle fibers. They form sphincters, hence found around orifices, e.g., orbicularis oris around oral cavity.

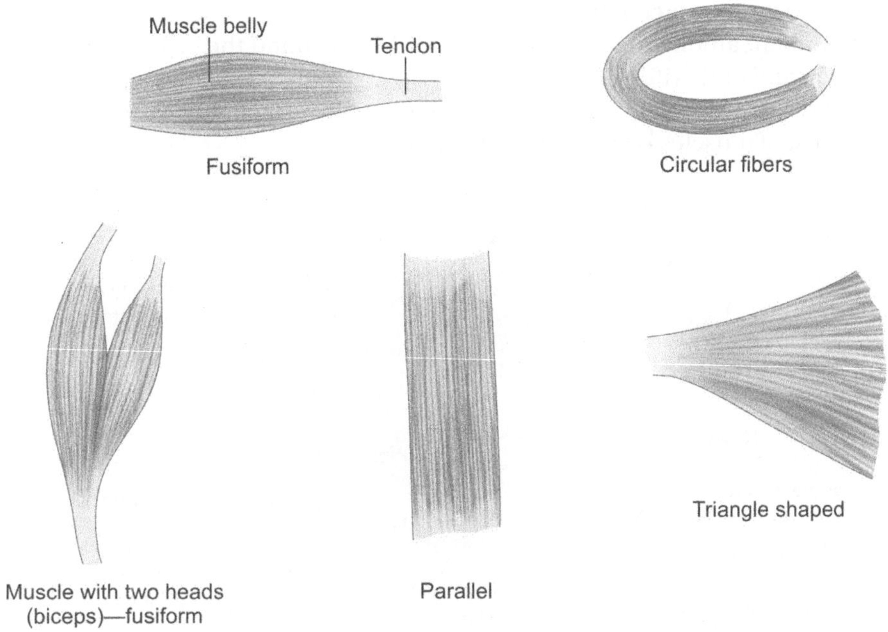

Fig. 7.26: Naming of muscles based on fiber arrangement.

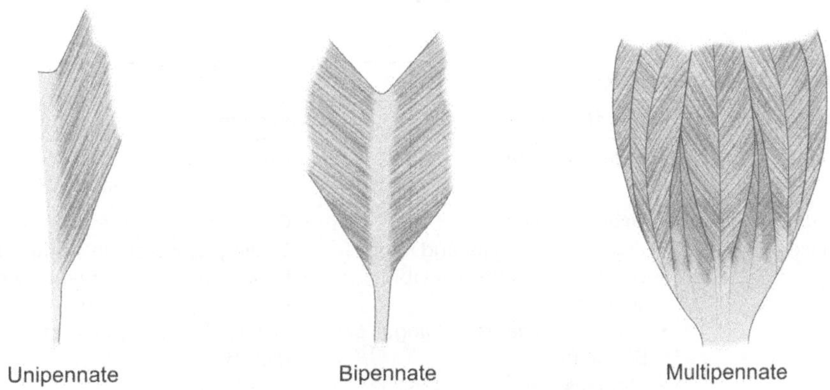

Fig. 7.27: Pennate arrangement of muscle fibers.

4. **Triangular**—fascicles arranged over broad area, e.g., trapezius.
5. **Pennate**—short fascicle and long tendon. It can be of three types **(Fig. 7.27)**.
   - Unipennate—fascicles along one side of the tendon—as in lumbricals.
   - Bipennate—fascicles arranged on both sides of the tendon, e.g., rectus femoris.
   - Multipennate—fascicles attach in oblique fashion to several tendons, e.g., deltoid.

25. Muscles of face/facial expression.

Ans.
- The muscles in the face are located in subcutaneous plane.
- **Origin**—fascia or any bone of the skull.
- **Insertion**—into the skin, hence they move the skin and not joints.

- **Nerve supply—facial nerve.**
- Prominent among them are the once which surround the orifices in face—ocular, nasal, and oral orifice.
- *Sphincters*—close the orifice; *Dilators*—open the orifice (**Fig. 7.28)**
- The list of muscles is given in the **Table 7.4.**

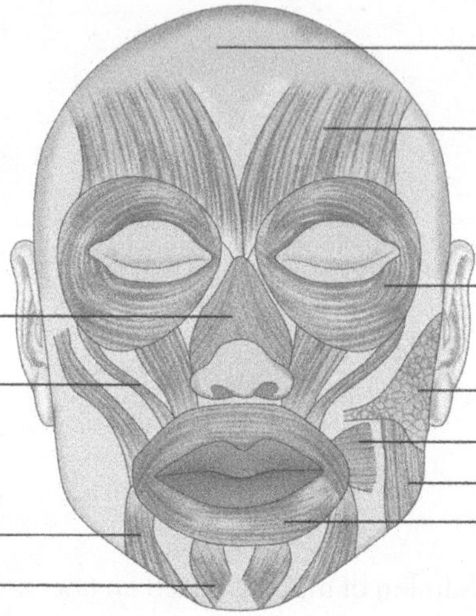

Fig. 7.28: Muscles of facial expression.

Table 7.4: Muscles of face.

Location	Name of the muscle	Comments
Scalp	**Occipitofrontalis**	• Draws scalp anteriorly • Wrinkles on forehead
Around the oral orifice	• **Orbicularis oris** • Zygomaticus major and minor • Levator and depressor labii superioris. • Levator and depressor anguli oris • Buccinator • Mentalis • Risorius	• Closes and protrudes the lips • Smiling- draws angle of mouth • Elevate upper lip, depress lower lip • Draws angle of mouth • Presses teeth against cheek, blowing mouth
Around the orbit	• **Orbicularis oculi** • Corrugator supercilii • Procerus	Closes the eyes by acting on eyelids—can be forceful or gentle closure
Neck	Platysma	Pouting of lips, may depress the mandible

- **Bell's or facial paralysis**—involves one side of face. It is due to involvement of facial nerve.

Etiology—inflammation of the nerve as in ear infection, trauma during ear surgery.

Patient—one half muscles of face paralyzed, manifest as—loss of wrinkles on forehead, inability to close the eyelid, drooling and difficulty in swallowing. Most of them recover spontaneously.

26. Muscles of mastication.

Ans. Mastication means chewing with the help of lower jaw. It occurs at temporomandibular joint.

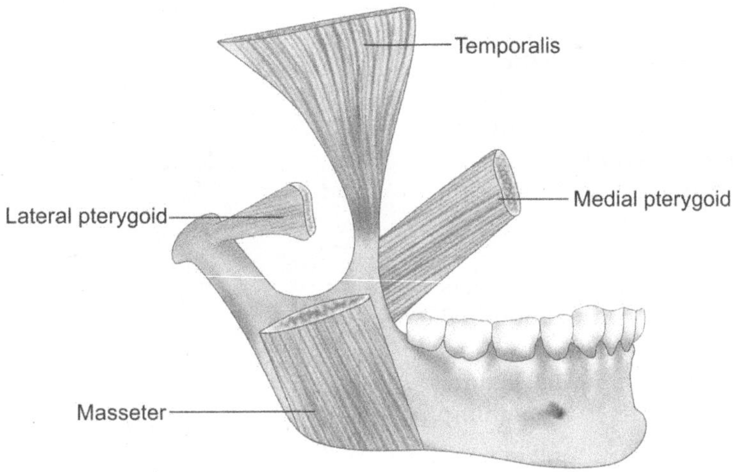

Fig. 7.29: Muscles of mastication.

- There are four muscles involved. Three of them help in closing the jaw and are very powerful—namely medial pterygoid, masseter and temporalis **(Fig. 7.29)**
- Lateral pterygoid helps to open the lower jaw.
- Medial and lateral pterygoids together help in side to side movements and protraction (mandible pulled backwards) at the TMJ. This crushes the food.
- **Nerve supply**—by mandibular nerve.
- **Attachments** are given in **Table 7.5**.

Table 7.5: Muscles of mastication.

	Origin	Insertion
Temporalis	Temporal fossa and temporal fascia	Coronoid process
Masseter	Zygomatic arch	Outer surface of ramus of mandible
Medial pterygoid	• Maxilla • Pterygoid process of sphenoid	Angle and ramus of mandible
Lateral pterygoid	Greater wing and pterygoid process of sphenoid	Neck of mandible

27. Pelvic diaphragm.

Ans.
- It is an important muscle in the pelvic cavity. It extends between pubis in front, behind by coccyx, on either side to the lateral pelvic wall.
- It is made of levator ani and ischiococcygeus.
- It is funnel-shaped, and separates pelvic cavity form perineum below it.
- Levator ani is composed of **three parts (Fig. 7.30):**
  1. Pubococcygeus
  2. Iliococcygeus
  3. Puborectalis
- **Origin**—pubis, ischial spine and pelvic fascia.

- **Insertion**—perineal body, coccyx, anal canal, urethra.
- **Nerve supply**—S2, S3, S4 spinal nerves.
- **Structures piercing the diaphragm**—urethra and anal canal, vagina in females.
- **Action/functions:**
  1. Maintains and supports the position of pelvic viscera.
  2. Important in various acts when intra-abdominal pressure increases—as in urination, defecation, childbirth, coughing, sneezing, vomiting.
  3. Has sphincteric action at—anorectal junction, urethra, and vagina.
  4. Maintains urinary and fecal continence.

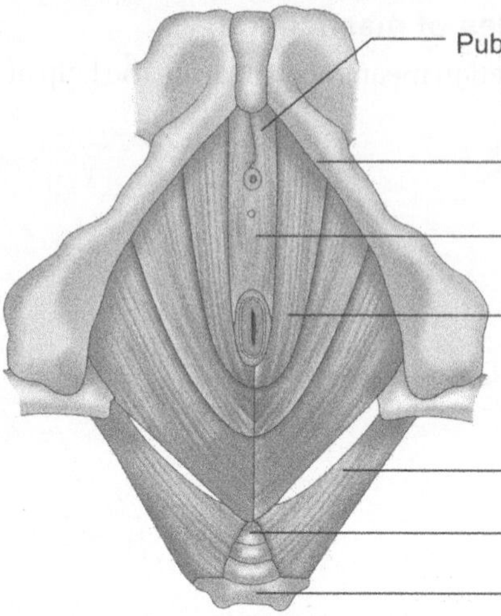

Fig. 7.30: Pelvic diaphragm.

28. Flexor retinaculum of hand.

Ans. Flexor retinaculum is a strong fibrous band of deep fascia extending across front of carpal bones (carpal tunnel). It prevents bow-stringing of flexor tendons.

Attachments (Fig. 7.31)

- Laterally to—tubercle of scaphoid, crest of trapezium.
- Medially to—hook of hamate, pisiform.
- Distal—continuous with palmar aponeurosis.

Relations (Fig. 7.32)

- Superficial—palmaris longus tendon, cutaneous branches of median and ulnar nerves and vessels.

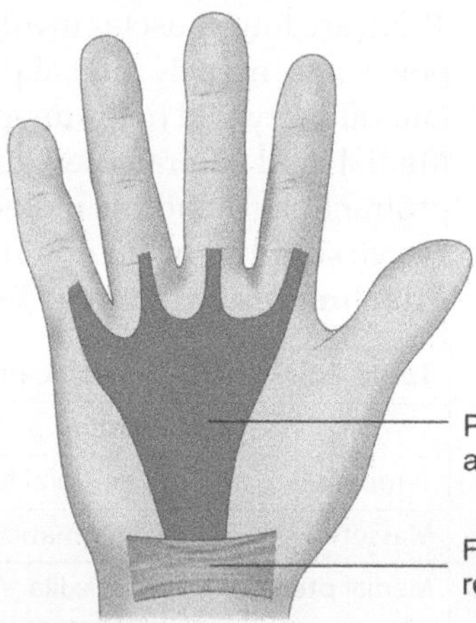

Fig. 7.31: Anterior view of flexor retinaculum.

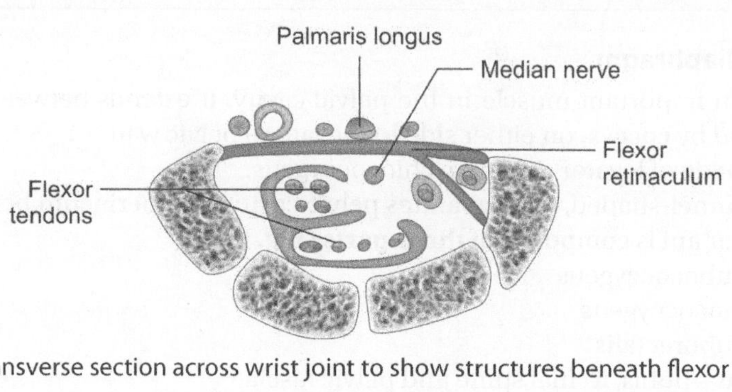

Fig. 7.32: Transverse section across wrist joint to show structures beneath flexor retinaculum.

- Deep—tendons of flexor digitorum superficialis, flexor carpi radialis longus, flexor digitorum profundus, flexor pollicis longus, median nerve.
- **Applied anatomy:** Compression of median nerve below the flexor retinaculum, i.e., in the carpal tunnel leads to carpal tunnel syndrome. This leads to pain, numbness and tingling of the affected hand.

SHORT ANSWERS 2 MARKS

29. Describe the terms origin, insertion and belly in relation to a skeletal muscle.

Ans. Any skeletal muscle has two ends **(Fig. 7.33)**.

- **Origin**—the muscle end attached to a stationary bone.
- **Insertion**—the tendon part of the muscle attached to a moving bone.
- The fleshy portion between these two is the **muscle belly**.

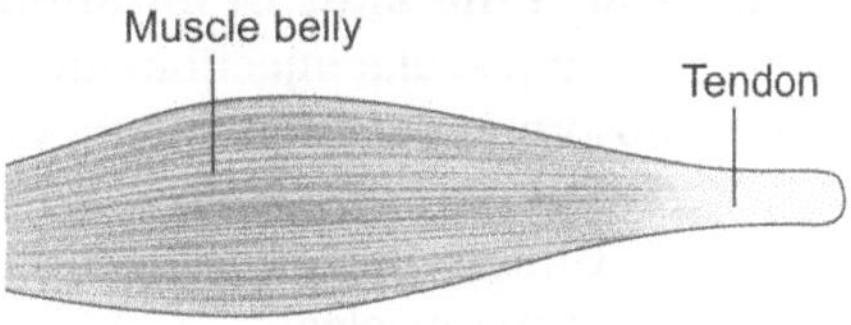

Fig. 7.33: Parts of a muscle.

30. What is a fascia and aponeurosis?

Ans. **Fascia**—it is dense, broad sheet of irregular connective tissue found lining the body wall and limbs, supports and surrounds the different muscles/muscle groups.

Aponeurosis—it is the broadened tendon of any flat muscle. It is the extension of connective tissue of muscle.

31. Name the connective tissue coverings of the muscle.

Ans. Three layer of connective tissue coverings extend from fascia of the muscle. It supports and protects the skeletal muscle. They are from outside to inside as follows:

- **Epimysium:** Covers entire muscle.
- **Perimysium:** Covers muscle fascicles.
- **Endomysium:** Covers individual muscle fibers.

The three connective tissue layers extend beyond the muscle in form of a **tendon**, that attaches it to the periosteum of the bone.

32. Differentiate the following terms.

Ans. a. **Tendon and aponeurosis**—tendon is round and cord like. Aponeurosis is broad and flat attachment of a muscle.

b. **Muscle origin and muscle insertion**—points of attachment of each muscle are its origin and insertion. The origin is the most stationary end of the muscle and the range of movement is greater at insertion.

33. Name any four flexors of forearm

Ans.
- The muscles in front of forearm are involved in flexion at wrist joint.
- They are arranged in superficial and deep layers.

Superficial group	**Deep group**
a. Pronator teres	a. Flexor pollicis longus
b. Flexor carpi radialis	b. Flexor digitorum profundus
c. Flexor carpi ulnaris	c. Pronator quadratus
d. Flexor digitorum superficialis	

- **Nerve supply**—median and ulnar nerves.

34. Name the muscles forming quadriceps femoris.

Ans.
- Quadriceps femoris is located in the anterior compartment of thigh.
- It causes extension at knee joint.
- Nerve supply by femoral nerve.
- The muscles are:
  a. Rectus femoris
  b. Vastus lateralis
  c. Vastus intermedius
  d. Vastus lateralis

35. Name the sites of intramuscular injections (Figs.7.34Ato D).

Ans. Intramuscular injections are given over the muscles which provide wide surface area for absorption of drugs and they are easily accessible. Sites of intramuscular injections are:
- Deltoid
- Gluteus maximus (over the gluteal area)
- Vasti muscles

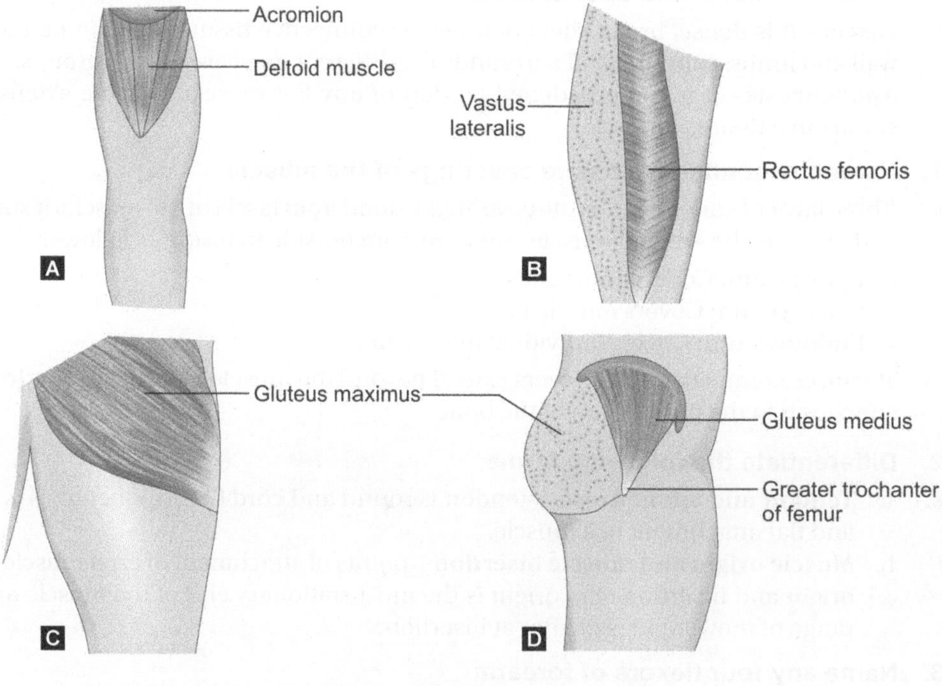

Figs. 7.34A to D: (A) Arm; (B) Thigh; (C) Gluteal region (dorsogluteal); (D) Lateral hip (ventrogluteal). (Source: https://www.nursingtimes.net/clinical-archive/assessment-skills/injection-technique-1-administering-drugs-via-the-intramuscular-route-23-07-2018/)

36. Features of muscles for facial expression.

Ans. Muscles of face are unique in many ways.
- They arise from fascia or bone of the facial skeleton, and inserted into the subcutaneous tissue of the face.

- They move the skin of face rather than the joint.
- They are arranged around the orifices—orbit and oral. So the muscles are arranged around these orifices. They are either constrictors or dilators of these orifices.
- They are supplied by facial nerve.

37. Contents of infratemporal fossa.

Ans. Infratemporal fossa is present over side of the head, below the zygomatic arch and behind the maxilla, front of ear. It has major structures namely:

- Mandibular nerve and its branches.
- Maxillary artery and its branches.
- Otic ganglion.
- Pterygoid venous plexus.

38. Name the layers of deep cervical fascia.

Ans. The entire neck structures are covered by connective tissue sheets which form well-defined fasciae. In some areas they are thin, and over some thick. They are important surgically.

The layers are:

- Investing layer
- Pretracheal layer
- Prevertebral layer
- Carotid sheath

39. Enumerate the subdivisions of anterior triangle.

Ans. The anterior triangle is in front of the sternocleidomastoid. It can be subdivided into four triangles:

1. Muscular triangle
2. Submandibular/digastric triangle
3. Carotid triangle
4. Submental triangle

40. Enumerate the contents of digastric triangle.

Ans. The digastric triangle is bounded by anterior and posterior belly of digastric, and lower border of mandible above. The contents include:

a. Submandibular gland
b. Submandibular lymph nodes
c. Mylohyoid nerve and vessels
d. Hypoglossal nerve

41. Inguinal canal.

Ans. It is a musculoaponeurotic passage extending from deep inguinal ring to superficial inguinal ring. Length—3.7-5 cm. **(Fig. 7.35)**.

Wall of the canal is formed by—external, internal oblique and transversus abdominis muscles.

Contents—spermatic cord in males, round ligament in females.

- Ilioinguinal nerve, genital branch of genitofemoral nerve.

Applied anatomy: Inguinal hernia can occur through the passage due to weakness in the anterior abdominal wall.

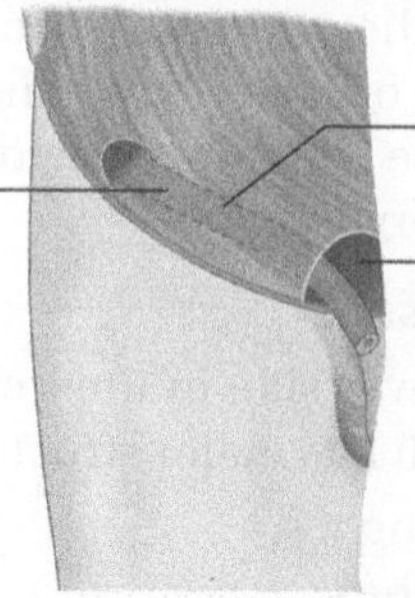

Fig. 7.35: Inguinal canal.

42. Name the anterior abdominal wall muscles.

Ans. The muscles include external, internal oblique, transversus abdominis muscles, pyramidalis and the rectus abdominis.

43. Name the muscles of mastication.

Ans.
- These muscles are attached to the mandible and act at the temporomandibular joint.
- The three muscles involved in **closing the jaw** are *medial pterygoid, masseter and temporalis.*
- The *lateral pterygoid muscle* is a **depressor** (opening the jaw) of the mandible.
- These are supplied by mandibular nerve.

44. What are the actions of anterior abdominal wall muscles?

Ans.
- Protect abdominal viscera.
- Flex the vertebral column.
- Helpful in expiratory efforts
- Important in acts of urination, defecation, child birth.
- Lateral flexion and rotation of the vertebral column.

45. Define perineum and its subdivisions.

Ans. Perineum is a diamond-shaped space at the pelvic outlet **(Fig. 7.36).**

Its **boundaries** are:

1. Anterior—pubic symphysis
2. Posterior—coccyx
3. Lateral—ischial tuberosities.

A transverse line between the two ischial tuberosities separates the perineum into two triangles:

1. Urogenital triangle in front
2. Anal triangle behind.

46. Rotator cuff muscles of shoulder joint.

Ans.
- These muscles located around the shoulder joint give stability and strength to it.
- They include—subscapularis, supraspinatus, infraspinatus and teres minor.
- They extend from scapula to humerus.
- Supraspinatus tendon is prone to wear and tear as it is between acromion and head of humerus.

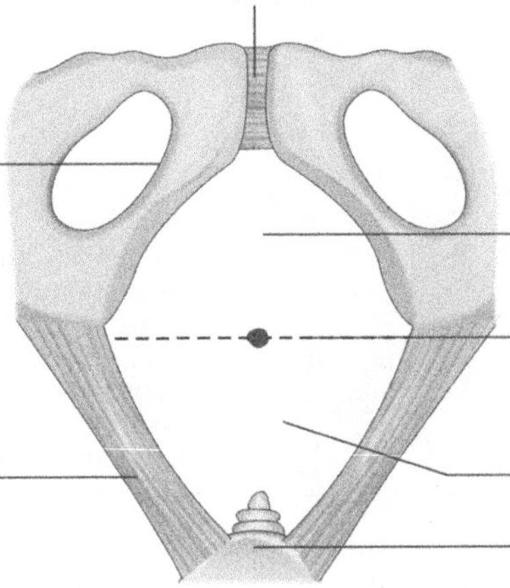

Fig. 7.36: Subdivisions of perineum.

- Inflammation of these tendons leads to rotator cuff tendinitis—pain during abduction and lateral rotation.

47. Name the structures passing deep to flexor retinaculum of hand.

Ans. Flexor retinaculum is a band of deep fascia extending across front of carpal bones. It prevents bow-stringing of flexor tendons.

Structures passing beneath it are (Fig. 7.31B):

- Tendons of flexor digitorum superficialis, flexor carpi radialis longus, flexor digitorum profundus, flexor pollicis longus.
- Median nerve.

Applied anatomy—median nerve maybe compressed in carpal tunnel syndrome.

48. Name the thenar and the hypothenar muscles.

Ans. Thenar muscles move the thumb and hypothenar muscles move little finger. They are located within the hand.

Thenar muscles—abductor pollicis, flexor pollicis brevis, abductor pollicis.

Hypothenar muscles—abductor digiti minimi, flexor digiti minimi, adductor digiti minimi.

49. Contents of rectus sheath.

Ans. Rectus sheath is formed by interlacing of fibers of aponeurosis of the flat muscles of the abdomen. It contains **(Fig. 7.22)**:

- Rectus abdominis muscle
- Pyramidalis
- Superior and inferior epigastric vessels
- Lower five intercostal nerves and subcostal nerves

50. Layers of the anterior abdominal wall.

Ans. There are nine layers in the anterior abdominal wall from superficial to deep **(Fig. 7.37):**

1. Skin.
2. Camper's fascia—superficial fatty layer.

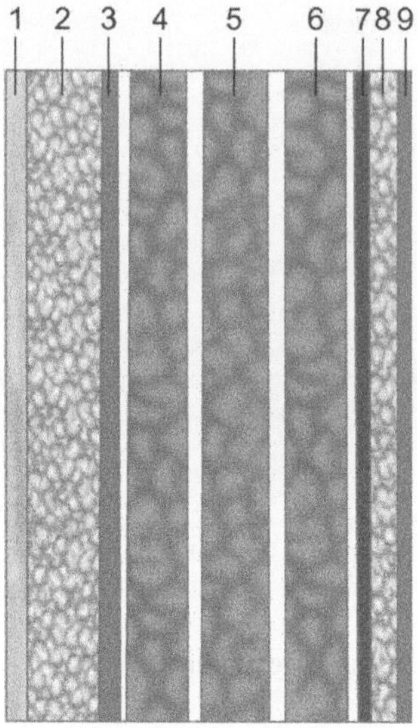

Fig. 7.37: Layers of anterior abdominal wall.

3. Scarpa's fascia—deep membranous layer.
4. External oblique muscles.
5. Internal oblique muscles.
6. Transversus abdominis.
7. Fascia transversalis.
8. Extraperitoneal fat
9. Parietal peritoneum.

51. Name the muscles which assist in respiration.

Ans.
- *Inspiration*—thoracoabdominal diaphragm, external intercostal muscle. Accessory muscles—sternocleidomastoid, scalene, pectoralis minor.
- *Expiration*—internal intercostal muscle.

Accessory muscles—flat muscles of the anterior abdominal wall.

52. Define an intercostal space and mention its contents.

Ans. *Refer* **Figures 7.38 and 7.39.**

The space between the upper and lower ribs is called intercostal space. It contains:
- External intercostal
- Internal intercostal
- Transverse thoracis
- Intercostal nerves and vessels

Contents of intercostal space are: intercostal artery and vein, intercostal nerve.

53. Perineal body.

Ans.
- It is a fibromuscular body anterior to anal orifice.
- Several perineal muscles are inserted into it, including few fibers of levator ani.
- The perineal muscles function to control—urination and ejaculation in males; urination and compressing vagina in females.

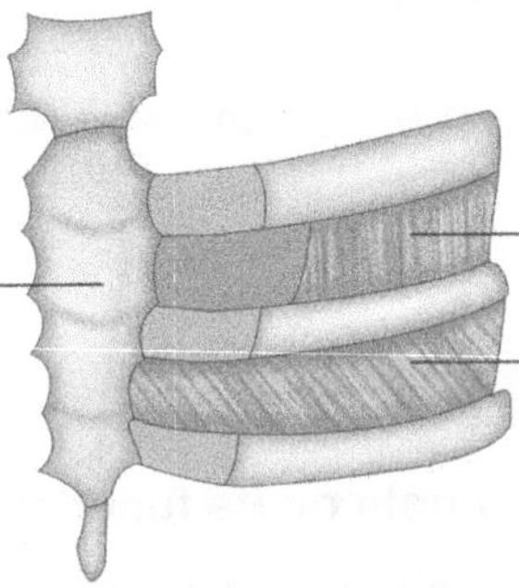

Fig. 7.38: Intercostal muscles.

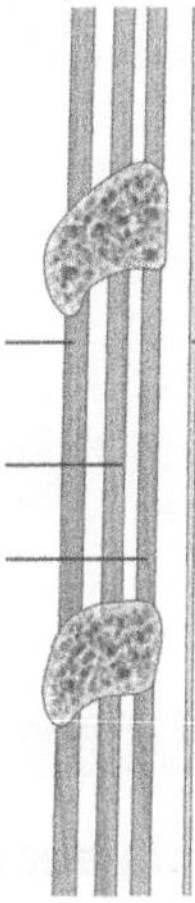

Fig. 7.39: Contents of intercostal space. (IC: intercostal muscle)

- Significance: Integrity of perineal body and muscles of perineum is required for continence and during childbirth. Perineal body may get damaged during delivery of the baby.
- Surgical incision across perineum during delivery is called episiotomy.

Notes:

- **Muscle hypertrophy**—it is the muscle growth occurring after birth by increase in size of existing fibers. It results from exercise, or effect of certain hormones like growth hormone.
- **Muscle atrophy**—it is the decrease in the size due to loss of myofibrils. It can be due to *disuse* (bed-ridden, those with casts) or interruption of nerve supply-*denervation* atrophy.
- **Rigor mortis**—it is a state of rigidity of the human body after death, due to loss of ATP following death. It begins in 3-4 hours after death, and disappears after 24 hours.
- **Duchenne muscular dystrophy**—it is a genetic condition caused due to mutation of gene coding dystrophin gene. It is X-linked recessive disorder. It leads to progressive weakness of muscles in the body.
- **Intramuscular injection**: is a common mode used to deliver drugs for rapid absorption. This penetrates the skin, subcutaneous tissue and then enters deep within the muscle. The drug is absorbed by the blood vessels in the muscle. Common sites include: Gluteus medius, deltoid, vasti muscles. Care should be taken to avoid blood vessels or nerves in the vicinity.
- **Dysphagia**—means difficulty in swallowing. Causes may be infections, cancer in the head and neck region or esophagus, due to weakness of muscles involved in deglutition (swallowing).
- **Hernia**—it is an abnormal protrusion of a structure or any organ. This is due to weakness of the muscles. It leads to a swelling in the inguinal region. Surgery is done to reduce the swelling, and repairing the defect. The various types include—inguinal, femoral, epigastric, lumbar hernias.
- **Superficial ring**—is a defect in the external oblique aponeurosis.
- **Deep inguinal ring**—is a defect in transversalis fascia.

8
CHAPTER

Integumentary System

LONG ESSAYS — 10 MARKS

1. Explain about the different layers of skin. Add a note on its function.

Ans. Skin is the outermost covering of the body and also the largest sensory organ. It is made up of **two layers**—(1) an outer epidermis and (2) an inner dermis. A third layer beneath it is called hypodermis which is nothing but subcutaneous layer of fat **(Fig. 8.1)**.

Epidermis—it is lined by stratified squamous keratinized epithelium. It is made of four to five layers of epithelial cells. They are stratum basale, stratum spinosum, stratum granulosum, stratum lucidum and stratum corneum. Details about each layer of epidermis is given in **Table 8.1**.

In thin skin, stratum lucidum is absent. Thick skin has all the five layers, found only in the palm and soles.

Cells of epidermis are called **keratinocytes**. They manufacture and store keratin. **Keratin** is a protein that gives hair, nails, and skin their hardness and water resistant properties.

Inner dermis—consists of connective tissue, blood vessels, nerves and lymphatics. Other skin appendages are also located namely sweat glands, sebaceous glands. Dermis again is divided into two layers—papillary and a deeper reticular layer.

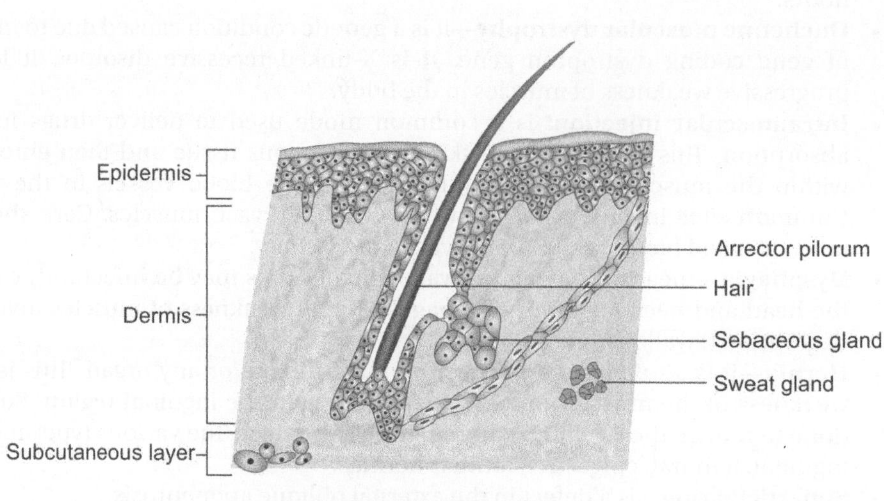

Fig. 8.1: Layers of skin.

Table 8.1: Description of different layers of skin, and function of different cell types.

Layer of epidermis (from deep to superficial)	Type of cell and its features	Functions
Stratum basale—single layer of cuboidal cells	i. Basal or the cuboidal cells—rest on the basement membrane. They are called keratinocytes. ii. Merkel cell iii. Melanocyte iv. Langerhans cell	i. Act as stem cells ii. Receptors for touch iii. Melanin synthesis—melanin pigment gives color to skin and hair. It also protects from UV light from sun iv. Antigen presenting cell
Stratum spinosum—9–10 layers thick	i. Keratinocytes—cells appear to have spines as they are attached by desmosomes at their cell membrane ii. Langerhans cell—skin macrophages	• Synthesize keratin—protective • Release lamellar granules—contains water repelling glycolipid, making skin waterproof Phagocytose bacteria, foreign particles and dead skin cells
Stratum granulosum—3–5 layer of cells	Keratinocytes—nuclei and other organelles begin to degenerate	Synthesize fibrous keratin and keratohyalin granules
Stratum lucidum	Translucent layer, made of dead, flattened cells	Protein eleidin that is lipid rich which is responsible for transparency
Stratum corneum—15–30 layer cell thick	Dry, dead layer	• Protects against bacteria • Prevents dehydration • Mechanical protection to the underlying layers

i. **Papillary layer**—loose connective tissue with elastic and collagen fibers, connective tissue cells; blood vessels, nerve endings. Finger-like projections called dermal papillae project into overlying epidermis.
ii. **Reticular layer**—it is thicker, made of dense, irregular connective tissue. It is rich in blood vessels, nerves. Elastic fibers are responsible for elasticity, whereas collagen fibers provide tensile strength and hydration to the skin.

Functions of skin:

a. Protection
b. Sensory organ
c. Thermoregulation
d. Vitamin D synthesis

SHORT ESSAYS 5 MARKS

2. Hair.

Ans. Hair is an appendage of skin. It is made of columns of dead, keratinized cells. Hair is absent over palms, soles, and fingers.

Hair consists of two main parts:

1. **Hair root**—located in the dermis.
2. **Hair shaft**—is exposed to the surface **(Fig. 8.2)**.

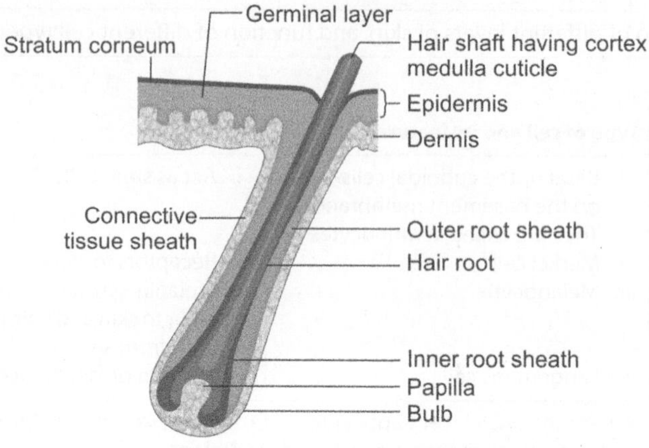

Fig. 8.2: Scheme to show some details of a hair follicle.

The **root** is embedded in the dermis. The enlarged lower part is called the **Bulb**. The bulb is invaginated by connective tissue of dermis called **hair papilla**. Around the bulb, is a tubular sheath of cells called **hair follicle**. The hair follicle is responsible for the production and growth of hair.

The hair papilla is surrounded by layers of keratinocytes called **matrix**. They also contain melanocytes, responsible for the hair color. The cells in the matrix undergo keratinization as the cells migrate upwards to form cuticle.

The **shaft** is the visible part of hair. The layers in the shaft are: cuticle, cortex, and medulla. Medulla has vacuolated cells and cortex has cuboidal cells. Cuticle has flat squamous cells and is the outermost layer.

Hair growth begins by proliferation of keratinocytes in the hair bulb. As new cells are produced, hair shaft is pushed up the skin surface. The external hair visible outside is completely made of dead cells filled with keratin, hence does not have sensation.

The root of the hair receives the opening of sebaceous gland on its side and forms **pilosebaceous unit.**

Arrector pili muscle attaches from the root of the hair to the dermis-epidermal junction.

Hair growth occurs in three phases—anagen, catagen and telogen.

- Anagen—hair cells multiply at the root, pushing the shaft upwards. Duration is 2–7 years.
- Catagen—lasts 2–3 weeks and is transitory phase.
- Telogen phase—lasts for 2–4 months. Hair follicle is at rest. No new growth occurs.

At end of telogen, new hair growth starts, old hair is shed off.

Function—protection, sensory input, thermoregulation, and communication.

Example—scalp hair, eyelashes, eyebrows, hair in nose and ears.

Clinical condition: If the passage of sebum from the sebaceous gland is blocked, it will accumulate leading to pus formation. The condition is called acne vulgaris. It affects the hair follicle, inflammation and accumulation of dead cells, and sebum called comedones.

3. Nail.

Ans. Nail is an accessory structure of the skin. It consists of dead, keratinized epithelium that is tightly packed and hard. It has two main parts—nail bed, nail body and also a free edge.

Location—on the dorsal aspect of the distal phalanx of the finger.

Nail bed—Figures 8.3 and 8.4

- Provides mechanical support to the tip of fingers.
- Back-supports while picking up small objects.
- Nail bed is composed of dead keratinocytes.
- It is rich in blood vessels, hence pink in color except at the lunula which is white.

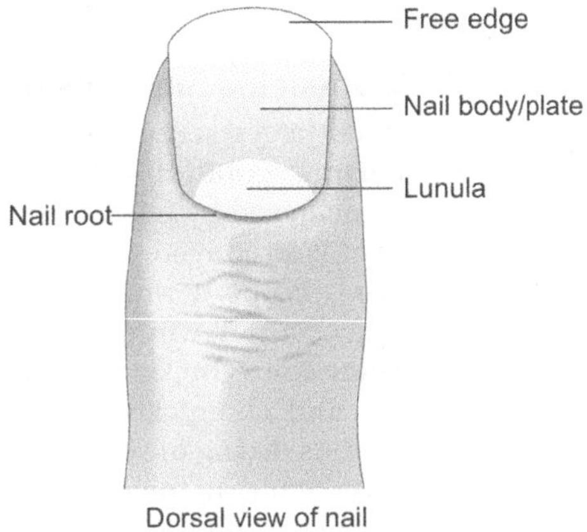

Fig. 8.3: Parts of nail.

Nail body (plate)—cell multiplication occurs from stratum basale. Deeper to this is the dermis, acts in supporting the nail plate.

- **The lateral nail fold** overlaps the nail on lateral side.
- Proximal portion of nail is overlapped by **eponychium** and beneath the nail distally is the **hyponychium**.

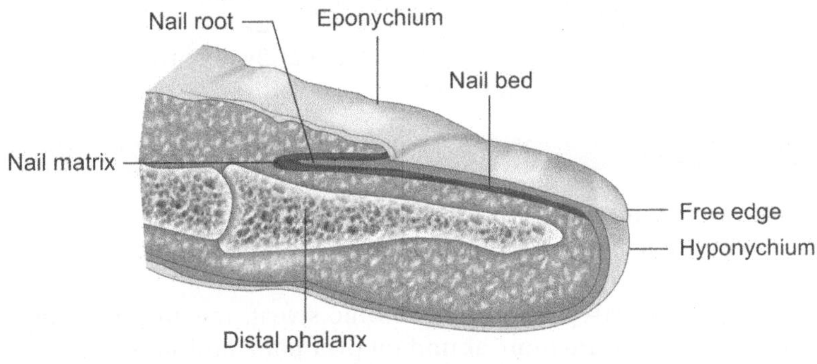

Fig. 8.4: Structures of nail.

4. Difference between thin and thick skin.

Ans. *Refer* **Table 8.2.**

Table 8.2: Differences between thick and thin skin.

Thick skin	Thin skin
Stratum corneum is thick making epidermis thicker layer	Stratum corneum is thinner
Stratum lucidum present	Stratum lucidum absent
Abundant sweat glands	Sweat and sebaceous glands are present in the dermis
Hair follicles absent	Hair follicles present
Sensory receptors more dense	Few sensory receptors

contd..

contd..

Thick skin	Thin skin
Epidermal ridges and dermal papillae are well developed	Epidermal ridges and dermal papillae are scanty (less in number)
Examples: skin of palm and soles	Examples: skin over arm, forearm, face, etc.

5. Write about the functions of skin.

Ans. Skin is the largest sensory organ. It has multiple functions apart from protection. They are:
- **Thermoregulation**—skin is involved in maintaining constant body temperature. It is achieved by means of sweat glands and blood vessels. In hot climate, excess sweat is produced; when this sweat evaporates skin surface cools down. Blood vessels in the dermis vasodilate which increases heat loss from the body. Vice-versa occurs in winter.
- **Protection**—the keratin layer of the skin protects form abrasion, microbes, dust, heat and chemicals. Lipids in the keratin layer prevent dehydration. Sebum prevents drying of skin. Melanin protects from harmful sunrays. Langerhans cells prevent entry of microbes.
- **Reservoirs of blood**—dermal blood vessels contain 8–10% of blood vessels in the body.
- **Synthesis of vitamin D**—with the help of sunlight.
- **Cutaneous sensation**—various receptors are present which help in perceiving touch, pressure, pain, temperature senses.
- **Excretion**—along with the sweat that evaporates, salt, CO_2, urea and ammonia are also excreted from the body.
- **Absorption**—lipid soluble substances are readily absorbed form the skin surface; like drugs, chemicals, vitamins, etc.

SHORT ANSWERS — 2 MARKS

6. Sweat glands of the skin.

Ans. Skin is rich in sweat glands which are important in thermoregulation. They are of two types:

i. Merocrine **glands**—produces hypotonic sweat, meant for cooling the body by evaporation. They are more abundant over palm and soles.

ii. Apocrine **sweat glands**—they are associated with hair follicles, e.g., armpit and genital areas. They are larger than merocrine sweat glands. Secretion contains water, salt and organic compound which decompose upon bacterial action. This results in peculiar odor.

7. Sebaceous glands of the skin.

Ans. They are oil producing glands found in the skin all over the body except palm and soles. They are associated with hair follicle. They become active at adolescent age as their functions are hormone-dependent.

Product—sebum that is made of lipids.

Function—lubrication of dry stratum corneum, waterproof, has antibacterial properties. It prevents water loss in low-humidity environments.

8. Name the layers of skin.

Ans. Skin is the largest sensory organ and covers the outer surface of the body. It consists of two basic layers:

i. **Epidermis**—has five layers of cells namely; stratum basale, spinosum, granulosum, lucidum and corneum.
ii. **Dermis**—is divided into papillary and deeper reticular layer.
Both these rest on the **subcutaneous layer**.

9. Name the appendages of the skin.

Ans. The appendages of the skin are—hair, nails, sweat glands and sebaceous glands and sensory receptors.

10. Mention some age-related changes in the skin.

Ans.
a. Thinner epidermis—due to reduced mitosis, metabolic activity, blood circulation, hormonal levels, and muscle strength.
b. Dermis—it is responsible for elasticity and resilience. They are reduced in old age.
c. Accessory structures—have lowered activity. Hair and nails become thin. Sweat and sebum production is reduced. Person is intolerant to extreme heat. Immunity is lowered due to loss of Langerhans cells. Melanocytes also decrease leading to paler skin.
d. Wrinkling of skin—due to reduced collagen and elastic production in the dermis, weakened muscles below the skin and inability to retain water.

11. What is integumentary system?

Ans. This system includes skin, hair, sebaceous and sweat glands, nails and skin receptors.

12. Name the cell types in the epidermis.

Ans. The cells found in epidermis include: **Keratinocytes** are the predominant ones—they are found in all layers of epidermis. They are synthesized in the basal layer, undergo differentiation as they migrate towards stratum corneum. They produce keratohyalin granules which along with dead keratinocytes form the protective stratum corneum. They also synthesize lamellar granules which act as waterproof sealant.

Others cells are:

- **Melanocytes**—responsible for color.
- **Langerhans cells**—for immune responses.
- **Merkel cells**—receptor for touch.

13. What are lines of cleavage (or the tension lines)?

Ans. They are fine lines aligned in a similar direction due to orientation of collagen fibers in the dermis of the skin. It is due to the direction of pull by the underlying structures like bony prominences, joints, and muscles. Surgical incisions along the cleavage lines results in minimal scarring. If the incision cuts across these tension lines, a wide scar results due to cutting of collagen fibers.

14. Write the factors responsible for color of the skin.

Ans. The principal factor responsible for skin color is **melanin**. Melanin is a yellow-red or brown-black pigment produced by **melanocytes**. Melanin pigment is transferred to other keratinocytes. It also helps to prevent harmful effects of ultraviolet rays of the sun. The factors responsible for skin color include:

a. Thickness of dermis and epidermis
b. Three pigments are responsible for skin color—melanin, hemoglobin and carotene.
c. Underlying blood vessels and their vascularity also influence the color of the skin.

d. Number of melanocytes is same in all individuals. The difference in skin color is due to the amount and concentration of melanin in the melanocytes.
   - Dark skinned persons have more melanin in the epidermis. Hence the skin color varies from light brown to black.
   - Light skinned individuals have very low melanin; skin color varies from pink to red depending upon the amount of hemoglobin.

e. Carotene is a yellow-orange pigment. It is precursor of vitamin A. It is located in stratum corneum, dermis and subcutaneous layer during excess intake of carotene rich foods (carrot).

15. Mention the different types of hair.

Ans. There are three types of hairs from fetus to adult:

1. **Lanugo hair**—very fine, downy, nonpigmented hairs. They are the first to appear, found covering the whole body. Hair follicles start appearing around 12 weeks in fetal life.
2. **Terminal hair**—they are long, coarse, heavily pigmented hair. The lanugo hairs over the eyebrow, eyelashes and scalp are shed after birth and replaced by these terminal hairs.
3. **Vellus hair**— they are short, fine, pale hairs. They are the predominant ones found all over the body.

Notes:

- Due to its location skin is vulnerable to trauma, environmental pollutants, sunburn, infections.
- It reflects emotions.
- Inspection of skin gives clue to various diseases:
  a. Bluish skin—cyanosis (due to hypoxia).
  b. Yellow skin—jaundice (due to increase in bilirubin, liver disorder).
  c. Certain dermatological conditions.
- Largest organ by weight—7% of body weight (4.5–5 kg).
- Covers an area of 22 square feet.
- Normal thickness—1-2 mm. Thinnest—eyelid (0.5 mm); thickest—palm and soles (4 mm).
- Skin graft—healthy skin is transferred to cover a large wound as in extensive burns. Autograft or isograft—skin from the same person.
- Skin cancer—can occur due to damage by UV radiation. Basal cell carcinoma (78%) is the most common followed by squamous cell carcinoma and malignant melanoma.
- Early detection of skin cancer is vital.
- Skin burn—is a tissue damage caused by harmful substances. It includes excess heat, electricity, radioactivity or corrosive substances. Burns are graded as per severity:
  i. First degree—only epidermis is involved (mild sunburn, hot water falling on hand)
  ii. Second degree—epidermis and part of dermis involved. There is redness, blister formation, pain. Skin appendages are not involved.
  iii. Third degree or full thickness burn—epidermis, dermis and subcutaneous tissue involved. It requires skin grafting.
- Ulcer—is a discontinuity in skin. It results due to various conditions like in diabetes, bedridden patients (decubitus ulcer).

9
CHAPTER

Nervous System

LONG ESSAYS 10 MARKS

1. Classify nervous system. Explain about gross features of cerebrum.

Ans. The nervous system controls all parts of the body. It chiefly consists of neurons and neuroglia.

Nervous system is broadly classified into central and peripheral nervous system. In addition, enteric nervous system is also included **(Fig. 9.1 and Flowchart 9.1).**

- Central nervous system (CNS) is made chiefly of brain and spinal cord—they contain neurons.
- Peripheral nervous system (PNS) consists of cranial and spinal nerves—made of axons.
- Functionally, it is classified as somatic, autonomic and enteric nervous systems.

Cerebrum:

- Cerebrum is located within the skull, protected by the meninges. It weighs 1.2–1.4 kg. It is made of up to 100 billion neurons.

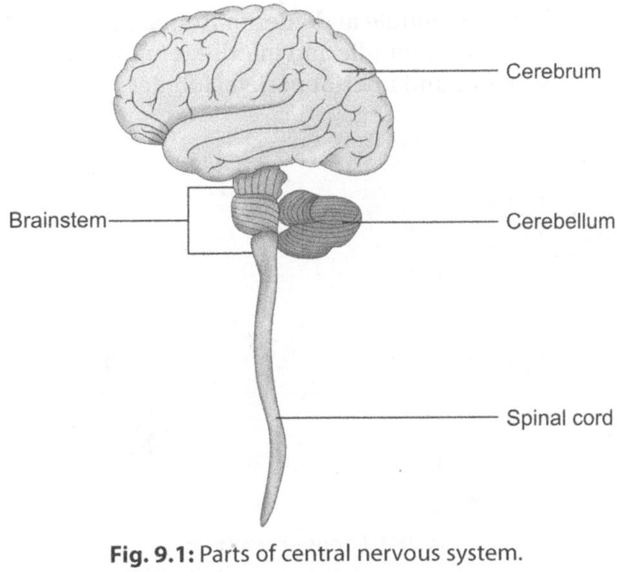

Fig. 9.1: Parts of central nervous system.

Flowchart 9.1: Classification of nervous system (NS).

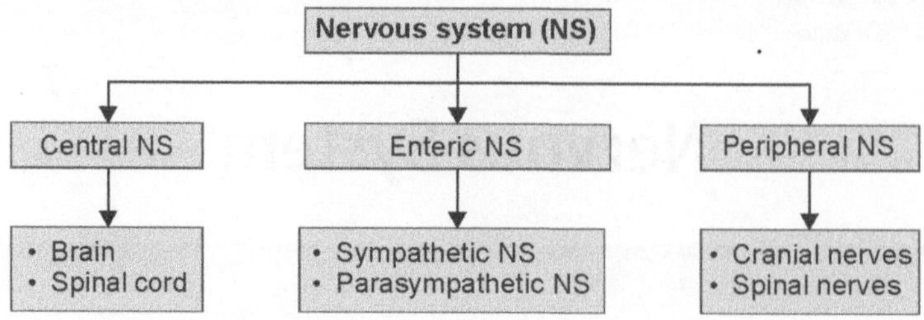

- It is the largest portion of the brain, and made of two cerebral hemispheres. It has an outer cortex, containing neurons, and inner white matter made of axons.
- The right and left hemispheres are separated by a prominent longitudinal fissure. They are connected by corpus callosum.

Lobes of the cerebrum are four in number. They are frontal, parietal, occipital and temporal lobes.

- It has **three poles**—frontal, occipital and temporal **(Fig. 9.2)**
- **Three surfaces**—superolateral, superomedial and inferior surfaces. The three borders are—superomedial, inferomedial and inferolateral **(Fig. 9.3)**.
- The surface of cerebrum is thrown into elevations **(gyri)** and depressions **(sulci)**. This arrangement helps to increase the surface area to accommodate more neurons.

Important sulci (Figs. 9.4 and 9.5)

- Central sulcus—separates the frontal and parietal lobes.
- Precentral gyrus—is in front of the central sulcus.
- Postcentral gyrus—is behind the central sulcus.
- Lateral sulcus—is a large one in between frontal, parietal and temporal lobes.
- Intraparietal sulcus—within the parietal lobe.
- Parieto-occipital sulcus—separates the parietal and occipital lobes.

Important gyri (Figs. 9.5 and 9.6)

- Frontal lobe—superior, middle and inferior frontal gyri.
- Temporal lobe—superior, middle and inferior temporal gyri.
- Parietal lobe—superior and inferior parietal lobules.

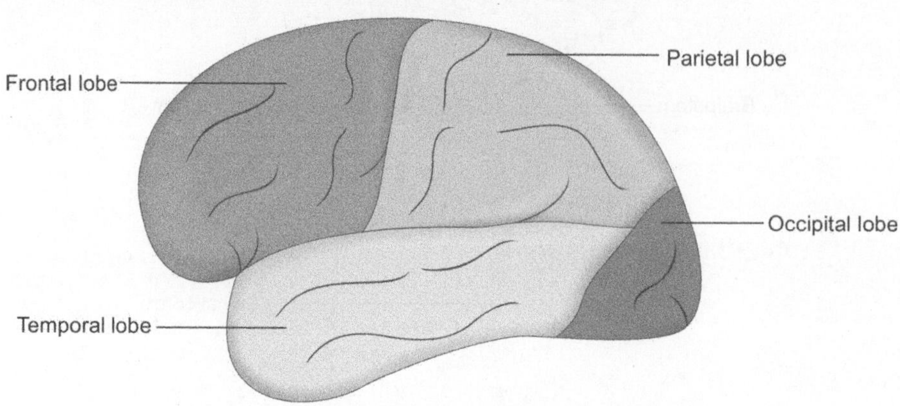

Fig. 9.2: Lobes of cerebrum.

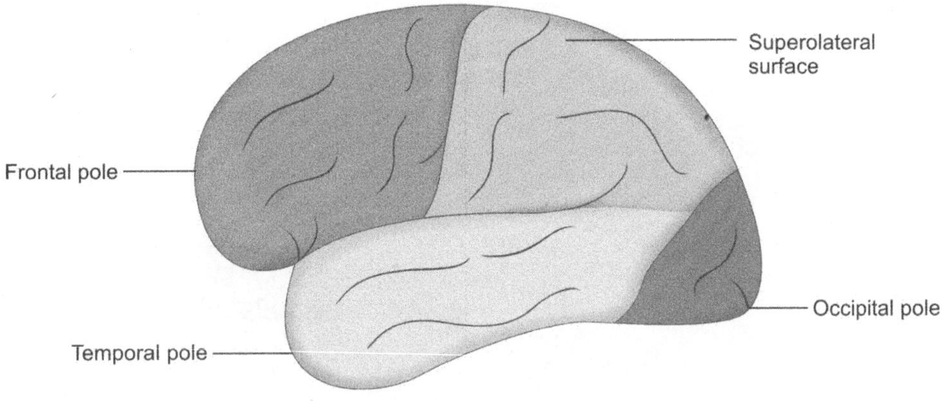

Fig. 9.3: Parts of cerebrum.

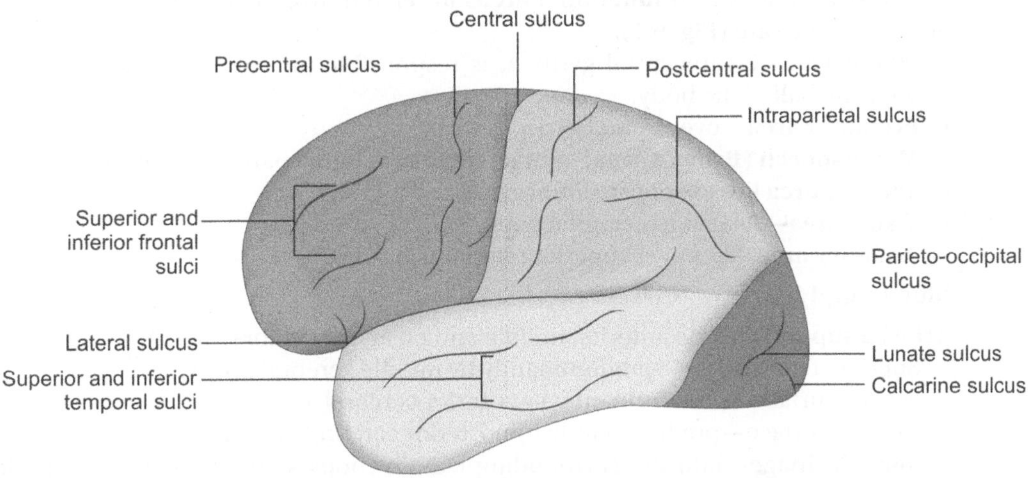

Fig. 9.4: Sulci on superolateral surface.

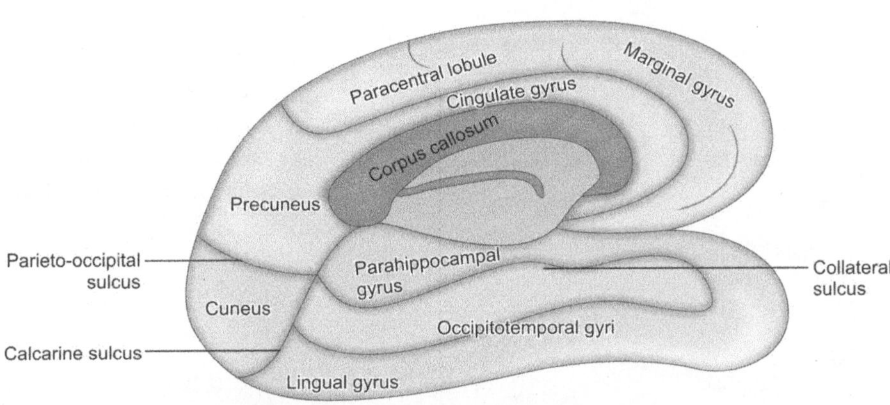

Fig. 9.5: Medial surface of cerebrum—sulci and gyri.

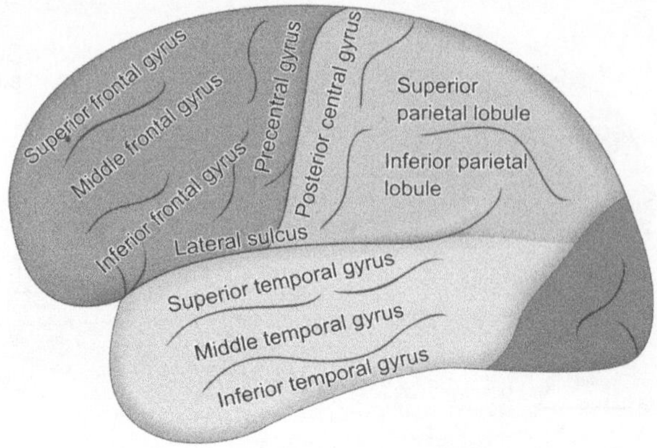

Fig. 9.6: Gyri on superolateral surface of cerebrum.

Scientists have localized **functional areas** in relation to sulci and gyri. Some of the important once are **(Fig. 9.7)**:

- **Motor area**—in precentral gyrus. It is responsible for voluntary movements of opposite half of the body.
- **Premotor area**—over frontal gyri.
- **Motor speech (Broca's area)—for speech**, over initial part of lateral sulcus.
- **Sensory area** lies over postcentral gyrus.
- **Visual area**—related to occipital pole.
- **Auditory area**—lies over superior temporal gyrus.

Blood supply:

Arterial supply is by the anterior, middle and posterior cerebral arteries.

- Superolateral surface—predominantly by middle cerebral artery.
- Medial surface—predominantly by anterior cerebral artery.
- Inferior surface—predominantly by posterior cerebral artery.

Venous drainage—into the surrounding Dural venous sinuses, then into superior sagittal sinus and finally into internal jugular vein.

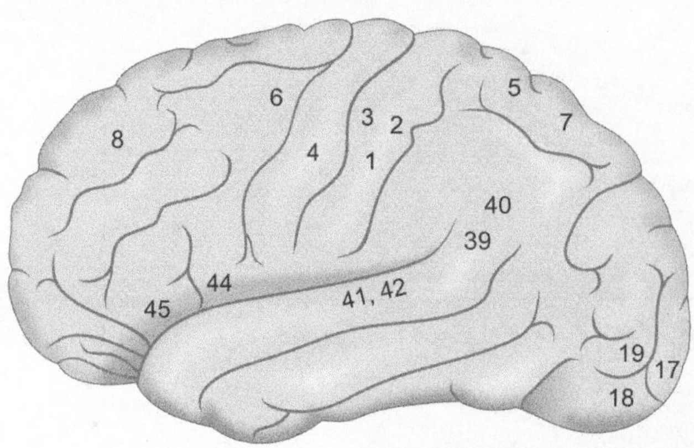

1. Area 4—primary motor area
2. Area 3, 1, 2—primary sensory area
3. Area 44, 45—Broca's speech area
4. Area 41, 42—auditory area
5. Area 17, 18, 19—visual area

Fig. 9.7: Functional areas of the cerebrum.

2. Describe the spinal cord in detail.

Ans. Spinal cord is a part of the CNS, cylindrical in shape which gives rise to spinal nerves.

Location and extent—vertebral canal, from the level of upper border of C1 vertebra to lower border of L2. In infants it extends till L3 or L4.

Length—42-45 cm in adults: **Diameter**—1.5 cm in the cervical region.

It presents two **enlargements—cervical and lumbar**. Cervical enlargement is caused due to the more number of neurons meant to supply the upper limb. Lumbar enlargement is formed due to the neurons supplying lower limb.

External features (Fig. 9.8)

i. **Anterior median fissure**—is a wide, midline groove on the ventral aspect cord.
ii. **Posterior median sulcus**—is a narrow groove on the dorsal side of the cord.
iii. Each half of the spinal cord again consists of **anterolateral sulcus**, through which ventral roots of nerves emerge, and
iv. **Posterolateral sulcus** through which, dorsal roots emerge.

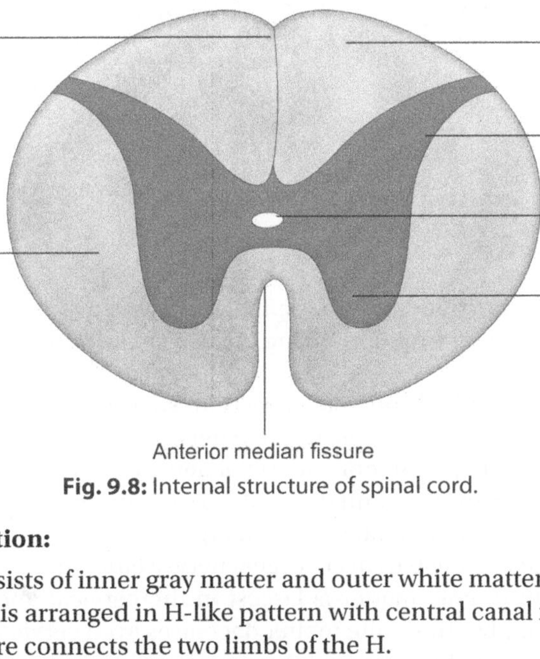

Fig. 9.8: Internal structure of spinal cord.

Internal organization:

- Spinal cord consists of inner gray matter and outer white matter.
- The gray matter is arranged in H-like pattern with central canal in the middle.
- Gray commissure connects the two limbs of the H.
- The gray matter consists of neuronal cell bodies, their dendrites and neuroglia.

Gray matter—gray matter of each half is again divided into **anterior (ventral) gray horn** and **posterior (dorsal) gray horn.**

- The *ventral gray horn* contains *somatic motor neurons* meant to supply skeletal muscles, whereas the *dorsal horn* consists of *sensory neurons.*
- In between is the **lateral horn** containing autonomic motor nuclei, and is restricted to thoracic and lumbar regions.

White matter is similarly organized into three columns on either side:

i. Anterior (ventral) white column,
ii. Lateral white column, and
iii. Posterior (dorsal) white column.

Each column has named tracts, each having specific origin and destination with specific function. They can be either **sensory (ascending tracts)** and motor **(descending)** tracts.

Conus medullaris (Fig. 9.9): Terminal portion of spinal cord is conical in shape, ends at the level of L1-L2. From its tip, an extension of pia mater called **filum terminale** continues downwards till the coccyx.

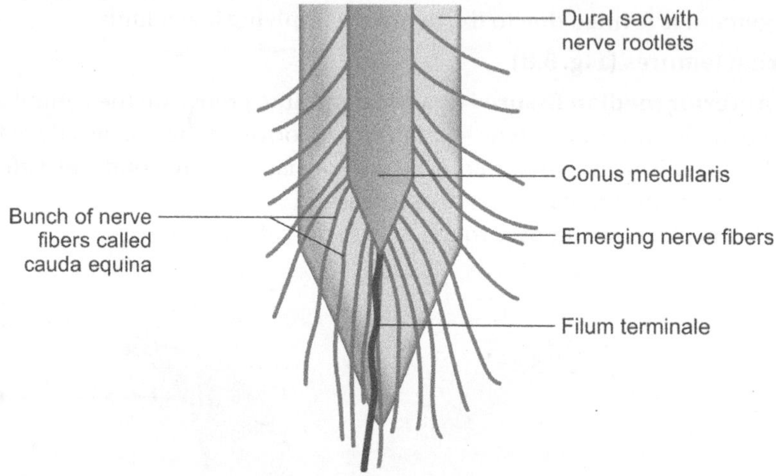

Fig. 9.9: Conus medullaris.

Cauda equina: Caudally, the spinal cord is surrounded by longer spinal nerves around the filum terminale, giving horse-tail like appearance. Hence called as cauda equina.

Regions of the spinal cord—it consists of **five regions (Fig. 9.10):**

1. Cervical—8 pair of cervical spinal nerves emerge.
2. Thoracic—12 pair if thoracic spinal nerves emerge.
3. Lumbar—5 pair of lumbar spinal nerves emerge.
4. Sacral—5 pair of sacral nerves emerge.
5. Coccygeal—one pair of coccygeal nerves emerge.

The amount of gray matter is largest in the cervical and lumbar segments as they supply the limbs. The white matter decreases from cervical to sacral region.

Spinal segment: The region of the spinal cord giving rise to a pair of spinal nerves is called a spinal segment.

Spinal nerves (Fig. 9.11):

- There are **31 pair of spinal nerves,** hence 31 spinal segments.
- Spinal nerve is formed by the union of ventral and dorsal nerve roots.
- **Dorsal root is sensory (afferent)** in function and possess dorsal root ganglion.
- **Ventral root is efferent or motor** in function.

Note: Spinal nerves emerge through the respective intervertebral foramina. Since spinal cord is shorter than the length of the vertebral column, lower thoracic level onwards, the nerves have to travel longer distance to emerge out through the respective intervertebral foramina.

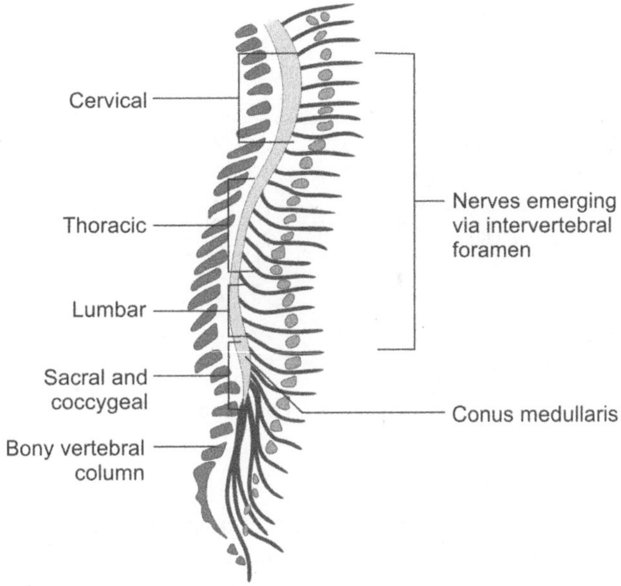

Fig. 9.10: Spinal cord regions and spinal nerves emerging from intervertebral foramen.

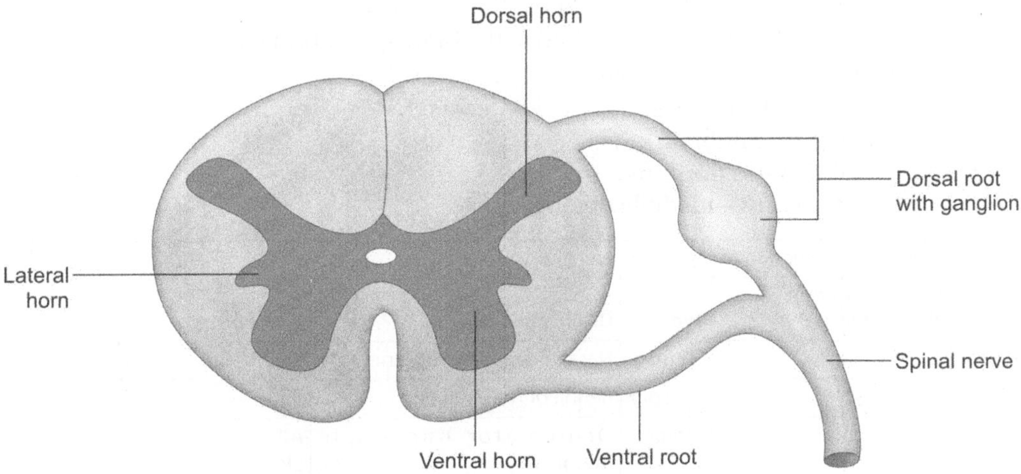

Fig. 9.11: Formation of spinal nerve.

Protection to the spinal cord:

1. Vertebral column.
2. **Spinal meninges (Fig. 9.12)**
   - Outer dura mater—it is a thick strong layer of irregular connective tissue.
   - Middle arachnoid mater—it is web-like, made of cells and loosely arranged collagen and elastic fibers.
   - Pia mater—innermost layer, firmly adherent to the cord. It consists of cells, connective tissue with collagen and elastic fibers. Rich in capillaries. Its derivatives include ligamentum denticulatum and filum terminale.

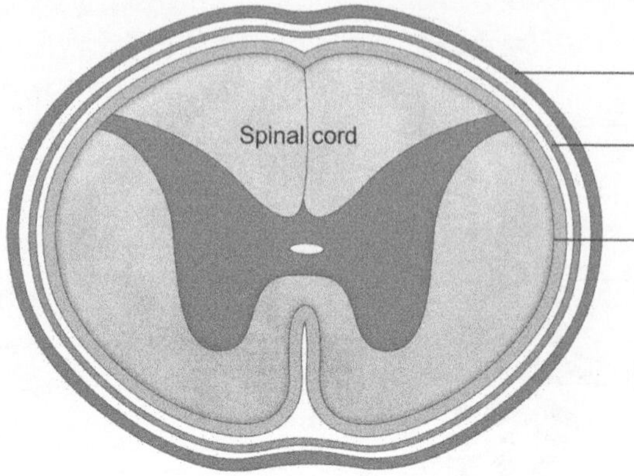

Fig. 9.12: Coverings of spinal cord.

3. Vertebral ligaments.
4. Cerebrospinal fluid.

Blood supply to the cord—is by anterior and posterior spinal arteries. They arise from vertebral arteries. Venous drainage is by internal vertebral venous plexuses.

3. List the cranial nerves in order. Mention their central and peripheral connections.

Ans. Cranial nerves are twelve in number. They are sensory, motor or mixed. Except the first and second, others are attached to the brainstem **(Table 9.1)**.

- Attachment of cranial nerves
  a. 1, 2—to the forebrain
  b. 3 and 4—midbrain
  c. 5, 6, 7, 8—to the pons
  d. 9, 10, 11, 12—medulla oblongata.

Table 9.1: Description of cranial nerves.

Sl. No.	Name of the cranial nerve	Type	Origin and nuclei	Function
1.	Olfactory	Sensory	Nasal mucous membrane	Smell
2.	Optic	Sensory	Retina of the eyeball	Vision
3.	Oculomotor	Motor	Oculomotor nucleus in midbrain	All extraocular muscles, except LR, SO
4.	Trochlear	Motor	Trochlear nucleus in midbrain	Superior oblique muscle of eye
5.	Trigeminal	Mixed	• Pons—motor nucleus in the midbrain • Sensory nucleus in the brainstem	• Muscles of mastication. • Sensory supply to face
6.	Abducent	Motor	Abducent nucleus in pons	Lateral rectus muscle of eye
7.	Facial	Mixed	Facial nucleus in pons	• Muscles of face • Taste sensations from the anterior 2/3rd of tongue • Secretomotor to salivary glands

Contd...

Contd...

Sl. No.	Name of the cranial nerve	Type	Origin and nuclei	Function
8.	Vestibulocochlear	Sensory	• Cochlear nuclei in pons • Vestibular nuclei in the medulla	• Cochlear part—for hearing • Vestibular part—for equilibrium
9.	Glossopharyngeal	Mixed	• Nucleus ambiguous for muscle • Nucleus tractus solitarius for taste • Both are in medulla	• Stylopharyngeus—a muscle of pharynx. • Taste sensations from posterior 1/3rd of tongue • Sensory to tongue, tonsil and pharynx
10.	Vagus	Mixed	• Nucleus ambiguous for muscle • Nucleus tractus solitarius for taste • Both are in medulla	• Motor—muscles of soft palate, pharynx and larynx • Cardiac muscle • Smooth muscle of GI tract
11.	Spinal accessory nerve	Motor	• Nucleus ambiguous for muscle • In medulla	• Trapezius • Sternocleidomastoid
12.	Hypoglossal	Motor	Hypoglossal nucleus in medulla	Muscles of tongue

4. Describe the location, parts, external features, nuclei and blood supply of cerebellum. Add a note on its functions and applied anatomy.

or

Describe the structure and functions of cerebellum.

Ans. Cerebellum is a part of the hindbrain. It is mainly involved in coordination of muscular movements. Lesions to cerebellum or its connections results in the triad of symptoms namely—ataxia, nystagmus and intention tremors.

Location—it is located in the posterior cranial fossa, below the tentorium cerebelli, behind the pons and medulla.

Anatomical parts (Figs. 9.13 and 9.14):

1. It consists of **two hemispheres (right and left)** united by a median portion called **vermis.**
2. **Three fissures**—horizontal fissure, primary fissure and posterolateral fissure.
3. **Three lobes**—anterior, posterior, and flocculonodular lobes.
4. **Two surfaces**—superior and inferior.

Structure (Fig. 9.15):

- It has an outer cortex or the gray matter and inner white matter.
- Cortex is highly folded in a leaf-like pattern called folia.
- Inner white matter is arranged in a branching tree-like pattern called **Arbor vitae cerebelli.**
- It also contains **cerebellar nuclei (Fig. 9.16)** in the core namely—**dentate, globose, fastigii, and emboliform**. These nuclei receive information from neurons in the gray matter and send it to the higher centers.

Histology of the cerebellar cortex—it consists of three layers from superficial to deep.

1. Outer molecular layer—stellate and basket cells.
2. Middle Purkinje cell layer—made of single row of large, Purkinje neurons.
3. Inner granular layer—granule and Golgi cells.

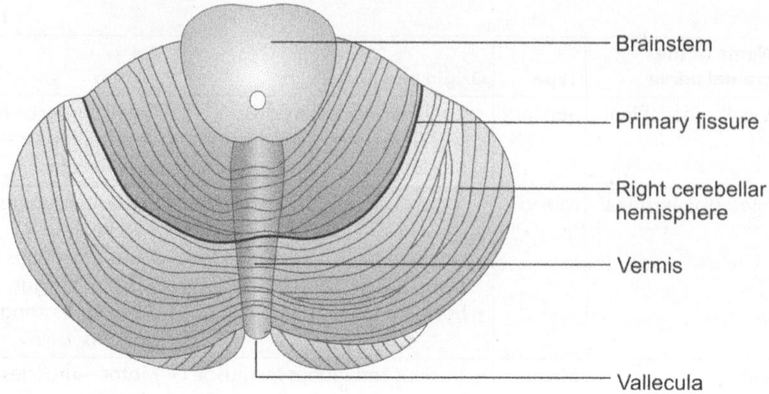

Fig. 9.13: Cerebellum.

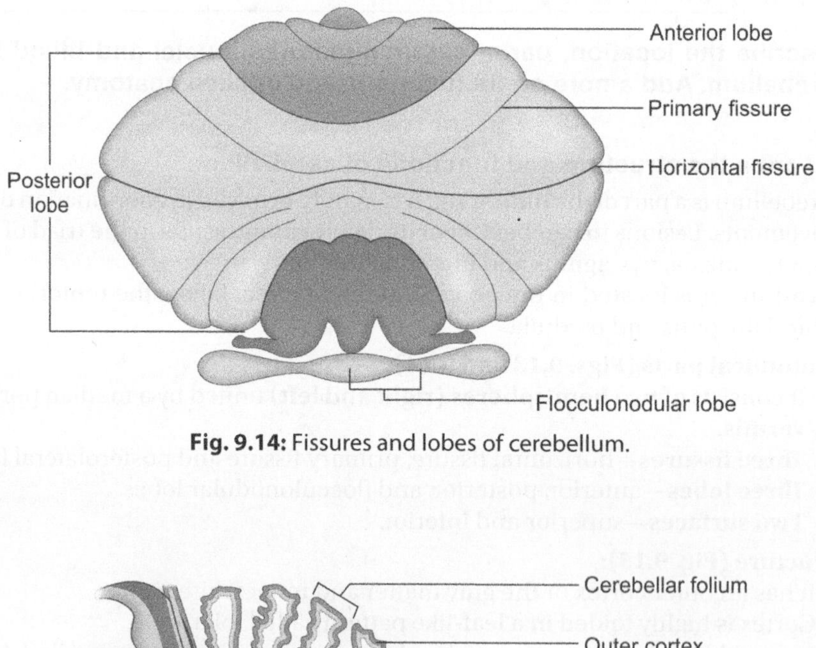

Fig. 9.14: Fissures and lobes of cerebellum.

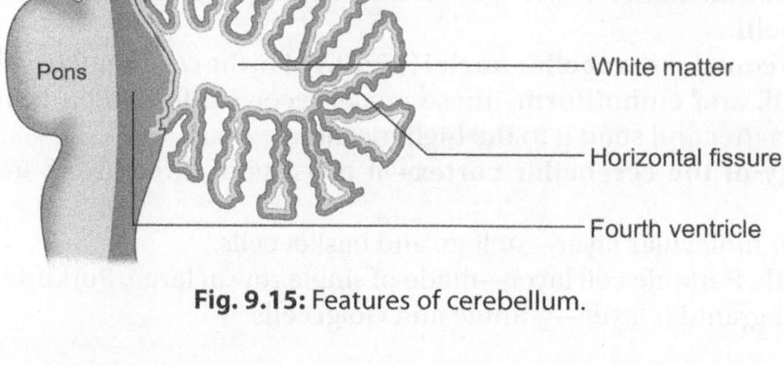

Fig. 9.15: Features of cerebellum.

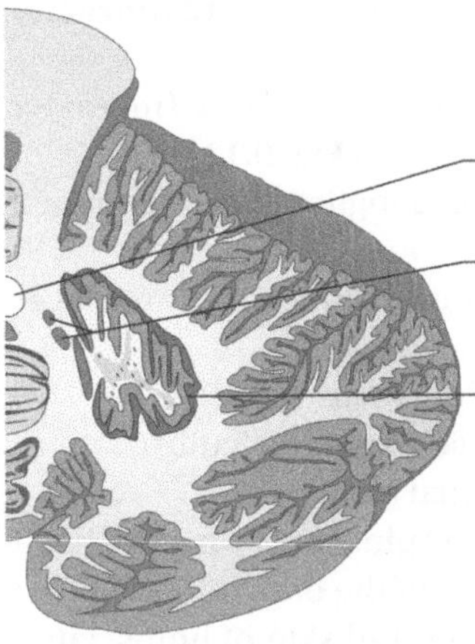

Fig. 9.16: Nuclei of cerebrum.

Cerebellar peduncles: They are bundles of axons which connect the cerebellum to the brainstem.

- **Superior cerebellar peduncle**: Afferents from Purkinje neurons are conveyed to the red nucleus and thalamus.
- **Middle cerebellar peduncle:** Fibers from pontine nuclei travel via the middle peduncle to reach the cortex of cerebellum.
- **Inferior cerebellar peduncle**: It connects nuclei in medulla to the cerebellum.

Blood supply:

- **Arterial supply**—superior cerebellar arteries (from basilar artery), anterior and posterior inferior cerebellar arteries (from vertebral arteries).
- **Venous drainage**—into the adjacent dural venous sinuses.

Functions:

- Maintenance of equilibrium.
- Maintenance of muscle tone and posture.
- For coordination and smooth movements.

Applied anatomy: Lesion in the cerebellum results in the following:

- Ataxia—loss of coordination of skeletal muscles.
- Hypotonia—loss of muscle tone.
- Tremors.
- Involuntary movement of eye (nystagmus).
- Inability to perform rapid alternating movements.
- Slurred speech (dysarthria)

5. Describe a spinal nerve (peripheral nerve).

Ans.
- Spinal nerve is attached to the spinal cord and is part of peripheral nerve system (PNS).
- They consist of parallel arranged axons with neuroglia, covered by connective tissue coverings.
- Spinal nerves connect CNS to their target organs like muscles, glands, and sensory receptors.

31 pair of spinal nerves are present—**8 cervical, 12 thoracic, 5 lumbar, 5 sacral and 1 coccygeal.**

- They are connected to spinal cord by anterior (motor) and posterior (sensory) nerve roots. Hence it is a mixed nerve **(Fig. 9.11).**
- The anterior root also carries preganglionic sympathetic fibers, meant to supply blood vessels and sweat glands.

Connective tissue coverings: They are arranged in three layers from outside to inside **(Fig. 9.17):**

1. **Epineurium**—covers group of nerve fasciculi.
2. **Perineurium**—covers individual nerve fasciculi.
3. **Endoneurium**—covers individual axons.

Distribution of spinal nerves: Each spinal nerve trunk divides into:

- **Dorsal ramus**—supplies muscles of the back and the skin over it.
- **Ventral ramus**—supplies muscles and skin of limbs, lateral and ventral aspect of trunk.
- **Meningeal branch**—supplies vertebrae, vertebral ligaments and blood vessels.

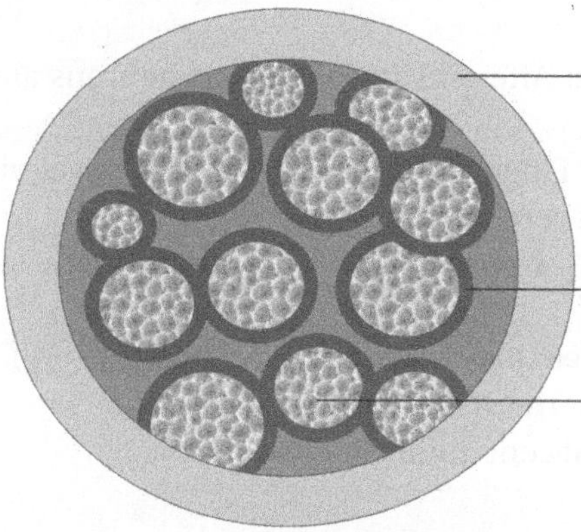

Fig. 9.17: Coverings of spinal nerve.

6. Draw neat labeled diagram of a neuron.

or

Describe the structure of neuron with the help of diagram.

Ans. Neurons are the structural and functional unit of nervous system. It is involved in generation of nerve impulses. It is made of three basic parts—cell body (somata), dendrites and axons **(Fig. 9.18).**

Cell body—consists of a central nucleus, cytoplasm enclosed in cell membrane. The cell organelles are as follows:

- Golgi complex—for packaging synthesized proteins.
- Mitochondria—provides energy.
- Ribosomes—protein synthesis.
- Rough endoplasmic reticulum called **Nissl bodies or (granules)**—site of protein synthesis.
- Lysosomes.

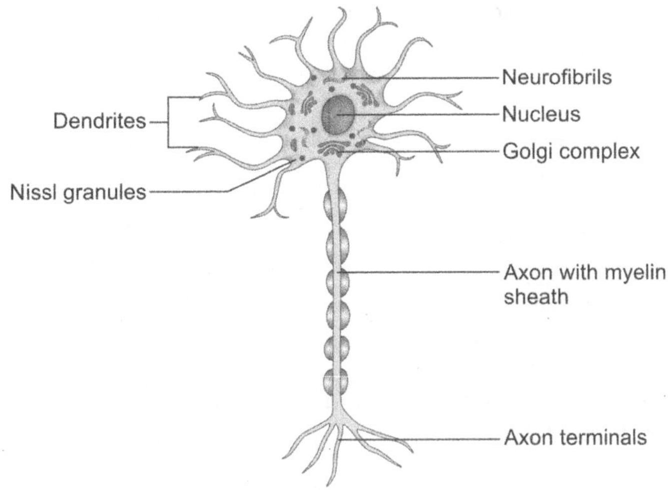

Fig. 9.18: Structure of neuron.

- Cytoskeleton:
  - **Neurofibrils**—provide support to the cell and maintain cell shape.
  - **Microtubules**—involved in transport of substances between cell body and axon.
- **Lipofuscin pigment**—aging pigment, yellow in color.

Nerve fiber includes—axon and dendrite.

Dendrites are multiple. They are branch-like tree. Dendrites transmit impulses towards the neuron. They possess receptors for neurotransmitters.

Axon—is single, long, cylindrical processes. They carry impulses away from the body. it begins at cone-shaped axon hillock or the initial segment. It has central axoplasm enclosed in the axolemma (plasma membrane). They have insulated covering of myelin sheath which is made of lipids. Myelin is produced by Schwann cell.

Note: The outer cell membrane of a Schwann cell is called the neurilemma. The fact that axons in the brain and cord have no neurilemma is clinically significant because it plays an essential part in the regeneration of cut and injured axons. Therefore, the potential for regeneration in the brain and spinal cord is far less than it is in the peripheral nervous system.

7. Describe neuroglia.

Ans. Neuroglia are the **non-nervous** cell types of the nervous system.

- They cannot generate impulses.
- Smaller than neurons.
- More numerous (5–25 times).
- Capable of dividing.
- In case of injury/disease, they multiply and occupy the space of neurons.
- Brain tumors derived from glial cells are **Gliomas.**

Classification of neuroglia:

Classification of neuroglia is shown in **Flowchart 9.2**.

Flowchart 9.2: Classification of neuroglia.

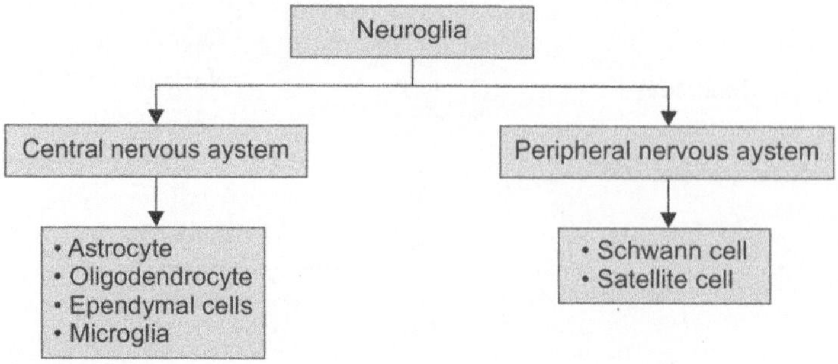

The details of the characteristics and functions of various types of neuroglia is discussed in **Table 9.2**.

Table 9.2: Characteristics and functions of neuroglia.

Type of neuroglia	Location	Types	Characters	Function
1. Astrocytes	CNS	• Fibrous • Protoplasmic	Processes contact blood capillaries, neurons and pia mater	• Support neurons • Forms blood-brain barrier
2. Oligodendrocyte	CNS	–	Lining of axons in CNS	Formation of myelin sheath in CNS
3. Microglia	CNS	–	Most numerous cell type	• Function as phagocytes • Involved in fibrosis after nervous tissue damage
4. Ependymal cells	CNS	Cuboidal to columnar, possess microvilli and cilia	They line cavities of ventricles of CNS	Involved in production of CSF
5. Schwann cells	PNS		Encircle PNS axons	Myelin production in PNS
6. Satellite cells	PNS		Surround cell bodies of PNS ganglia	• Insulation • Metabolic exchange

8. Brachial plexus.

Ans. It is a nerve plexus formed by the union of ventral rami of C5-8 and T1.

Location:

a. Posterior triangle—supraclavicular part.

b. And in the axilla—is the infraclavicular potion. Here it forms the three cords—medial, lateral and posterior cords. Cords gives rise to branches that are motor and sensory.

Distribution: Skin and muscles of upper limb, shoulder scapular muscles, and pectoral muscles, serratus anterior.

Its formation is complex and described to consist of various parts—roots, trunks, divisions, cords, and finally branches **(Table 9.3)**.

Table 9.3: Formation and branches of brachial plexus.

Roots	Trunks	Divisions	Cords	Branches
C5 C6	Upper	Anterior Posterior	Lateral cord—union of anterior division of upper and middle trunk	1. Lateral pectoral nerve 2. Lateral root of median nerve* 3. Musculocutaneous nerve
C7	Middle	Anterior Posterior	Medial cord—anterior division lower trunk	1. Medial pectoral nerve 2. Medial root of median nerve* 3. Medial cutaneous nerve of arm 4. Medial cutaneous nerve of forearm 5. Ulnar nerve*
C8 T1	Lower	Anterior Posterior	Posterior cord—posterior division of all the three trunks	1. Upper subscapular nerve 2. Lower subscapular nerve 3. Nerve to latissimus dorsi 4. Axillary nerve* 5. Radial nerve*

*nerves of clinical significance

Applied anatomy:

- Lesion of upper trunk leads to *Erb's paralysis.*
- Damage to lower trunk results in *Klumpke's paralysis.*
- Radial nerve in axilla or middle of arm—wrist drop.
- Axillary nerve compression—deltoid paralysis.

9. Describe lumbar plexus.

Ans. **Formation**—ventral rami of L1-L4 roots

Location—in the posterior abdominal wall, in relation to psoas major muscle.

Branches: *Refer* **Table 9.4.**

Table 9.4: Branches and distribution of lumbar plexus.

Nerve	Distribution
Iliohypogastric	Abdominal wall muscles, buttock
Ilioinguinal	Abdominal muscles, skin over external genitalia and medial aspect of thigh
Genitofemoral	Cremaster muscle, external genitalia
Lateral cutaneous nerve of thigh	Lateral aspect of thigh
Femoral nerve—largest nerve of lumbar plexus	Muscles of anterior compartment of thigh, hip and knee joint
Obturator nerve	Muscles of medial compartment of thigh, hip and knee joint

10. Sacral plexus.

Ans. **Formation**—ventral rami of L4, L5, S1 to S4.

Location—anterior to sacrum.

Branches—*Refer* **Table 9.5.**

Table 9.5: Branches and distribution of sacral plexus.

Name of the nerve	Distribution
Muscular branches • Superior and inferior gluteal nerves • Nerve to piriformis, quadratus femoris, obturator internus, gemelli	 • Gluteal muscles • Respective muscles
Posterior cutaneous nerve of thigh	Skin of posterior aspect of the thigh
Pudendal nerve	Muscles of the perineum, skin over external genitalia
Sciatic nerve	
• Tibial component • Common peroneal component	• Muscles of the calf (posterior compartment of leg • Muscles of sole of foot • Muscles of the anterior and lateral compartment of leg

11. Name the ventricles of brain. Add a note on cerebrospinal fluid (CSF) circulation.

Ans. Ventricles of the brain are cavities inside CNS lined by ependyma. They are **(Fig. 9.19)**:

1. Lateral ventricles—cavities in the cerebral hemisphere (telencephalon).
2. Third ventricle—cavity of diencephalon (thalamus).
3. Cerebral aqueduct—cavity of midbrain.
4. Fourth ventricle—cavity of the hindbrain (between brainstem and cerebellum).

CSF is an interstitial fluid that circulates through the ventricles and the subarachnoid space. It is clear and transparent.

Function: (i) Protect the brain and spinal cord from physical and chemical injuries, (ii) Homeostasis, (iii) Medium of exchange of nutrients and waste products.

Production—by *choroid plexuses* in the lateral, third and fourth ventricle. Choroid plexus is a network of blood capillaries in relation to ventricles of the brain. They are covered by ependyma joined by tight junctions. It filters the blood plasma to produce CSF.

Absorption: CSF is finally drained into superior sagittal sinus via arachnoid granulations, thus entering the venous circulation.

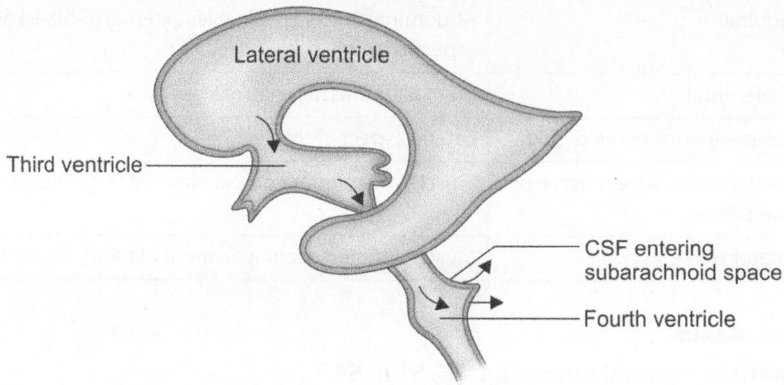

Fig. 9.19: Flow of CSF in the ventricles of brain (arrow indicate pathway of CSF drainage).

Total volume: 80–150 mL.

Content: Water, protein, glucose, lactic acid, ions, white blood cells.

Circulation of CSF: Circulation of CSF is depicted in **Flowchart 9.3**.

Flowchart 9.3: Circulation of cerebrospinal fluid.

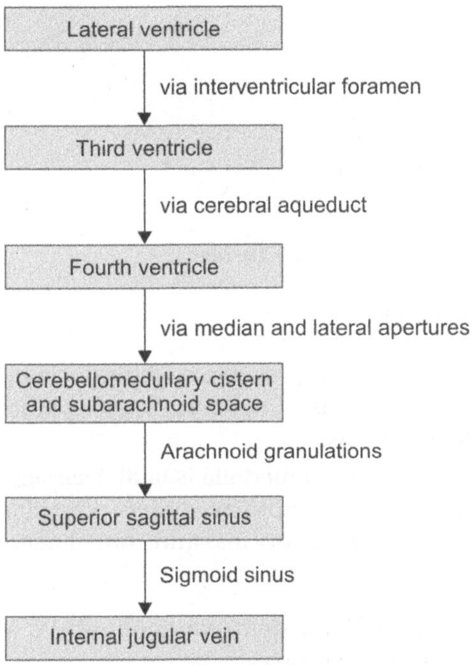

Applied anatomy: Any defect in *production or drainage* of CSF leads to excess CSF pressure leading to a condition called **hydrocephalus.** In newborns and infants, head bulges in hydrocephalus as fontanelles are yet to fuse.

12. Describe about medulla oblongata.

Ans. Medulla oblongata is a part of brainstem. It is a continuation of spinal cord, and continues above with the pons.

Location—in the posterior cranial fossa, in front of cerebellum.

External features (Fig. 9.20):

- Anterior—two elevations—pyramid medially and olive laterally. Medial to olive, hypoglossal nerve emerge out. Lateral to olive, 9th, 10th, 11th cranial nerves emerge out.
- Pontomedullary junction—6th, 7th and 8th cranial nerves attached.
- Posterior—fasciculus gracilis medially and fasciculus cuneatus laterally.
- Upper part of medulla forms floor of fourth ventricle containing vagal and hypoglossal triangle and vestibular area.

Important functional areas:

1. Reticular formation
2. Pyramid—carries corticospinal tract

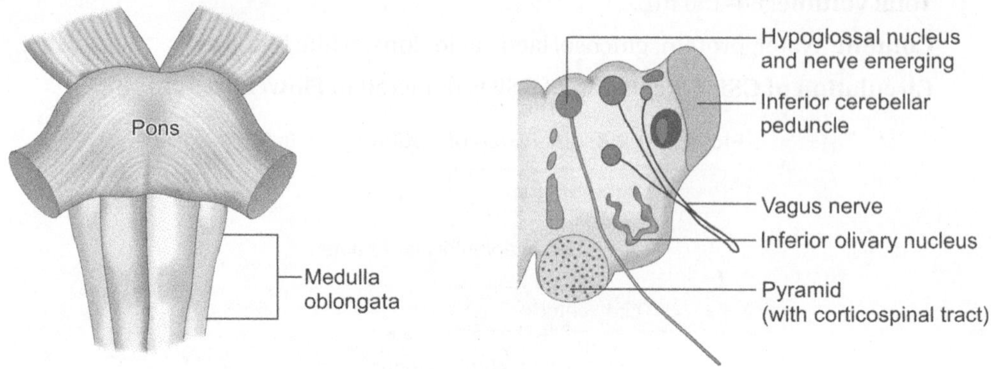

Fig. 9.20: Medulla.

3. Cardiovascular center
4. Respiratory center
5. Others—centers for vomiting, hiccup, deglutition, cough
6. Nuclei gracilis and cuneatus—for touch, pressure, vibration and proprioception.
7. Gustatory nucleus—for taste.

Applied anatomy: Any injury to medulla is fatal. Damage to the vital centers results in immediate death. Other symptoms due to vascular lesion are—paralysis of contralateral side of body, or sensory loss and cranial nerve involvement.

13. Pons.

Ans. **Pons** (= bridge) is a part of brainstem, continues above with the midbrain. It forms upper half of floor of fourth ventricle.

Location—in the posterior cranial fossa, in front of cerebellum.

External features (Fig. 9.21):

- Ventral surface is smooth and continues laterally as middle cerebellar peduncle. Trigeminal nerve is attached here.
- Dorsal surface—forms floor of fourth ventricle, containing facial colliculus. It is caused by facial nerve winding around the abducent nucleus.

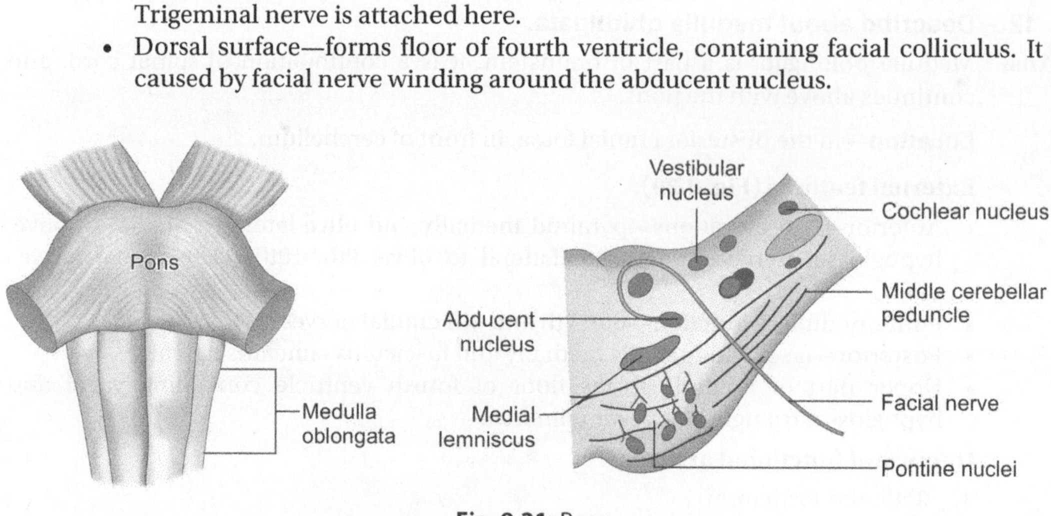

Fig. 9.21: Pons.

Important functional features:

- Corticospinal tract intermingles with pontine nuclei.
- Cranial nerve nuclei—trigeminal, abducent, facial, and vestibulocochlear.
- Reticular formation—pontine respiratory center.

14. Midbrain.

Ans. Midbrain (mesencephalon) connects pons to diencephalon. It contains a central cavity lined by ependyma called cerebral aqueduct. It contains cranial nerve nuclei and tracts.

Location:

- **Ventral aspect** of the midbrain contains bundles of axons of corticospinal tract called cerebral peduncles.
- **Dorsal part** is called the tectum—contains four rounded elevations, the superior and inferior colliculi.

Important functional regions (Fig. 9.22):

- Superior colliculus—for processing visual stimuli and reflexes.
- Inferior colliculus—for processing auditory stimuli and reflexes.
- Cranial nerve nucleus—oculomotor and trochlear nerve nuclei.
- Red nucleus—connects with cerebellum and cerebral cortex for coordinating muscular movements.
- Substantia nigra—it is related to basal nuclei. Any lesion here leads to Parkinson's disease.

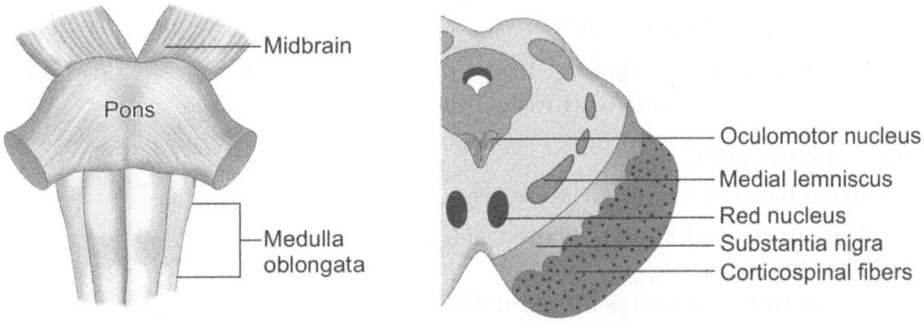

Fig. 9.22: Midbrain.

15. Internal capsule.

Ans. Internal capsule is a collection of white matter, which extend from all parts of the cerebral cortex and connect to the brainstem and spinal cord.

- It is the best example for projection fibers.
- It has both ascending and descending tracts.

It has the following parts (Fig. 9.23):

- Anterior limb.
- Genu.
- Posterior limb.
- Retrolentiform part.
- Sublentiform part.

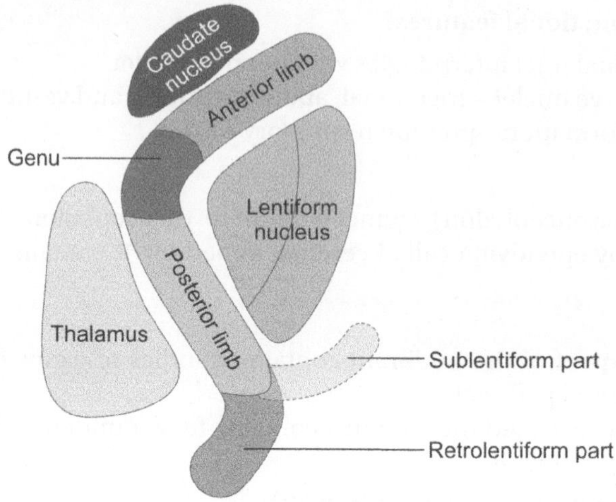

Fig. 9.23: Parts of internal capsule.

Relations:

1. Lateral—lentiform nucleus.
2. Medial—anterior limb to caudate nucleus, posterior limb to thalamus.
3. Superior—continues as corona radiate fibers.
4. Inferior—enters midbrain.

Blood supply: From circle of Willis.

Applied anatomy: Any damage in the internal capsule leads to widespread damage, including motor and sensory involvement.

16. Corpus callosum.

Ans.
- Largest band of commissural fibers.
- Connects the right and left cerebral hemispheres.
- **Parts (Fig. 9.24):**
  - Rostrum—connects the frontal lobes
  - Genu—connects the frontal lobes.
  - Trunk—connects temporal and parietal lobes.
  - Splenium—connects the occipital lobes.

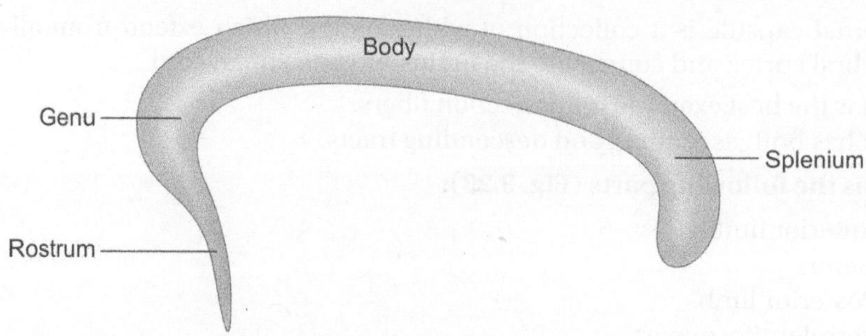

Fig. 9.24: Parts of corpus callosum.

- **Functions:**
  - Transfer of speech functions.
  - Transfer of learning and memory.

17. White matter of cerebrum.

Ans. White matter of cerebrum is nothing but the axons. It is organized into named fibers which are of three types **(Fig. 9.25):**

1. **Commissural fibers**—connects the identical parts of two cerebral hemispheres, e.g., corpus callosum, anterior and posterior commissures, hippocampus.
2. **Association fibers**—connects two different areas within the same hemisphere, e.g., superior and inferior longitudinal hemispheres, cingulum.
3. **Projection fibers**—they connect cerebral hemispheres to different parts of CNS, e.g., internal capsule, fornix, fimbria.

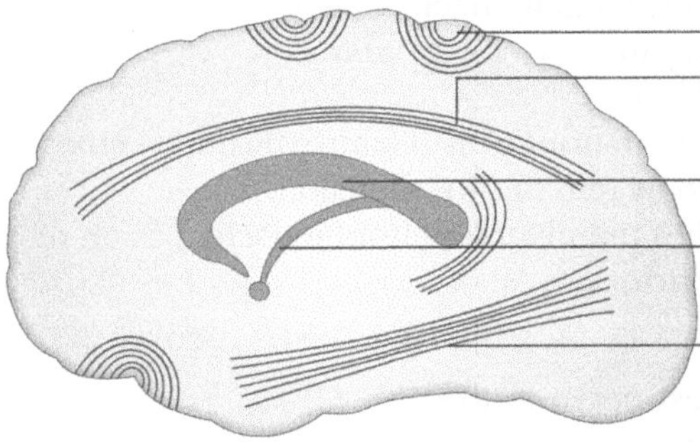

Fig. 9.25: White matter of cerebrum.

18. Major nerves of the upper limb.

Ans. There are four major branches of brachial plexus supplying the upper limb **(Fig. 9.26).**

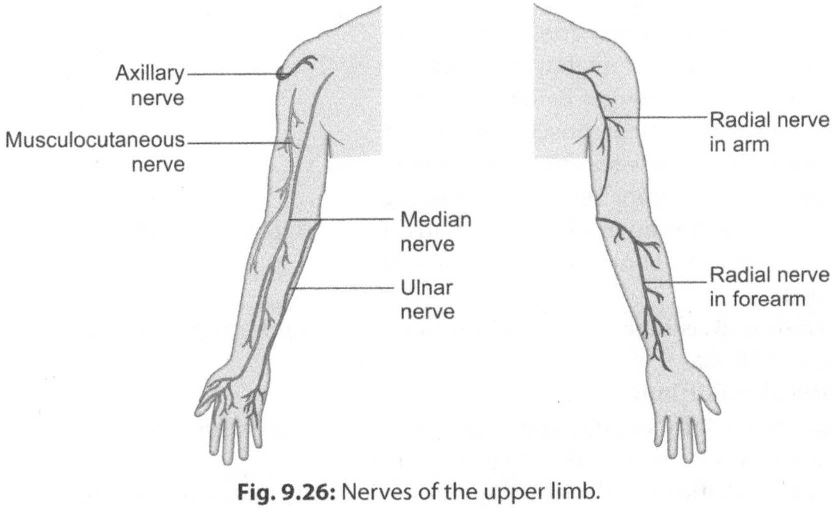

Fig. 9.26: Nerves of the upper limb.

They are:

A. **Median nerve**—this is the nerve supplying:
- Flexors of forearm.
- Muscles acting on the thumb.
- Cutaneous supply to medial 3 1/2 fingers and palm.
- Lesion of the nerve results in—tingling and numbness over palm, inability to flex fingers.

B. **Radial nerve**—this is the nerve which supplies:
- Extensors of elbow joint.
- Extensors of wrist joint.
- Skin over dorsum of the hand.
- Lesion of the nerve results in—*wrist drop.*

C. **Ulnar nerve**—this nerve supplies:
- Small muscles of the hand.
- Skin over medial one and half fingers.
- Lesion of the nerve results in—*claw hand.*

D. **Musculocutaneous nerve**
- This supplies muscles in front of arm (cause flexion at elbow joint).
- Lesion—leads to elbow remains in extension.

E. **Axillary nerve**—supplies mainly the deltoid muscle. Lesion of the nerve leads to inability to abduct the arm.

19. Sciatic nerve.

Ans. Sciatic nerve is the thickest nerve in the body. It has two components:
- Tibial component.
- Common peroneal component.

Root value: L4-5, S1 to S4.

Location: The main trunk emerges from the pelvis to enter the *gluteal region.* Then it enters the back of thigh and supplies the hamstring muscles **(Fig. 9.27).**

Course and relations: The sciatic nerve enters the gluteal region via greater sciatic nerve. It emerges below piriformis and runs on—gemelli muscles, obturator internus, quadratus femoris. Then enters thigh, giving branches to hamstring muscles. At the apex of popliteal fossa divides into tibial and common peroneal branches.

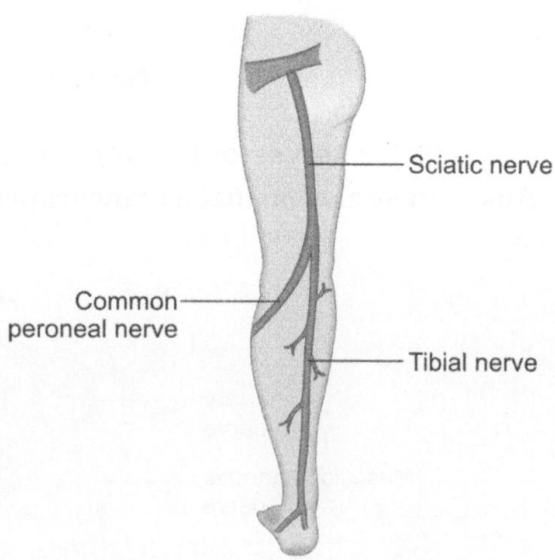

Fig. 9.27: Sciatic nerve in the back of lower limb.

Terminal divisions: It divides into tibial and common peroneal component in the popliteal fossa.

Clinical condition:

Sciatica—painful condition due to compression of sciatic nerve. Pain extends along buttocks, down to posterior thigh, leg and foot.

Injury to sciatic nerve leads to foot drop—inability to dorsiflex the foot.

SHORT ANSWERS 2 MARKS

20. Define gray and white matter of brain.

Ans.
- Gray matter comprises of cell body of neurons.
- White matter comprises of axons with or without myelin sheath.
- Cerebrum, cerebellum—gray matter is outside, white matter is inside.
- Spinal cord—gray matter is inside; white matter is outside.

21. Define sulci and gyri.

Ans. *Sulci* are depressions on the surface of cerebrum.

Gyri are elevations. They are formed so as to increase the surface area of the brain. More number of neurons can be accommodated in the sulci and gyri.

22. Name the parts of basal nuclei.

Ans. *Refer* **Figure 9.28.**
- The parts of basal nuclei are caudate nucleus, putamen and globus pallidus.
- Caudate nucleus is C-shaped and follows the curve of lateral ventricle.
- Putamen is located deep inside frontal and parietal lobe.
- The putamen with globus pallidus together forms the lentiform nucleus.

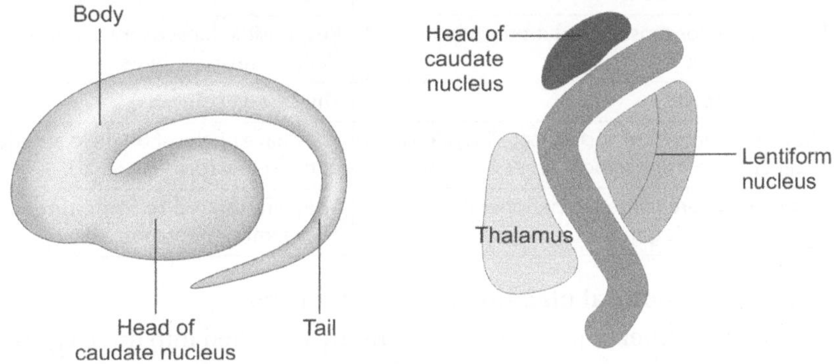

Fig. 9.28: Basal ganglia.

23. Name the parts of diencephalon.

Ans.
- Diencephalon is located deep inside the cerebrum and acts as link between it with the rest of the nervous system.
- It forms major part of the third ventricle.
- The components include: thalamus, hypothalamus, epithalamus (pineal gland), and the subthalamic nuclei.

24. Name the parts of the brainstem.

Ans. The midbrain, pons and medulla constitute brainstem. It connects brain with the spinal cord. They contain ascending and descending pathways, cranial nerve nuclei and reticular formation **(Fig. 9.22).**

Midbrain—is for visual, auditory and somatosensory perceptions.

Pons is mainly connected with cerebellum.

Medulla and pons contain very crucial cardiovascular and respiratory centers.

25. Differentiate ganglia and nuclei.

Ans. **Ganglia** (Ganglion—singular)—it is a collection of neuronal cell bodies outside the central nervous system, i.e., located within the PNS. It is closely related to cranial and spinal nerves, e.g., dorsal root ganglia of the spinal cord.

Nuclei—it is a collection of neuronal cell bodies inside the central nervous system, e.g., basal nuclei, and thalamus.

26. Name the connective tissue coverings of the nerve fiber.

Ans. *Refer* **Figure 9.17.**

Any nerve will be covered by protective three connective tissue coverings. They are:

- Epineurium—outermost covering.
- Perineurium—each nerve fasciculus has its own connective tissue covering.
- Endoneurium—this covers the individual axons.

27. Differentiate cranial and spinal nerves.

Ans. **Table 9.6** shows difference between cranial and spinal nerves.

Table 9.6: Differences between cranial and spinal nerves.

Cranial nerves	Spinal nerves
1. Attached to the brain	Attached to the spinal cord
2. Responsible for sensory and motor functions of head and neck	Responsible for sensory and motor function of skeletal muscles, joints
3. They are 12 pairs	They are 31 pairs
4. They have origin from nuclei located in brainstem except optic and olfactory nerves	They have nuclei of origin in anterior gray horn of the spinal cord
5. Some nerves are related to peripheral parasympathetic ganglia	They are related to sympathetic ganglia for autonomic innervation

28. Mention the structural classification of neurons.

Ans. Based on the number of processes, neurons are classified into three types:

1. **Multipolar neurons**—possess single axon and multiple dendrites, e.g., motor neurons in the anterior gray horn of the spinal cord.
2. **Bipolar neurons**—possess single dendrite and a single axon, e.g., bipolar neurons in retina and cochlea of inner ear.
3. **Unipolar neurons**—possess a common trunk which divides into a central and a peripheral process, e.g., dorsal root ganglion of the spinal cord.

29. Mention the functional classification of neurons.

Ans. The functional classification is based on the direction in which the nerve impulse is conveyed in relation to CNS.

- **Sensory (afferent) neuron**: It receives impulses from peripheral receptors and conveys towards CNS. Majority of them are unipolar neurons.
- **Motor (efferent) neuron**: It sends impulses from CNS and conveys towards periphery or target organs. Majority o**f them are multipolar neurons.**
- **Interneurons**: They are located within the CNS. They receive information from a sensory neuron and stimulate appropriate motor neuron. They are also multipolar in nature.

30. Differentiate nerve from tract.

Ans. Nerve is a collection of axons outside the CNS. For instance, cranial and spinal nerves.

Tract is an aggregation of axons in the CNS. They interconnect neurons of the brain and spinal cord.

31. Nerve plexus.

Ans. The ventral rami of spinal nerves form network called plexus. Numerous branches emerge from these plexus, destined to supply specific regions of the body.

Example: Brachial plexus supplying upper limb is formed by union of ventral rami of cervical C5 to C8 and T1 nerve roots. It supplies upper limb. Other plexuses are mentioned below.

- Cervical plexus—head and neck.
- Lumbar plexus—for lower limb.
- Lumbosacral plexus—pelvis and perineum, lower limb.
- Sacral plexus—pelvis and perineum, lower limb.
- Coccygeal plexus.

32. Phrenic nerve.

Ans.
- Phrenic nerve is a branch of cervical plexus.
- Its root value is C3, 4 and C5.
- It supplies the chief muscle of respiration, the diaphragm.
- Any injury to the phrenic nerve leads to diaphragmatic paralysis and breathing stops. The nerve may also be injured due to tumors in the mediastinum. Severance of the spinal cord above the level of origin of this nerve leads to respiratory arrest.

33. Dermatome.

Ans.
- The area of the skin supplied by a single spinal nerve is called dermatome.
- It is useful to locate the damaged spinal segment in any disease.
- In trunk, dermatomes are horizontal in orientation.
- Over the face, sensory supply by trigeminal nerve is also along dermatomal fashion.

Applied anatomy: In herpes zoster infection, the lesion involves dermatomes of one-half of the body.

34. Sciatic nerve.

Ans. It is a branch of sacral plexus. Its root value is L4,5, S1,2,3. It is the thickest nerve in the human body.

Location—gluteal region. Hence, one should be careful while giving intramuscular injections in this region **(Fig. 9.27)**.

It consists of two components—tibial and common peroneal component.

Main trunk of sciatic nerve supplies Hamstring muscles.

Applied anatomy—injury to the nerve results in sciatic nerve. Leads to pain over lower back and thigh. Common peroneal nerve is commonly involved leading to foot drop.

35. Name the meningeal layers and dural folds.

Ans. Brain is protected by cranium as well as three meningeal layers—dura, arachnoid and pia mater from superficial to deep. It also encloses the spinal cord.

Dura mater—it is a thick strong layer of irregular connective tissue. It is made of outer endosteal and inner meningeal layers. Four dural folds are formed by folding of inner meningeal layer. This divides the cranial cavity into compartments. The **dural folds are**—falx cerebri, falx cerebelli, tentorium cerebelli and diaphragma sellae. The two layers of the dura are fused except at the location of dural venous sinuses.

Middle arachnoid mater—it is web-like, made of cells and loosely arranged collagen and elastic fibers.

Inner pia mater—innermost layer, firmly adherent to the nervous tissue. It carries blood vessels.

36. Dural venous sinuses.

Ans. *Refer* **Figure 9.29.**

These are venous channels which are found in between the meningeal layers of dura mater. They are lined by endothelium supported by connective tissue. Tunica media is absent.

Function: Collect venous blood from brain as well as CSF drains into it. Finally the blood enters internal jugular vein.

Classification:

- **Paired**—transverse sinus, cavernous sinus, etc.
- **Unpaired**—superior and inferior sagittal sinus, straight sinus, etc.

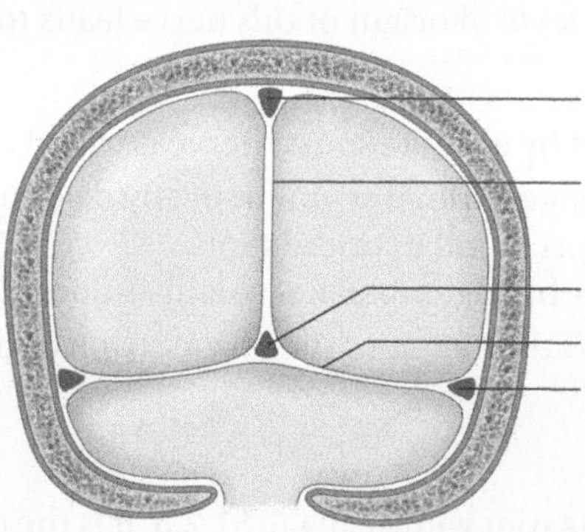

Fig. 9.29: Dural venous sinuses.

37. Name the branches of trigeminal nerve.

Ans. *Refer* **Figure 9.30.**

It is the fifth cranial nerve. The branches of trigeminal nerve are:

- Ophthalmic nerve—supplies the eyeball and surrounding structures, sensory to upper part of face.
- Maxillary nerve—supplies paranasal air sinuses, teeth of upper jaw, glands of nasal cavity, soft palate, nasopharynx, sensory to middle part of the face.
- Mandibular nerve—supplies muscles of mastication, salivary glands, sensations from lower part of the face.

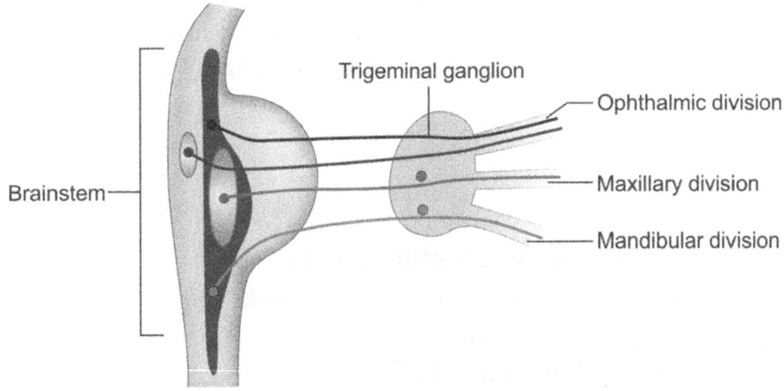

Fig. 9.30: Trigeminal nerve.

38. Name the neuroglial cells.

Ans. The neuroglial cells support the neurons. They are as follows:

- Astrocytes
- Oligodendrocytes
- Schwann cells
- Satellite cells
- Microglia
- Ependymal cells.

39. Name the dural folds.

Ans. The dura mater covering the nervous system is made of outer meningeal layer and inner endosteal layer. The meningeal layer is reflected between various parts of the brain forming dural folds. They accommodate venous sinuses **(Fig. 9.29)**:

- Falx cerebri
- Falx cerebelli
- Tentorium cerebelli
- Diaphragm sellae.

40. Name the structures forming blood-brain barrier.

Ans. Blood-brain barrier prevents entry of harmful substances from blood into the brain substance. It consists of:

- Tight junctions between the endothelial cells of the capillaries.
- Basement membrane of the capillaries.
- Processes of astrocytes.

The barrier is damaged due to trauma, inflammation, and toxins.

41. Name the parts of internal capsule.

Ans. Internal capsule is collection of axons. It belongs to projection fibers, extending from cerebral cortex to lower centers. Its parts are **(Fig. 9.23):**

- Anterior limb
- Genu
- Posterior limb
- Retrolentiform part
- Sublentiform part.

42. Name the parts of corpus callosum.

Ans. Corpus callosum is the largest band of commissural fibers. It connects the right and the left cerebral hemisphere. It has the following parts:

- Rostrum
- Genu
- Body
- Splenium

43. Name the cranial parasympathetic ganglia.

Ans. There are four cranial ganglia in the head and neck. They are:

1. Ciliary ganglion—supplies sphincter papillae.
2. Otic ganglion—supplies parotid gland.
3. Submandibular ganglion—supplies submandibular and sublingual salivary glands.
4. Pterygopalatine ganglion—supplies mucosal glands of nasal cavity, soft palate and pharynx.

44. Components of basal ganglia.

Ans. Basal ganglia/nuclei are a part of the **extrapyramidal system**. It consists of **(Fig. 9.28):**

1. Caudate nucleus—has a head, body and tail.
2. Lentiform nucleus—consists of Putamen and Globus pallidus.
3. Claustrum.
4. Amygdaloid nucleus.

45. What is cauda equina?

Ans. *Refer* **Figure 9.9.**

It is an aggregation of nerve fibers around the filum terminale that resembles the tail of a horse. It is around the caudal end of the spinal cord. It consists of lumbar, sacral and coccygeal spinal nerves. Compression of cauda equina leads to cauda equina syndrome.

46. Define lumbar puncture.

Ans. Lumbar puncture (spinal tap) is a procedure wherein a long needle is inserted into the subarachnoid space for following reasons:

- Diagnostic—done to withdraw the cerebrospinal fluid (CSF).
- To inject anesthetic agents for spinal anesthesia.
- For radiological procedures—like myelography.
- Therapeutic—to inject chemotherapeutic agents.

Level—between L3 and L4 spine or L4 and L5 spines (since spinal cord ends at L2; spinal meninges and CSF extend till S2).

Structures pierced by the lumbar puncture needle:

1. Skin and subcutaneous tissue.
2. Supraspinous ligament.
3. Interspinous ligament.
4. Ligamentum flava.
5. Dura mater
6. Arachnoid mater and subarachnoid space.

47. Cerebellar peduncles.

Ans. Cerebellar peduncles attach the cerebellum to the brainstem and are three in number. It consists of white matter (axons).

1. Superior cerebellar peduncles—from cerebellum to red nucleus in midbrain.
2. Middle cerebellar peduncles—from pontine nuclei in pons to cerebellum.
3. Inferior cerebellar peduncles—from medulla oblongata to cerebellum. It carries sensory information from trunk, limbs, and vestibular apparatus.

Note:

Table 9.7 Shows receptors and sensation carried by the special senses.

Table 9.7: Receptors and sensation carried by the special sensory organs.

Sense organ	Specific receptor	Receptor type	Sense
1. Eye	Rods and cones	Photoreceptor	Vision
2. Ear	Organ of Corti Crista ampullaris	Mechanoreceptor Mechanoreceptor	Hearing Balance
3. Nose	Olfactory cells	Chemoreceptor	Smell
4. Taste buds in tongue	Gustatory cells	Chemoreceptor	Taste
5. Skin	Meissner's corpuscles Merkel's disc	Mechanoreceptor	Touch
	Free nerve endings	Mechanoreceptor	Pain, heat, cold
	Pacinian corpuscles Ruffini endings	Mechanoreceptor	Pressure

- Level of termination of spinal cord in different age groups:
  1. Fetus: Lower border of S3.
  2. At birth: Lower border of L3.
  3. Adults: Lower border of L1.
- Types of hemorrhages related to the skull and cranial cavity:
  1. Extradural—outside the dura mater. Most common cause is rupture of middle meningeal vein, beneath pterion.
  2. Subdural hemorrhage—it occurs beneath the dura mater.
  3. Subarachnoid hemorrhage—it occurs in subarachnoid space, which is filled with CSF. The common cause is the rupture of berry aneurysm.
  4. Intracerebral hemorrhage—is due to bleeding into the brain tissue (commonly called stroke).
- Anosmia—is loss of sense of smell.
- Diplopia—is double vision.
- Sensory supply to face by trigeminal, but motor supply to facial muscles is by facial nerve.
- Bell's palsy—is the paralysis of muscles of one half of face.
- Largest cranial nerve—trigeminal nerve.
- Longest cranial nerve—vagus nerve.
- The main cerebral vessels lie in the subarachnoid space.
- Medulla—contains respiratory and cardiovascular centers (called vital centers).
- Pyramidal tract is the collection of nerve fibers arising in the motor cortex of cerebrum (upper motor neuronal fibers), that carries motor information to the brainstem or spinal cord.
- Hypothalamus is the head ganglion of autonomic nervous system.
- Thalamus—final relay station for sensory modalities except olfaction.

10

CHAPTER

Special Senses

LONG ESSAYS — 10 MARKS

1. Describe the structure of eyeball with help of neat labeled diagram.

Ans. Diagram of structure of eyeball is shown in **Figure 10.1**.

- Eye is an organ of vision.
- Located in anterior part of orbit.

Anatomical parts:

- Two poles—anterior and posterior.
  - Anterior pole—center of cornea.
  - Posterior pole—near optic nerve attachment.
- Optic axis—line joining anterior and posterior pole.
- Equator—midway between poles.
- Lens:
  - Convex.
  - Attached to ciliary body by suspensory ligaments.
- Aqueous humor: Watery fluid between cornea and lens.
- Vitreous humor: Jelly-like, between lens and retina.

Eyeball consists of three layers—from outside to inside: fibrous, vascular and neural **(Fig 10.1)**

- Tenon's capsule/fascia bulbi—fascia around eyeball.

Fibrous layer consists of two parts:

1. Cornea—anterior 1/6, transparent.
2. Sclera—posterior 5/6, opaque.

1. Sclera:

- Thick, opaque and white fibrous membrane.
- Function:
  - Maintains shape of eyeball.
  - Gives attachment to extraocular muscles.
- Meets cornea at limbus (sclerocorneal junction).
- Canal of Schlemm—seen in sclera near limbus.
- Anterior part—visible in eye, covered with conjunctiva.
- Posterior part—covered with fascia bulbi, gives attachment to extraocular muscles.
- Weakest part—lamina cribrosa. Optic nerve pierces sclera at lamina cribrosa.

2. Cornea:
- Transparent.
- Avascular.
- More convex than sclera.
- Important refractory media.
- Five layers.
- Nutrition from:
  - Capillaries near its margin.
  - Aqueous humor.
  - Atmosphere oxygen in tear film on its surface.
- Inflammation—keratitis.

Vascular layer/uvea: Three parts—iris, ciliary body and choroid.

1. Iris
- Circular diaphragm between cornea and lens.
- Central aperture—pupil.
- Function—regulates entry of light into pupil.
- Contents—pigments, blood vessels and muscles.
- Muscles—sphincter pupillae and dilator pupillae.

2. Ciliary body
- Between iris and choroid.
- Secretes aqueous humor.
- It has ciliary processes which give attachment to suspensory ligament of lens.
- Contains ciliaris muscle (muscle of accommodation).

3. Choroid
- Brown in color.
- Extends from optic nerve to ciliary body.
- Contains blood vessels and melanocytes.
- Provides nutrition to outer layers of retina.
- Perichoroidal space—separates choroid and sclera.

Retina:
  - Consists of neural layer and pigment epithelium.
  - Photosensitive layer.
  - Macula lutea—yellow area near center.
  - Fovea centralis:
    - ¤ Central depressed area in macula.
    - ¤ Contains high concentration of cone cells.
- Optic disc—3 mm medial to macula. Also known as blind spot.
- Layers—10.
- Name of layers: Retinal pigment epithelium, rods and cones layer, outer limiting, outer nuclear (rods and cones cell bodies), outer plexiform, inner nuclear (bipolar, horizontal and amacrine cells nuclei), inner plexiform, ganglion cells, nerve fibers and internal limiting membrane.
- Limiting membranes—formed by Muller cells.
  Artery—central artery of retina.

SHORT ESSAYS 5 MARKS

2. Draw a neat labeled diagram of eyeball.

Ans. *Refer* **Figure 10.1.**

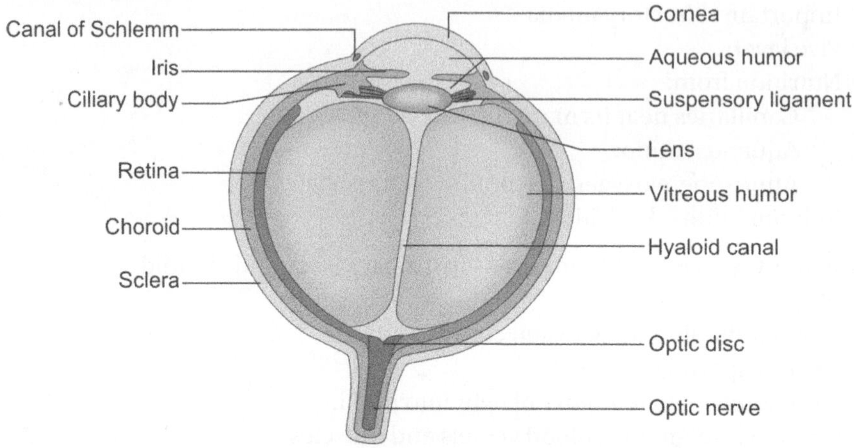

Fig 10.1: Section (sagittal) of eyeball.

3. Middle ear cavity.

Ans. *Refer* **Figure 10.2.**

- Also known as tympanic cavity.
- A small, air-filled cavity in the petrous temporal bone. It is situated between external and internal ear.
- Function—to amplify and conduct the sound waves from external to internal ear.
- Middle ear is fully developed at birth.
- Cavity of middle ear is lined with mucous membrane.

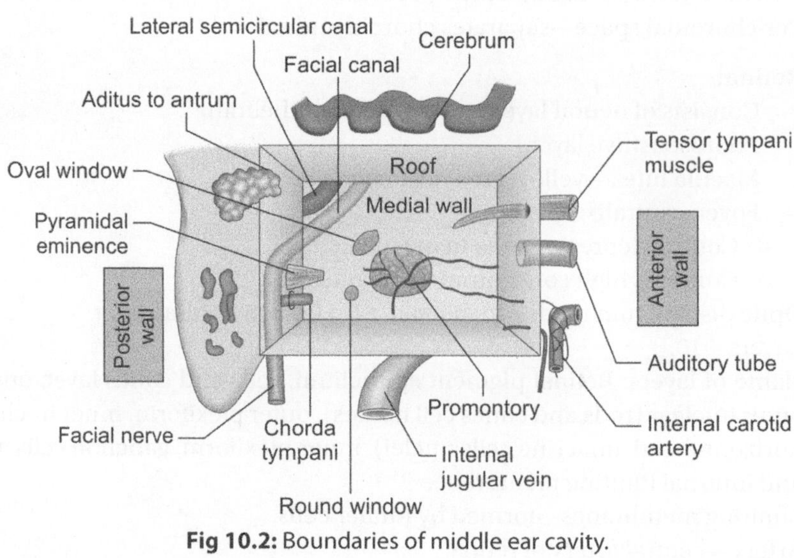

Fig 10.2: Boundaries of middle ear cavity.

- Shape—biconcave.
- Diameter:
  - Vertical and anteroposterior: 15 mm.
  - Transverse: Upper—6 mm; middle—2 mm; lower—4 mm.
- Contents of the middle ear:
  - Three ossicles—malleus, incus and stapes. Synovial joints are present between ossicles.
  - Two muscles—tensor tympani and stapedius.
  - Nerves—chorda tympani, facial nerve, caroticotympanic and tympanic branch of glossopharyngeal.
- Parts:
  - Epitympanum—above tympanic membrane.
  - Mesotympanum—opposite tympanic membrane.
  - Hypotympanum— below tympanic membrane.
- Boundaries:
  - Lateral (membranous) wall—formed by tympanic membrane.
  - Medial (labyrinthine) wall—between middle and internal ear. Consist of promontory, oval window (fenestra vestibule), round window (fenestra cochleae) and facial canal. Facial canal contains facial nerve. Promontory is round prominence due to first cochlear turn.
  - Roof (tegmental wall)—formed by tegmen tympani. Separates middle ear from middle cranial fossa.
  - Floor (jugular wall)—formed by jugular fossa. Separates cavity from superior bulb of internal jugular vein
  - Anterior (carotid) wall—has following structures from above downwards: canal for tensor tympani, auditory tube opening and carotid canal (with internal carotid artery).
  - Carotid canal with internal carotid artery.
  - Posterior (mastoid) wall—has following structures from above downwards: aditus to mastoid antrum, fossa incudis, pyramid and vertical part of facial canal. Pyramid contains stapedius muscle.

Applied anatomy

- Otitis media—middle ear infection.
- Otosclerosis—fixation of stapes can lead to hearing loss.

4. Parts of the ear.

Ans.
- Ear is an organ of hearing.
- Human ear consists of three parts **(Fig 10.3)**:
  1. **External ear:** Includes auricle (pinna) and external auditory (acoustic) meatus. Its function is to gather sound and conduct it to tympanic membrane.
     Tympanic membrane vibrates and sets the chain of ossicles to move.
  2. **Middle ear (tympanic cavity):**
     - Fully developed at birth. Small cavity in petrous bone. Connected to nasopharynx and mastoid antrum. It is lined with mucous membrane and contains air. It carries and amplifies sound from tympanic membrane to inner ear.

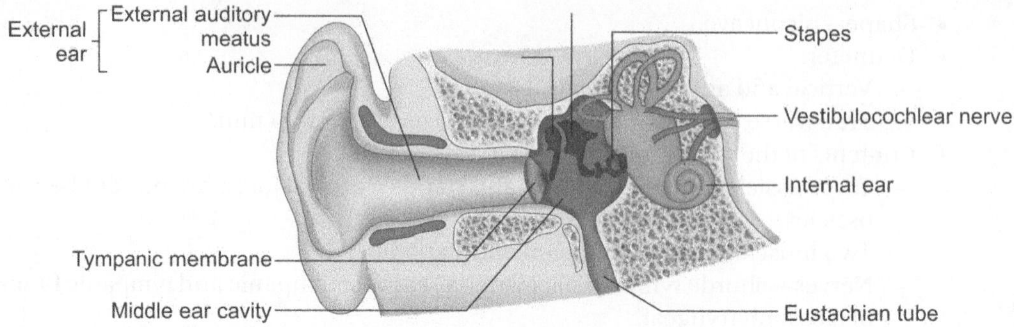

Fig 10.3: Structure of ear.

- ¤ Three ear ossicles are seen in middle ear: Malleus, incus and stapes. These ossicles are connected by synovial joints.
- ¤ The movement of ossicles sends impulses to inner organ of hearing—the cochlea.

3. **Internal ear:**
   - ¤ Converts sound into nerve impulse to be carried to brain by auditory nerve. It has outer bony and inner membranous labyrinth.
   - ¤ Parts of bony labyrinth are cochlea, vestibule and 3 semicircular canals.
   - ¤ Membranous labyrinth is filled with endolymph and its parts are cochlear duct, saccule, utricle and 3 semicircular ducts.
   - ¤ Cochlea is meant for hearing. It converts mechanical stimulus to electrical impulses.
   - ¤ The semicircular ducts, utricle and saccule—are responsible for balance.

5. External auditory meatus.

Ans. *Refer* **Figure 10.3.**

- S-shaped tube.
- Extends from concha of auricle to tympanic membrane. Closed at medial end by tympanic membrane.
- Lined by skin with ceruminous (sebaceous) glands which secrete ear wax.
- Length—2.5 cm. Shorter in infants.
- Parts—outer 1/3 cartilaginous and inner 2/3 bony.
- Two constrictions:
  1. At junction of cartilaginous and bony parts.
  2. Isthmus—in bony part, 2 cm from concha.

Applied anatomy

- Syringing of external acoustic meatus for wax removal can cause vomiting in children and heart failure in elderly. It occurs due to stimulation of vagus nerve.
- Tympanic membrane is examined by inserting auroscope (ear speculum) into external acoustic meatus. For this meatus should be straightened by pulling pinna upwards, backward and laterally.
- Inflammation of external acoustic meatus is very painful due to skin adherence to underlying tissue.

6. Tympanic membrane.

Ans. *Refer* **Figure 10.4**.

- Also known as eardrum.
- Oval membrane seen at medial end of external acoustic meatus.
- Separates middle ear from external ear.
- Diameter: Maximum: 9–10 mm; minimum: 8–9 mm
- It is placed obliquely at angle of 55°.
- Two surfaces: Outer and inner.
- Inner surface is convex, faces middle ear cavity and gives attachment to handle of malleus. Its most convex part is called as umbo.
- Three layers: Outer skin, middle fibrous and inner mucous.
- Divided into two parts: Pars flaccida and pars tensa. Middle fibrous layer is absent in pars flaccida which makes it lax.
- During examination of tympanic membrane using ear speculum, normally a cone of light is seen in anteroinferior quadrant.

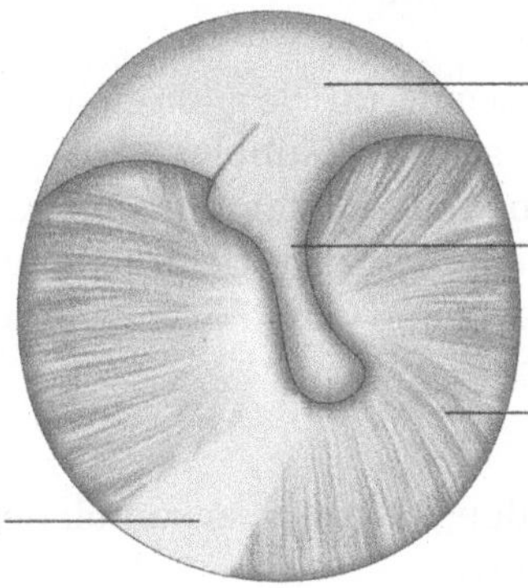

Fig. 10.4: Tympanic membrane.

Applied anatomy

- Myringotomy—a surgical incision is made on tympanic membrane to drain fluid or pus from middle ear.
- Myringoplasty—surgical repair of tympanic membrane perforation.

7. Internal ear.

Ans. *Refer* **Figure 10.5**.

- Converts sound vibrations into nerve impulses. These impulses are carried to brain by auditory nerve (vestibule-cochlear nerve).
- It has outer bony and inner membranous labyrinth.
- Bony labyrinth
  - Located in petrous temporal bone.
  - Perilymph fills space between bony and membranous labyrinths.
  - Parts—vestibule, cochlea and semicircular canals.
  - Cochlea—conical and looks like shell of a snail. It is spirally rotated 2¾ times around a central modiolus. On the inside, it is divided into scala vestibule and scala tympani.
  - Semicircular canals—form angle of 90° with each other and each canal is 2/3 of a circle. Three: anterior, posterior and lateral.

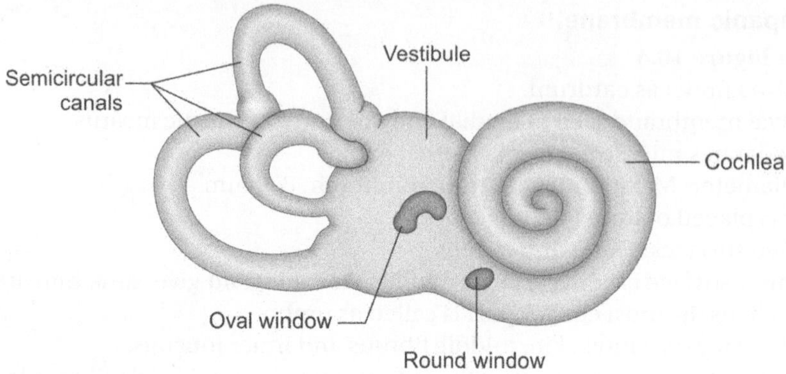

Fig. 10.5: Internal ear.

- Membranous labyrinth
  - Present inside bony labyrinth.
  - Filled with endolymph.
  - Parts: Cochlear duct, saccule, utricle and semicircular ducts.
  - Utricle and saccule are seen in vestibule.
  - Cochlear duct (scala media)—contains organ of Corti.
  - Organ of Corti—located on basilar membrane. It contains hair cells covered by tectorial membrane. Sound vibrations move hair cells and stimulate nearby cochlear nerve fibers.

Applied anatomy

Meniere's disease—occurs due to excess accumulation of endolymph. It causes dizziness, tinnitus and deafness.

SHORT ANSWERS 2 MARKS

8. Name the layers of eyeball.

Ans. It consists of following three layers from outside to inside:
1. Fibrous layer—sclera and cornea.
2. Vascular layer—uvea.
3. Retina—neural and pigment layer.

9. Auricle/pinna.

Ans.
- Function—to collect sound vibrations.
- Shaped like a trumpet.
- Structure—skin and elastic cartilage. Cartilage is absent in lobule.
- Muscles—extrinsic and intrinsic.
- Surfaces—external and internal.
- External surface is irregular with following features:
  - Helix.
  - Antihelix.
  - Concha—depressed area with tragus anteriorly and antitragus posteriorly.
  - Lobule—lower part with fibrofatty tissue.

10. Papillae of tongue.

Ans. The taste buds of the tongue are located in modifications of surface epithelium of tongue called papillae.

Role of papillae:

- Have taste buds within them.
- Provide frictional surface for food to stay in oral cavity during chewing food.

Types (Figs. 10.6A to C)

- Filiform—no taste buds. Provide mechanical support.
- Fungiform—are small, red colored. Have taste buds.
- Circumvallate—largest ones, in front of sulcus terminalis. Have plenty of taste buds.

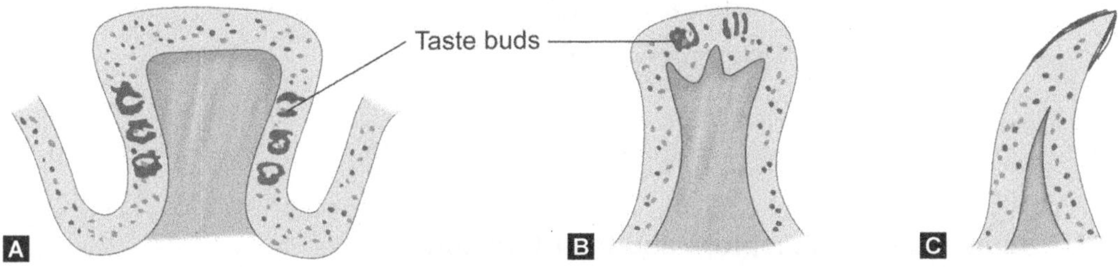

Figs. 10.6A to C: Papillae of tongue. (A) Circumvallate papilla; (B) Fungiform papilla; (C) Filiform papilla.

11. Name the accessory structures of eyes.

Ans. The accessory structures of the eye include the eyelids, eyelashes, eyebrows, the lacrimal (tear-producing) apparatus, and the extrinsic eye muscles.

12. Draw labeled diagram of lacrimal apparatus.

Ans. *Refer* **Figure 10.7**.

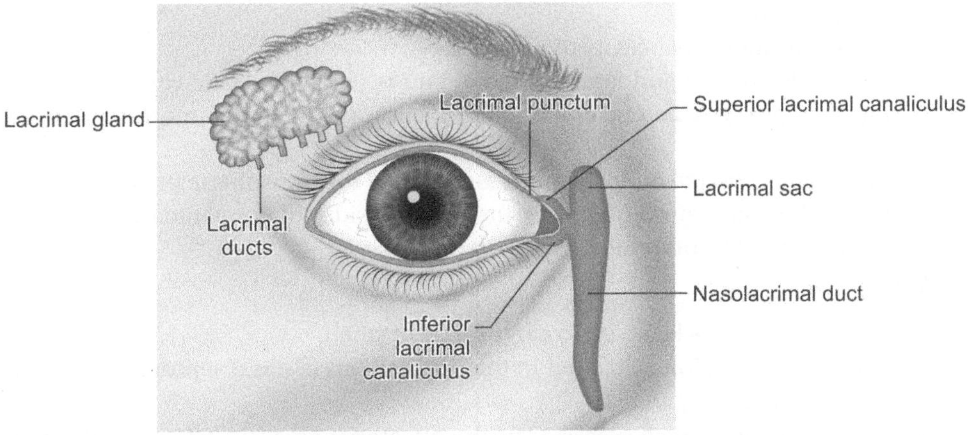

Fig. 10.7: Lacrimal apparatus.

13. Draw a flowchart for passage of tears (lacrimal fluid).

Ans. *Refer* **Flowchart 10.1**.

Flowchart 10.1: Passage of tears (lacrimal fluid).

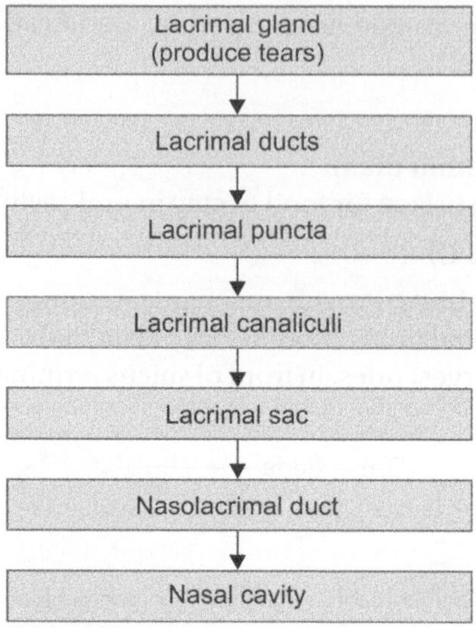

14. Name the photoreceptors and their function.

Ans.
- There are two photoreceptors in eye located in retina: Rods and cones
- Function of photoreceptors:
  - Rods—these are required for black and white vision, and work in low light.
  - Cones—these are required for colored vision and work in bright light. Three types of seen in eye: blue, green and red. Fovea centralis in retina is the area of highest visual acuity and contains only cones.

15. Eustachian tube.

Ans.
- Also known as pharyngotympanic tube.
- Length—3.6 cm.
- Connects middle ear cavity to pharynx.
- Two ends: Medial and lateral. Medial end is made of elastic cartilage and opens into nasopharynx. Lateral end is made of bone and opens in anterior wall of middle ear.
- Function—to make middle ear pressure equal to atmospheric pressure by passage of air. This maintains equal pressure on both sides of tympanic membrane and is required for its vibrations.

16. Olfactory region.

Ans.
- The olfactory area is meant to carry sense of smell.
- The olfactory region is located in the upper 1/3rd of nasal septum and lateral wall of nasal cavity.
- The sensation of smell is carried by the olfactory nerve (the first cranial nerve).
- Absence of ability to smell—anosmia.
- The receptors of olfaction are modified neurons, with capacity to regenerate.

Table 10.1 shows list of structures in the eyeball with function.

Table 10.1: List of structures in the eyeball with function.

Structure	Function
Cornea	Refraction of light
Sclera	Protects and maintains shape of eyeball
Iris	Controls entry of light into eye
Ciliary body	Secretes aqueous humor and contains ciliaris muscle for accommodation
Retina	Converts light to nerve impulses
Lens	Refraction
Anterior chamber	Aqueous humor present here maintains shape of eyeball and gives nutrition to lens and cornea
Vitreous body	Maintains shape of eyeball

Table 10.2 shows nerve supply of tongue.

Table 10.2: Nerve supply of tongue.

Sensory supply			Motor supply
Area of tongue	General sensation (pain and temperature)	Special sensation (taste)	Hypoglossal nerve supplies all muscles of tongue except palatoglossus (supplied by cranial accessory nerve)
Anterior two-third	Lingual nerve (from mandibular nerve)	Chorda tympani (from facial nerve)	
Posterior one-third	Glossopharyngeal nerve	Glossopharyngeal nerve	
Posterior most part	Vagus nerve	Vagus nerve	

Table 10.3 shows components of ear with their function.

Table 10.3: Components of ear with their function.

Component	Function
Auricle (pinna)	Gathers sound waves and direct to meatus
External auditory meatus	Conducts sound waves to tympanic membrane
Tympanic membrane	Vibrates to transmit sound waves to middle ear
Ear ossicles	Amplify vibrations from tympanic membrane and transmit to inner ear
Auditory tube	Maintains equal pressure on both sides of tympanic membrane
Cochlea	Converts sound vibrations to nerve impulses
Semicircular canals	Maintains head position in response to rotational movements
Utricle	Maintains static equilibrium
Saccule	Maintains static equilibrium

11
CHAPTER

Cardiovascular System

LONG ESSAYS — 10 MARKS

1. Describe the types of circulation.

Ans. Types of circulation:

a. **Pulmonary circulation (Fig. 11.1)**: Pulmonary circulation carries deoxygenated blood from the heart to the lungs. The right and left pulmonary arteries carries the deoxygenated blood from the right ventricle to the lungs. Oxygenated blood from the lung returns to the left atrium of the heart via the four pulmonary veins.

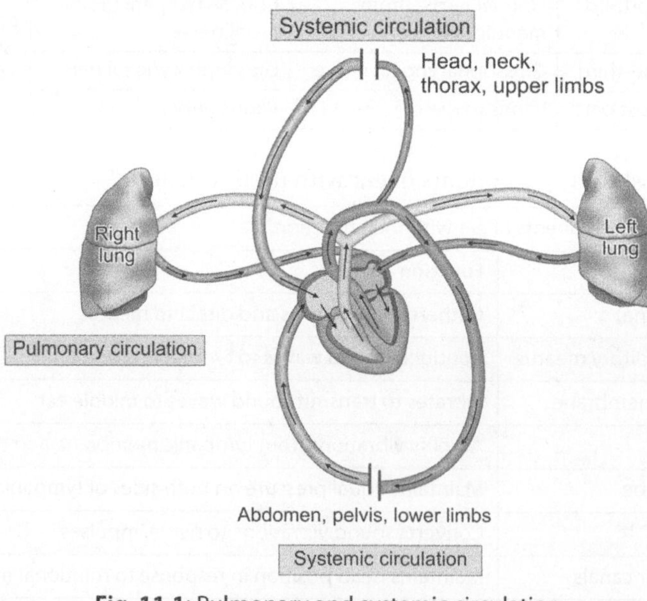

Fig. 11.1: Pulmonary and systemic circulation.

b. **Systemic circulation (Fig. 11.1)**: Branches from the aorta carries oxygenated blood to all the body tissues. The deoxygenated blood from the body returns to the right atrium of heart through the superior vena cava and inferior vena cava. Subdivisions of systemic circulation are coronary circulation, cerebral circulation and hepatic portal circulation.

- Coronary circulation: Heart receives its arterial supply through coronary arteries. Venous blood drains into the coronary sinus which in turn drains into right atrium **(Figs. 11.2 and 11.3)**.
- Cerebral circulation: Arteries that form the "Circle of Willis" supplies blood to the brain. The three arteries supply the cerebrum. They are anterior cerebral, middle cerebral and posterior cerebral arteries **(Fig. 11.3)**.
- Hepatic portal circulation **(Fig. 11.4)**: Venous blood from gastrointestinal organs are carried to the liver via the hepatoportal circulation.
  - ¤ Superior mesenteric vein drains the pancreas, stomach, small intestine, cecum, appendix, ascending colon and right two-third of transverse colon.
  - ¤ Venous blood from the left one-third of transverse colon, descending colon, sigmoid colon and rectum drains into the inferior mesenteric vein.
  - ¤ Inferior mesenteric vein drains into the splenic vein.
  - ¤ Venous blood from the spleen, stomach and pancreas drains into splenic vein.
  - ¤ Portal vein: Superior mesenteric joins with the splenic vein and forms the portal vein behind the neck of pancreas.
  - ¤ Portal vein receives the nutrient-rich blood from gastrointestinal organs. It gives rise to right- and left branch. Then it divides into capillaries and ends in the sinusoids of liver where metabolism takes place.

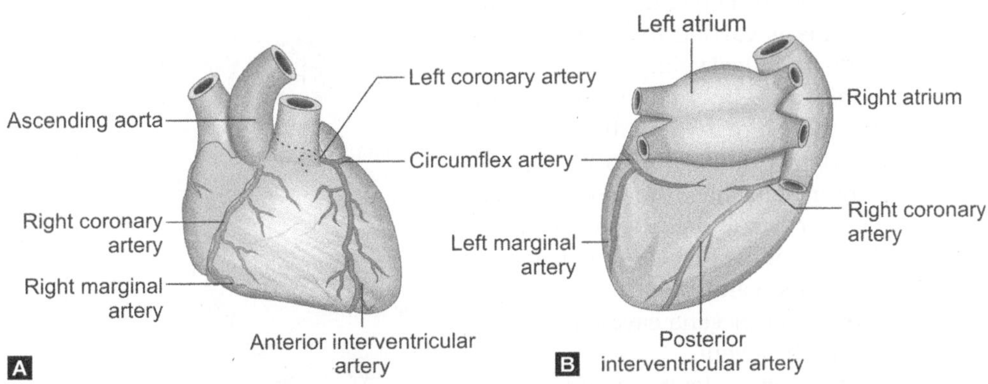

Figs. 11.2A and B: Arterial supply of heart. (A) Anterior surface; (B) Posteroinferior surface.

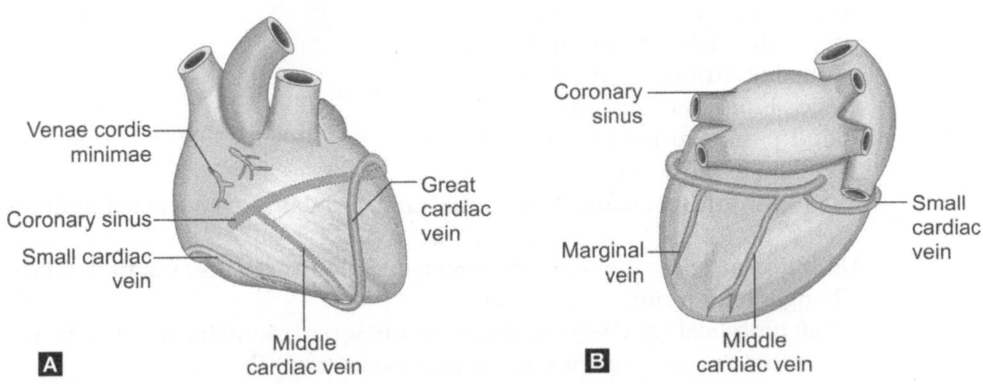

Figs. 11.3A and B: Venous drainage of heart. (A) Anterior surface; (B) Posteroinferior surface.

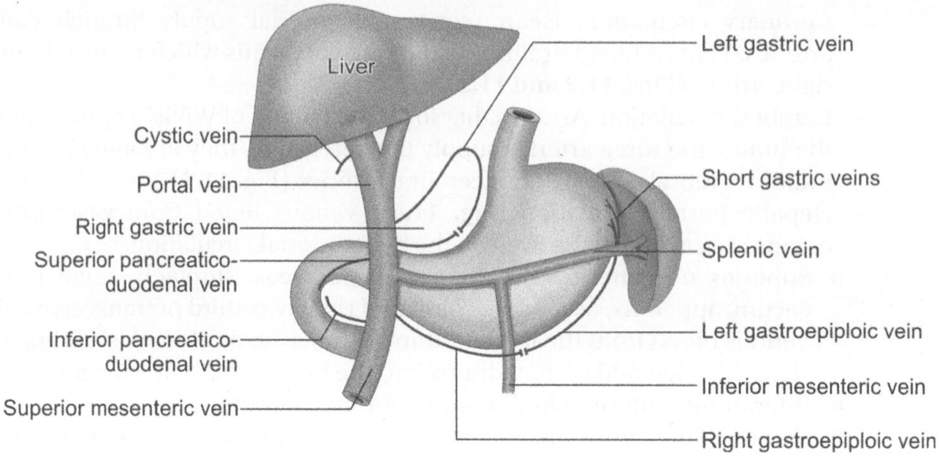

Fig. 11.4: Portal vein and its tributaries.

c. **Fetal circulation (Fig. 11.5)**: Deoxygenated blood from the fetus passes via the two umbilical arteries to the placenta. Oxygenated blood from the placenta is carried to the fetus by a single umbilical vein.

Umbilical vein: In the intrauterine life, there are two umbilical veins. The right umbilical vein disappears early in fetal life. The left umbilical vein persists and carries oxygenated blood from the placenta to the fetus.

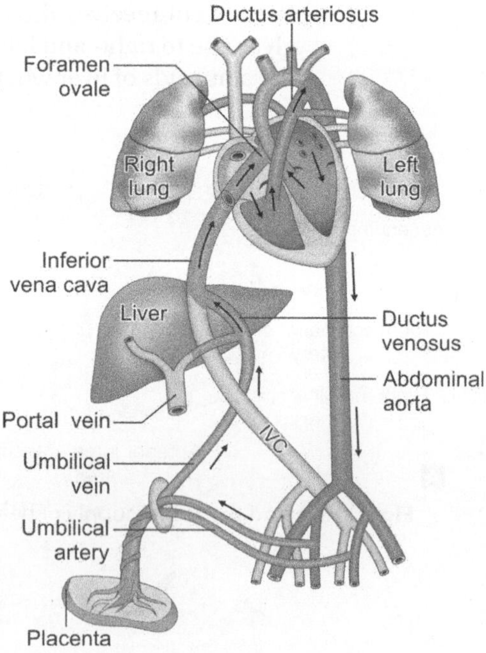

Fig. 11.5: Fetal circulation.

- Ductus venosus: Communicates the inferior vena cava and the left umbilical vein.
- Foramen ovale: It is an opening in the interatrial septum. Oxygenated blood from the inferior vena cava enters the right atrium and then to the left atrium via the foramen ovale. From the left atrium, the blood passes to the left ventricle and then to the aorta.
- Ductus arteriosus: It forms the communication between aorta and pulmonary artery.
- Umbilical arteries: They carry deoxygenated blood from the fetus to the placenta.
- Changes after birth:
  - ¤ Left umbilical vein becomes ligamentum teres (round ligament of liver).
  - ¤ Ductus venosus becomes ligamentum venosum.
  - ¤ Foramen ovale closes and forms fossa ovalis.

- Ductus arteriosus becomes ligamentum arteriosum.
- Umbilical arteries become medial umbilical ligaments.

Applied anatomy:

- Portocaval anastomosis: It is the anastomosis between the portal and systemic veins. In case of portal vein obstruction, the veins at the anastomosis become distended (*Refer Q. No. 55,* Short Answers).
- Patent ductus arteriosus: Ductus arteriosus remains open after birth. Deoxygenated blood from pulmonary artery mixes with the oxygenated blood in aorta.
- Atrial septal defect: Foramen ovale does not close at birth which results in mixing of venous blood in right atrium and arterial blood in left atrium.

2. Describe the coronary circulation (blood supply of the heart) under the following headings: Origin, course, branches, area of supply and its clinical anatomy.

Ans. A. Arterial supply (Fig. 11.2)

Heart is supplied by right and left coronary arteries which arise from the *aortic sinuses of the ascending aorta.*

- **Right coronary artery** arises from the anterior aortic sinus (right coronary sinus). It passes downwards in the atrioventricular groove and curves around the right side to lie on the coronary sulcus.

  Branches:
  1. Sinoatrial (SA) nodal branch
  2. Right marginal artery
  3. Atrial and ventricular branches
  4. Posterior interventricular artery: It is present in the posterior interventricular groove and anastomoses with the anterior interventricular branch of left coronary artery.
  5. Branch to interventricular septum.

  Area of supply:

  Right atrium, a part of left atrium, posterior surface of ventricles, posterior part of interventricular septum, SA node, AV node and bundle of His.
- **Left coronary artery**: Left posterior aortic sinus (left coronary sinus) gives rise to left coronary artery. It enters the atrioventricular groove by passing between the pulmonary trunk and left auricle. It gives rise to anterior interventricular and circumflex arteries, in the interventricular groove.

Branches:

1. Anterior interventricular artery: It is present in the anterior interventricular groove and winds around the apex of the heart to anastomose with the posterior interventricular artery.
2. Atrial and ventricular branches.
3. Circumflex artery: It passes in the atrioventricular groove and anastomoses with the right coronary artery. Left marginal artery arises from circumflex artery.
4. Branch to interventricular septum.

Area of supply: A part of left atrium, anterior surface of both the ventricles, anterior part of interventricular septum and bundle of His.

B. Venous drainage (Figs. 11.3A and B)

1. Coronary sinus: It is situated in the coronary sulcus. It receives many tributaries and finally terminates into the right atrium.
   Tributaries: Great cardiac vein, middle cardiac vein, small cardiac veins, oblique vein of left atrium (oblique vein of Marshall) and posterior vein of the left ventricle.
2. Anterior cardiac veins: These veins drains into the right atrium.
3. Venae cordis minimae: These are small veins that drain the myocardium. They drain into all the chambers of the heart.

Clinical anatomy

- **Angina pectoris:** Substernal constricting pain due to partial obstruction of the coronary arteries. It results in insufficient blood supply to the cardiac muscle. Pain might radiate to the left shoulder and medial side of the left arm.
- **Myocardial infarction (MI):** Obstruction of the coronary arteries lead to loss of blood supply to myocardium which might be fatal.
- **Coronary angiography:** It is a technique done to find out any obstruction in the coronary arteries. A catheter is passed through femoral or radial artery into the ascending aorta. Coronary arteries are injected with radiopaque dye and they can be visualized.
- **Coronary artery bypass grafting (CABG) surgery:** A graft is taken from great saphenous vein, radial artery or internal thoracic vein to connect the ascending aorta and the coronary artery.

3. Describe the chambers of heart.

Ans. Heart is muscular organ which consists of four chambers: Right and left atrium and right and left ventricles. Atria are situated above and posterior to the ventricles **(Fig. 11.6)**.

A. **Right atrium:**
   - *Right auricle* projects forward from the upper anterior part of the right atrium.
   - Coronary sinus, superior vena cava and inferior vena cava open into the right atrium. They drain deoxygenated blood from all parts of the body.

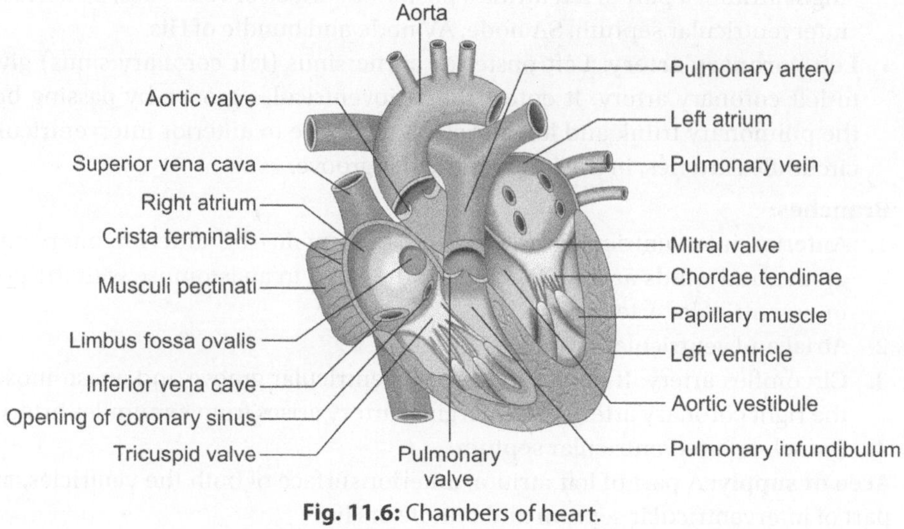

Fig. 11.6: Chambers of heart.

- *Sulcus terminalis* is a groove extending between the superior vena cava and inferior vena cava on the surface of right atrium.

  Interior of right atrium: It has three parts:
  a. Right atrium proper
  b. Sinus venereum.
  c. Tricupsid opening.

  Crista terminalis: A muscular ridge that separates the right atrium proper and sinus venereum on the interior of right atrium.

1. **Right atrium proper:**
   - In the anterior and lateral walls transverse muscular ridges called *musculi pectinati* are present. They arise from the *crista terminalis.*
   - Medial wall or the septal wall separates the right and left atrium. It has an oval depression called the *fossa ovalis*. This fossa has a prominent margin called limbus fossa ovalis.
2. **Sinus venereum:** It is the smooth part and the following veins open into it.
   a. Superior vena cava opens into it posterosuperiorly.
   b. Inferior vena cava opens posteroinferiorly and is guarded by a valve.
   c. Coronary sinus opens near the inferior vena caval opening and has a valve called **Thebesian valve.**
   d. Venae cordis minimae or Thebesian veins.
   e. Anterior cardiac veins.
3. **Tricuspid opening:** It connects the right atrium and ventricle. There are 3 cusps (anterior, inferior and septal) which gives attachment to chordae tendinae.

B. **Right ventricle:** Interior of the right ventricle has 2 parts: Inflowing and outflowing parts.
- Inflowing part:
  i. Muscular ridges called *trabeculae carneae* are present in the wall.
  ii. Conical muscular projections called *papillary muscles* are connected to tricuspid cusps by chordae tendinae.
  iii. There are three papillary muscles: Anterior, posterior and septal papillary muscles. *Moderator band* connects the anterior papillary muscle and the septal wall. Right bundle of His passes through the moderator band.
- Outflowing part: Pulmonary trunk arises from the smooth part called the infundibulum. Pulmonary opening has 3 valves (2 anterior and 1 posterior).

C. **Left atrium:** Left auricle projects from the upper part of left atrium. The posterior wall of the atrium is pierced by four pulmonary veins.
- Interior:
  - Two parts: Rough anterior part and smooth posterior part.
  - Musculi pectinati are present in the anterior part.
  - Venae cordis minimae and the four pulmonary veins open into the smooth posterior part.

Mitral opening: It connects the left atrium and ventricle. There are 2 cusps (anterior and posterior) which gives attachment to chordae tendinae.

D. **Left ventricle:** The wall is very thick as it has to pump blood through aorta to the body.
- Inflow part:
  - Trabeculae carneae are present in the wall.
  - Two papillary muscles: anterior and posterior

¤ Papillary muscles are connected to the bicuspid valve through chordae tendinae.

- Outflowing part: *Aortic vestibule* is the smooth part just below the aortic opening. *Aortic opening* has three valves (2 posterior and 1 anterior).

Applied anatomy

Septal defects: Small openings seen in the septa due to congenital defects. It can involve atrial or ventricular septum or both. Due to the defect, deoxygenated blood mixes with oxygenated blood leading to cyanosis and breathing difficulty and various other symptoms. The two types of septal defects are atrial septal defect (ASD) and ventricular septal defect (VSD).

4. Draw a neat labeled diagram of external features of heart. Describe the right atrium in detail.

Ans. **External features:** *Refer* Q. No. 5, Short Essays

Right atrium: *Refer* Q. No. 3, Long Essays

SHORT ESSAYS — 5 MARKS

5. Describe the external features of heart.

Ans. Heart is a muscular organ, conical in shape. It is situated in the middle mediastinum.

Parts (external features) (Figs. 11.7A and B)

- It has an apex and base (posterior surface).
- Anterior and inferior surfaces, right and left lateral surfaces.
- It has four margins: Right, left, inferior, superior.

Apex is formed by left ventricle. Apex beat is felt 9 cm from the midline in the left 5th intercostal space.

Base or posterior surface: Formed by right atrium and small part of left atrium. Oblique vein of Marshall is seen on posterior surface of left atrium.

Anterior surface or sternocostal surface:

- It is mainly formed by right atrium and right ventricle and also by a small part of left ventricle and left auricle.
- Coronary sulcus separates the right atrium and right ventricle.

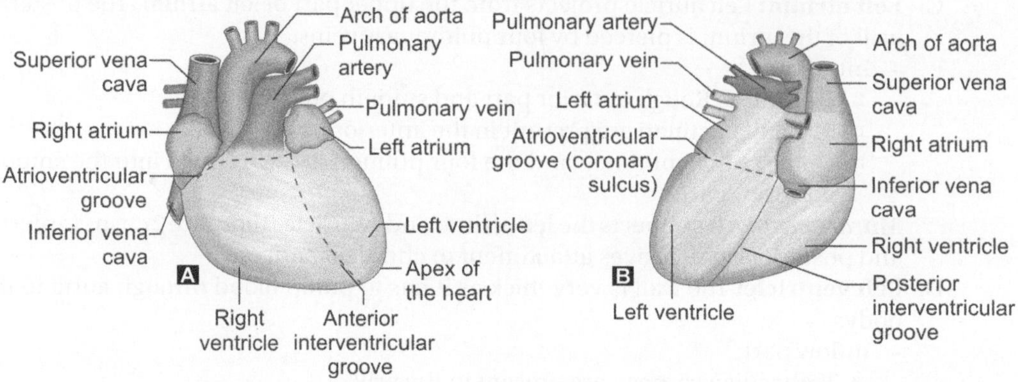

Figs. 11.7A and B: External features of heart (A) Anterior surface; (B) Posteroinferior surface.

- Anterior interventricular groove is present between the ventricles and it lodges anterior interventricular artery and great cardiac vein.

Inferior or diaphragmatic surface:
- Greater part is formed by left ventricle and small part by right ventricle.
- Posterior interventricular groove is seen between the ventricles and it lodges posterior interventricular artery and middle cardiac vein.

6. Structure of wall of the heart.

Ans. Heart consists of three layers—epicardium, myocardium and endocardium.
- **Epicardium**: It is the visceral layer of serous pericardium.
- **Myocardium**: It is the middle layer formed by cardiac muscle fibers. Cardiac muscle is a striated muscle. These muscle fibers branch and intercalated discs are seen between two adjoining muscle fibers. Nucleus is oval in shape and is located in the center of the muscle fiber. The muscle fibers are attached to *fibrous skeleton of heart.*
- **Endocardium**: It is the innermost layer. It consists of thin layer endothelium which prevents clotting of blood.

7. Aorta.

Ans. Aorta is the largest vessel that arises from the left ventricle of the heart. All parts of the body receives oxygenated blood from the aorta.

It has four parts (Fig. 11.8):
1. Ascending aorta
2. Arch of aorta
3. Descending (thoracic) aorta and
4. Abdominal aorta.

Ascending aorta: It arises from the left ventricle at the level of left 3rd costal cartilage and passes upward, forward to the right 2nd costal cartilage. There are three dilatations at the root of the ascending aorta called *aortic sinuses (1 anterior and 2 posterior).*

Anterior aortic sinus: It gives rise to right coronary artery.

Left posterior aortic sinus: It gives rise to left coronary artery.

Arch of aorta: It connects the ascending and descending aorta. It is situated *in the superior mediastinum* posterior to the sternal manubrium. It extends from left 2nd costal cartilage to the left side of T4 vertebra.

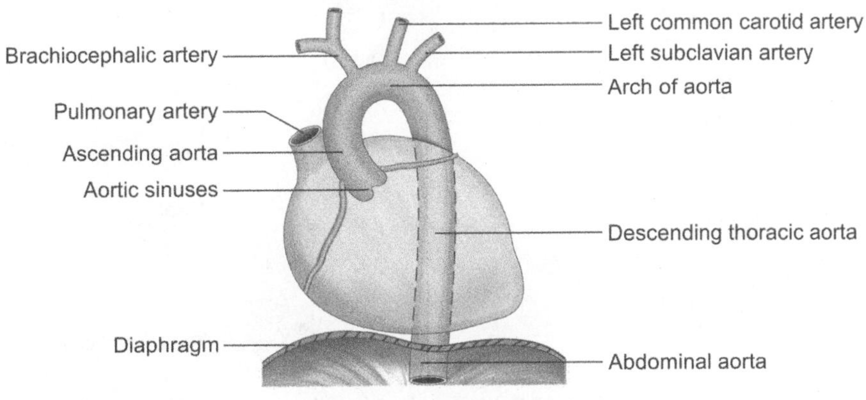

Fig. 11.8: Aorta.

Branches: It gives *three branches.*

1. Brachiocephalic artery: It gives rise to right common carotid artery and subclavian artery.
2. Left common carotid artery
3. Left subclavian artery.

Descending (thoracic) aorta: Arch of aorta continues as thoracic aorta at the lower border of T4 vertebra. It enters the abdomen through aortic opening of the diaphragm at the level of T12 vertebra and continues as abdominal aorta.

Branches: Pericardial arteries, posterior intercostal arteries, subcostal arteries, esophageal arteries, bronchial arteries, mediastinal arteries and superior phrenic arteries.

Abdominal aorta: ***Refer Q. No. 45, Short Answers.***

8. Pericardium.

Ans. Pericardium is a fibroserous sac. It covers the heart **(Fig. 11.9)**.

Subdivisions: Outer fibrous pericardium and Inner serous pericardium.

A. **Fibrous pericardium:** It is a fibrous sac. At its apex, it fuses with the adventitial layer of great vessels, the aorta, pulmonary artery and superior vena cava. Its base is attached to the central tendon of the diaphragm. Anteriorly sternopericardial ligaments extends between the sternum and pericardium.
B. **Serous pericardium:** It is a closed serous sac which has two layers: Visceral and parietal layers. The visceral layer is adherent to the heart. The parietal layer lines the inner surface of fibrous pericardium.

Pericardial sinuses (Fig. 11.10): Pericardial cavity has two recesses (spaces): They are transverse and oblique sinuses.

- Transverse sinus is the recess between the venous end and arterial end of the heart
- Oblique sinus is seen on the posterior aspect of heart bounded by pulmonary veins and inferior vena cava.

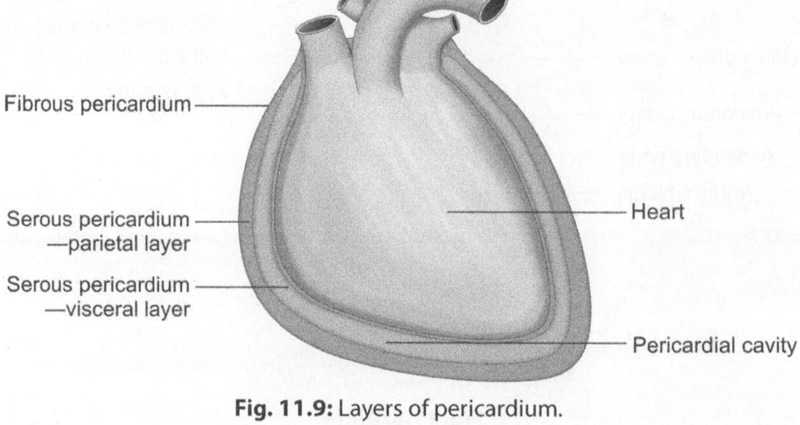

Fig. 11.9: Layers of pericardium.

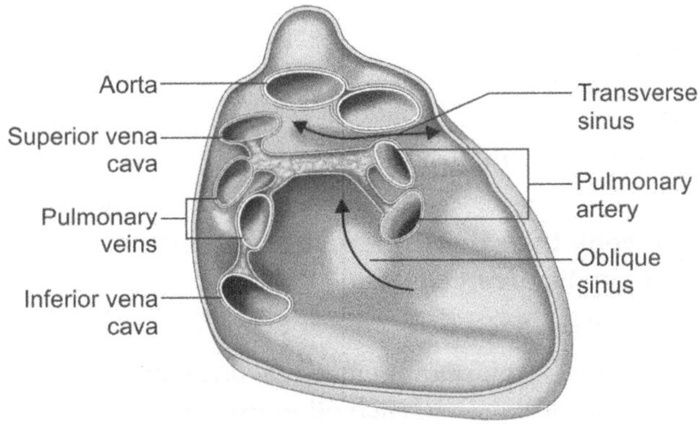

Fig. 11.10: Pericardial sinuses.

Arterial supply:

1. Pericardial and pericardiophrenic branches from internal thoracic artery
2. Superior phrenic arteries
3. Bronchial, esophageal and mediastinal branches from thoracic aorta.

Venous drainage: Corresponding veins drain into azygos, hemiazygos, internal thoracic and superior phrenic veins.

Nerve supply:

- Fibrous and parietal layer of serous pericardium: By phrenic nerve
- Visceral layer of serous pericardium: By cardiac plexuses.

Applied anatomy:

- Pericarditis: Inflammation of pericardium.
- Pericardial effusion: Collection of fluid in the pericardial cavity.
- Pericardiocentesis: Aspiration of fluid from the pericardial cavity.

9. Classify blood vessels according to their structure.

Ans. **Structure of a blood vessel (Table 11.1, Figs. 11.11 and 11.12):** Blood vessel consists of **three layers**—tunica intima, tunica media and tunica adventitia.

1. **Tunica intima** (interna)—is the innermost endothelial layer. Internal elastic lamina, a thin layer elastic fibers is seen between the tunica intima and tunica media.
2. **Tunica media**—is the middle smooth muscle layer which is thicker in arteries than in veins. In large arteries, elastic fibers are also present in addition to muscular fibers.
   External elastic lamina, a thin layer of elastic fibers is seen between the tunica media and tunica adventitia.
3. **Tunica adventitia** (externa)—is the outermost connective tissue layer with elastic and collagen Gibers. In large veins, longitudinally arranged smooth muscle fibers are also present.

Classification:

Artery:

a. Small-sized artery

b. Medium-sized **(muscular)** artery
c. Large-sized **(elastic)** artery.

Vein:

a. Small-sized vein
b. Medium-sized **(muscular)** vein
c. Large-sized vein.

10. Difference between the structure of vein and artery.

Ans. *Refer* **Table 11.1** and **Figures 11.11 and 11.12.**

11. Dural venous sinuses.

Ans.
- Dura mater has two layers: Outer endosteal layer and inner meningeal layer.
- Both the layers are adherent to each other except in certain places where it is filled with blood. These spaces are called dural venous sinuses. These sinuses do not have smooth muscle fibers or valves.

Dural venous sinuses are classified into paired and unpaired sinuses **(Figs. 11.13 and 11.14).**

Paired sinuses:

1. Cavernous sinuses: They are seen on either side of sphenoid bone.
2. Sphenoparietal sinuses are present on the lesser wings of the sphenoid bone.

Table 11.1: Difference between the structure of vein and artery.

Feature	Artery	Vein
Tunica intima	Well-defined internal elastic lamina	Internal elastic lamina is absent
Tunica media	• Thick with smooth muscle fibers • Well-defined external elastic lamina • Large (elastic) artery has more elastic fibers	• Thinner with few layers of smooth muscle fibers • Internal elastic lamina is absent
Tunica adventitia	Thinner than tunica media	• Thickest layer • Large-sized vein has longitudinally oriented smooth muscle fibers
Examples	• Medium-sized (muscular) artery: Radial artery, tibial artery • Large (elastic) artery: Aorta, pulmonary artery	• Medium-sized (muscular) vein: Cephalic vein, small saphenous vein • Large-sized vein: Superior and inferior vena cava

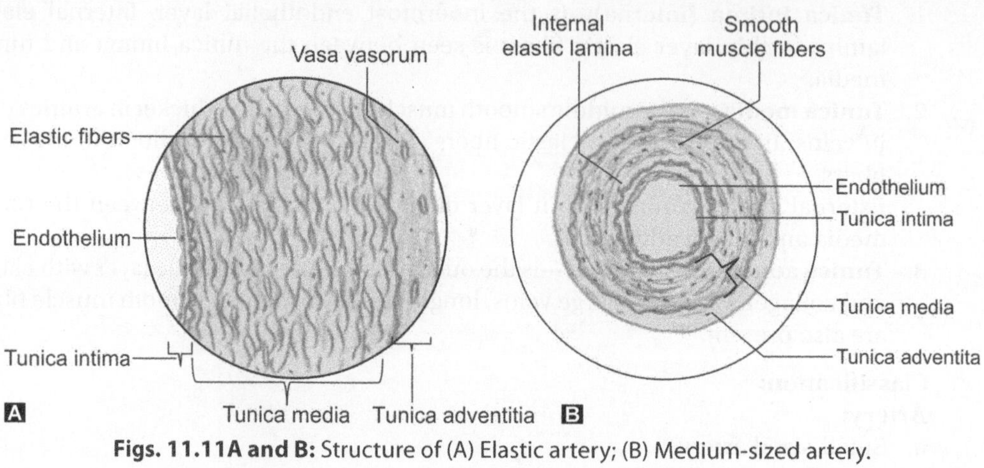

Figs. 11.11A and B: Structure of (A) Elastic artery; (B) Medium-sized artery.

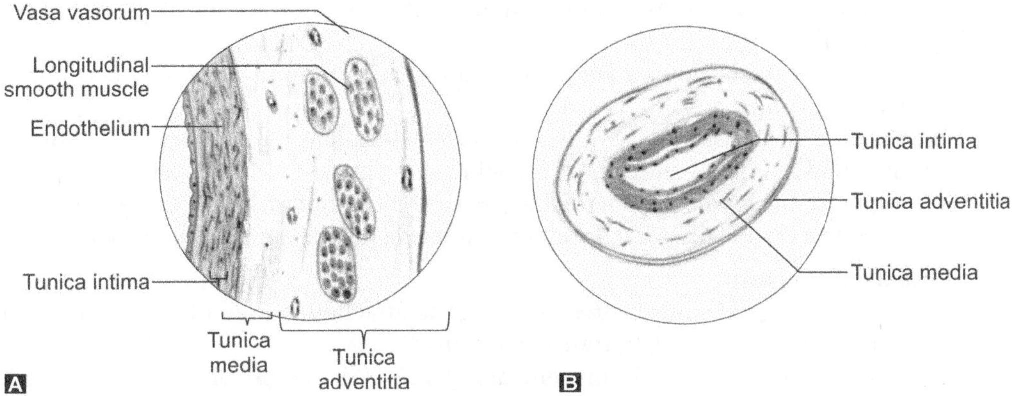

Figs. 11.12A and B: Structure of (A) Large-sized vein; (B) Medium-sized vein.

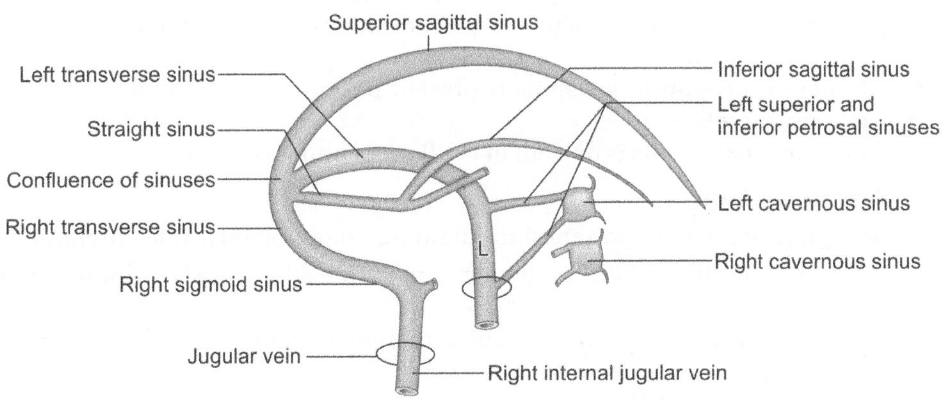

Fig. 11.13: Dural venous sinuses.

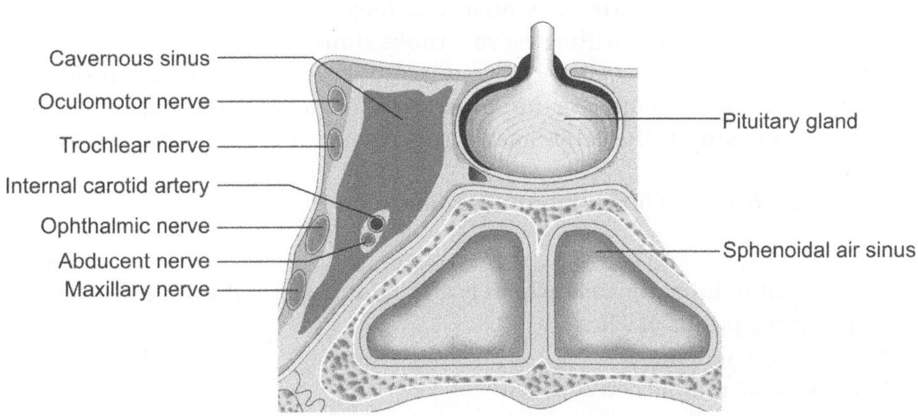

Fig. 11.14: Cavernous sinus.

3. Superior petrosal sinuses are seen along the superior border of petrous part of temporal bone.
4. Inferior petrosal sinuses are present along the inferior border of petrous part of temporal bone.
5. Transverse sinuses are seen in the transverse sulcus of occipital bone along the attached margin of tentorium cerebelli.
6. Sigmoid sinuses are present in the groove of the temporal and occipital bone in the posterior cranial fossa. It continues as internal jugular vein in the jugular foramen.

Unpaired sinuses:

1. Superior sagittal sinus is present along the attached margin of falx cerebri and is continuous with the right transverse sinus.
2. Inferior sagittal sinus is present along the free margin of falx cerebri and is continuous with the left transverse sinus.
3. Straight sinus is seen at the junction of tentorium cerebelli and posterior border of falx cerebri.
4. Occipital sinus—in the attached margin of falx cerebelli.
5. Anterior intercavernous sinus is present anterior to the pituitary gland in the diaphragma sellae.
6. Posterior intercavernous sinus is present posterior to the pituitary gland in the diaphragm sellae.
7. Intercavernous sinus is present in the floor of pituitary fossa.

12. Cavernous sinus.

Ans. Cavernous sinus is an important sinus draining venous blood inside the cranial cavity.

- Situation—in the middle cranial fossa on either side of the body of the sphenoid bone.
- Its interior is traversed by trabeculae thereby dividing the sinus into cavernous spaces—hence the name.

  Relations (Fig. 11.14):
  - Medially —sphenoidal air sinus and pituitary fossa with pituitary gland
  - Laterally—from above downwards, oculomotor, trochlear and ophthalmic branch of trigeminal nerve are present.
  - Internal carotid artery, sympathetic plexus around the artery and abducent nerve are present within the cavernous sinus.
- **Significance**: The cranial nerves and internal carotid arteries are inside the sinus. Hence any inflammation of the sinus, leads to cranial nerve palsies.
- **Regions drained**: The orbit, nasal cavity, meninges, frontal and temporal regions of cerebrum.
- **Eventually drains into**—internal jugular vein.

Tributaries:

1. Superior ophthalmic vein which is also connected to the anterior facial vein and pterygoid plexus of veins
2. Central vein of retina
3. Superficial middle cerebral vein
4. Anterior middle meningeal vein
5. Sphenoparietal sinus.

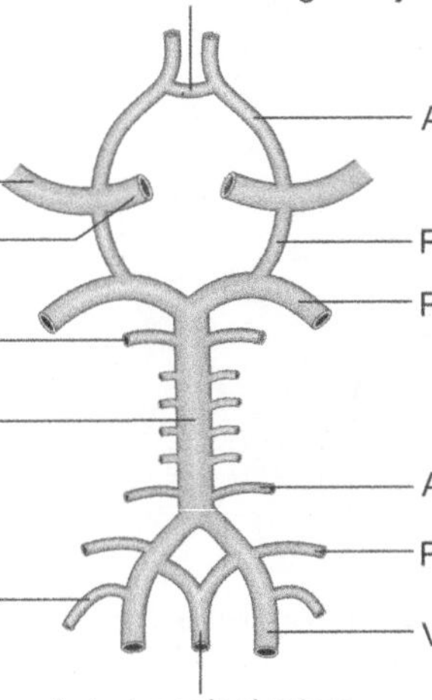

Fig. 11.15: Circle of Willis.

Applied anatomy:

1. Infection from the face can spread to cavernous sinus through the superior ophthalmic vein leading to thrombosis of the sinus.
2. Thrombosis of cavernous sinus will also affect the oculomotor, trochlear and abducent nerves.
3. Carotid-cavernous fistula can occur due to any trauma affecting this region.

13. Circle of Willis—formation, area of supply and applied anatomy.

Ans. Circle of Willis is an arterial circle. It is situated at the base of the brain **(Fig. 11.15)**.

Formation:

Anteriorly—anterior communicating artery.
Anterolaterally—anterior cerebral arteries.
Laterally—posterior communicating arteries.
Posteriorly—posterior cerebral arteries.

Area of supply: Cerebrum, thalamus, corpus striatum, internal capsule, choroid plexus of third and lateral ventricles.
Applied anatomy:
Hemiplegia: Obstruction of blood flow to internal capsule due to thrombosis results in paralysis of one-half of the body.

14. Arterial supply of face.

Ans. Face is supplied by facial artery, ophthalmic artery and superficial temporal artery **(Fig. 11.16)**.

- *Facial artery:* It is a branch of external carotid artery. It is *the main artery* that supplies face. It enters face in front of the masseter muscle. Branches: Inferior labial artery, superior labial artery, lateral nasal artery and angular artery.
- *Ophthalmic artery*: It is a branch of internal carotid artery. It gives supraorbital and supratrochlear arteries in the face.

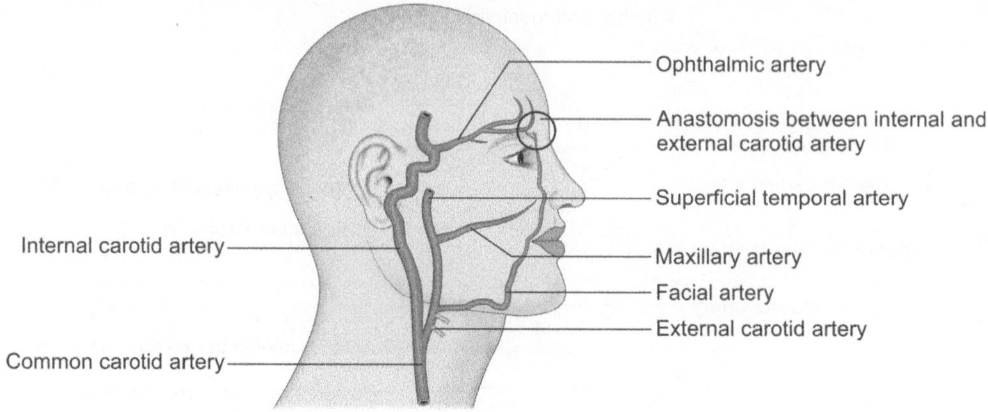

Fig. 11.16: Arteries of face.

- *Superficial temporal artery*: It is also a branch of external carotid artery. It gives rise to transverse facial artery which supplies the face.
- *Maxillary artery* gives rise to buccal and infraorbital branch.

Applied anatomy:

- Branches of facial artery freely anastomoses with the branches of opposite side of face.
- There is anastomosis between branches of internal carotid artery and external carotid artery.

15. External jugular vein.

Ans. External jugular vein is formed by the union of posterior auricular vein and posterior division of retromandibular vein at the level of angle of mandible **(Fig. 11.17).**

- It is superficial and is covered by platysma muscle, superficial fascia and skin. It passes downwards and backwards superficially across the sternocleidomastoid muscle.
- Near its termination it pierces the deep cervical fascia and ends in the subclavian vein.
- It drains the face and neck.

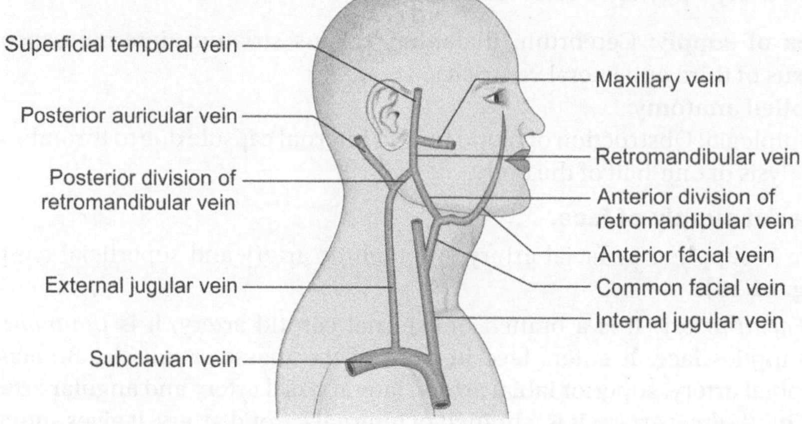

Fig. 11.17: External and internal jugular vein.

Applied anatomy: As the vein is firmly adherent to the deep cervical fascia, in case of any cut injury, the vein will not be able to retract. Thus air can be sucked into the open vein leading to air embolism which might be fatal.

16. Internal jugular vein.

Ans.
- *Sigmoid venous sinus* continues as internal jugular vein within *the jugular foramen* **(Fig. 11.17).**
- It passes downwards in the neck enclosed within the carotid sheath.
- It joins with the subclavian vein and forms the brachiocephalic vein, posterior to the medial end of clavicle.
- It drains the dural venous sinuses and face.

Tributaries:
1. Inferior petrosal sinus
2. Lingual vein
3. Common facial vein
4. Occipital vein
5. Superior and middle thyroid veins
6. Pharyngeal veins
7. Cochlear vein.

Applied anatomy:
- Venous pressure can be recorded.
- Used for catheterization.
- In congestive cardiac failure, venous pressure increases and the vein becomes dilated.

17. Inferior vena cava.

Ans. Formation and course (Fig. 11.18):
- Right and left common iliac veins unite to form inferior vena cava at the level of L5 vertebra.
- It passes upwards and through the vena caval opening of the diaphragm and terminate into the right atrium at the level of right 6th costal cartilage.

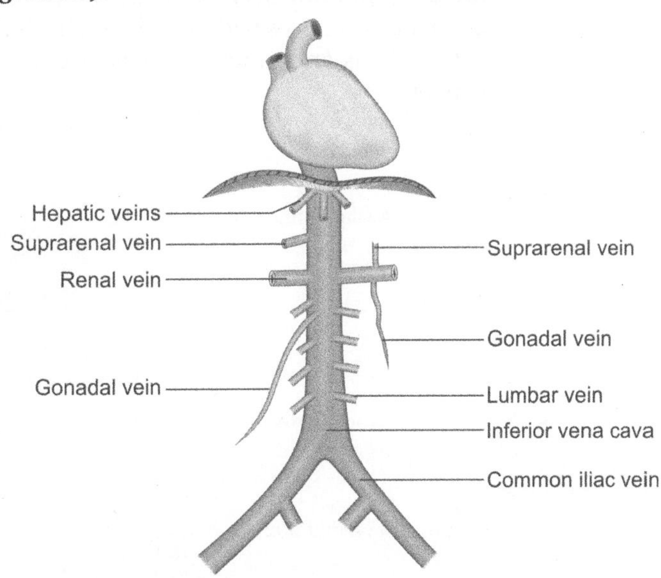

Fig. 11.18: Inferior vena cava and its tributaries.

Relations:
- Anteriorly: Right lobe of liver, epiploic foramen, first part of duodenum, head of pancreas, third part of the duodenum and right common iliac artery.

- Posteriorly: Lumbar vertebrae and right lumbar arteries, liver, second part of duodenum.

Tributaries:

a. Common iliac veins
b. Four pairs of lumbar veins
c. Renal veins
d. Right gonadal vein
e. Right suprarenal vein
f. Inferior phrenic veins
g. Hepatic veins.

Applied anatomy:

- Obstruction of inferior vena cava due to thrombosis leads to edema of lower limbs.
- During pregnancy, compression of inferior vena cava by the enlarged uterus can cause edema of ankle and foot and also temporary varicose veins.

18. Name the arteries of the upper limb.

Ans.
- Arteries of the upper limb are—axillary artery, brachial artery, radial artery, ulnar artery, superficial and deep palmar arch **(Fig. 11.19).**
- **Axillary artery**: It is the continuation of subclavian artery. Axillary artery supplies the axilla.
- **Brachial artery:** It is the continuation of axillary artery. It divides into ulnar and radial artery in the cubital fossa.
- **Ulnar and radial arteries** divide into superficial and deep branches which forms two arterial arches in the palm to supply the digits.
  - The **superficial palmar arch** is mainly formed by superficial branch of the ulnar artery which anastomoses with the superficial branch of radial artery.
  - The **deep palmar arch** is mainly formed by the deep branch of radial artery which anastomoses with deep branch of ulnar artery.
- Princeps pollicis and radialis indicis arteries supply the thumb and index finger respectively.

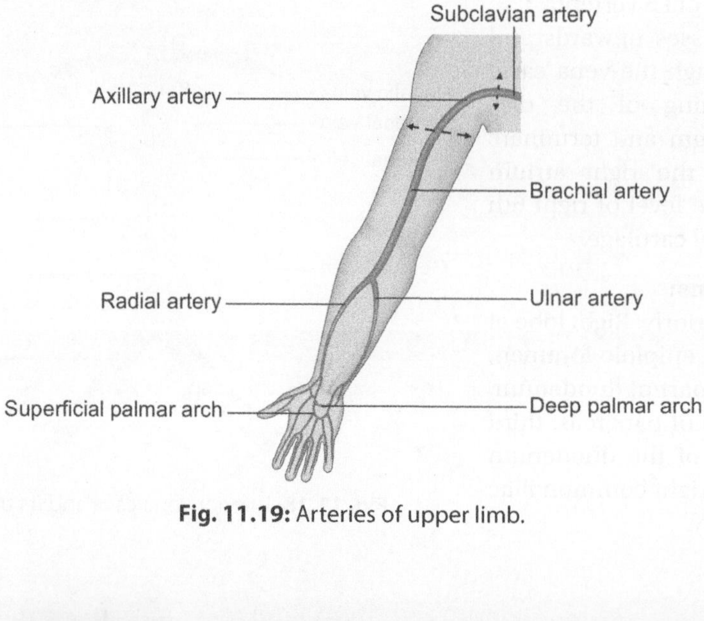

Fig. 11.19: Arteries of upper limb.

19. Axillary artery.

Ans. Axillary artery is the *continuation of subclavian artery* **(Fig. 11.20)**.

- Location: In the axilla.
- Extent: Outer border of first rib to the lower border of teres major muscle.
- It is divided into three parts by the pectoralis minor muscle.
- Distribution: To the upper limb, thoracic wall, breast, scapula and associated muscles.

Relations:

- Brachial plexus is closely related to the first and second part of the artery.
- Second part is related to medial, posterior and lateral cords of brachial plexus.
- Axillary vein is seen medially.

Parts and its branches:

- First part: It lies medial to the pectoralis minor muscle and gives rise to superior thoracic artery.
- Second part: It lies posterior to pectoralis minor and gives rise to two branches. They are acromiothoracic and lateral thoracic arteries.
- Third part: It lies lateral to the pectoralis minor muscle and gives rise to three branches. They are subscapular, anterior circumflex humeral and posterior circumflex humeral arteries.

Note: Scapular anastomosis is an important one as it connects branches of subclavian with axillary artery. If there is any block in axillary artery, blood reaches the upper limb via scapular anastomosis..

20. Brachial artery.

Ans. Axillary artery continues as the brachial artery from the lower border of teres major muscle **(Fig. 11.20)**.

Extension: From lower end of teres major muscle to the level of neck of radius. It terminates by dividing into ulnar and radial arteries.

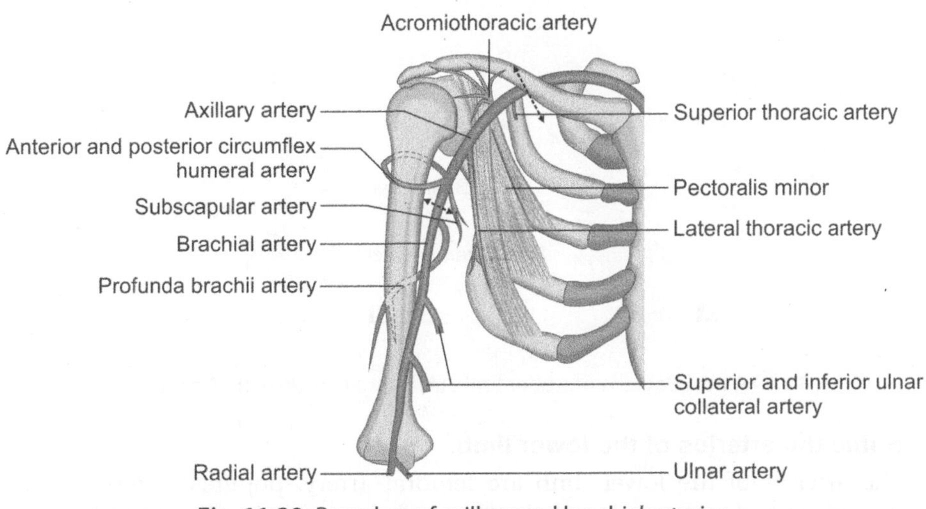

Fig. 11.20: Branches of axillary and brachial arteries.

Branches:

- Profunda brachii artery
- Superior ulnar collateral artery
- Nutrient artery to humerus
- Inferior ulnar collateral artery
- Terminal branches: Ulnar artery and radial artery.

Applied anatomy:

- Brachial artery pulsations can be felt in front elbow medial to biceps brachii tendon.
- Site for measuring blood pressure.

21. Name the veins of upper limb.

Ans. Veins of the upper limb drain into the axillary vein **(Figs. 11.21A and B)**.

- **Dorsal venous arch** drains venous blood from the digits. Medial end of the arch forms the basilic vein and the lateral end forms the cephalic vein.
- **Median cubital vein**: Cephalic and basilic vein are connected by median cubital vein in the cubital fossa.
- **Cephalic vein** continues upwards and drains into axillary vein.
- **Basilic vein** continues as axillary vein.
- **Axillary vein** continues as the subclavian vein.
- In the palm: Superficial and deep palmar venous arches.
- In the forearm: Radial and ulnar vein (deep veins).
- In the arm: Brachial vein (deep vein).

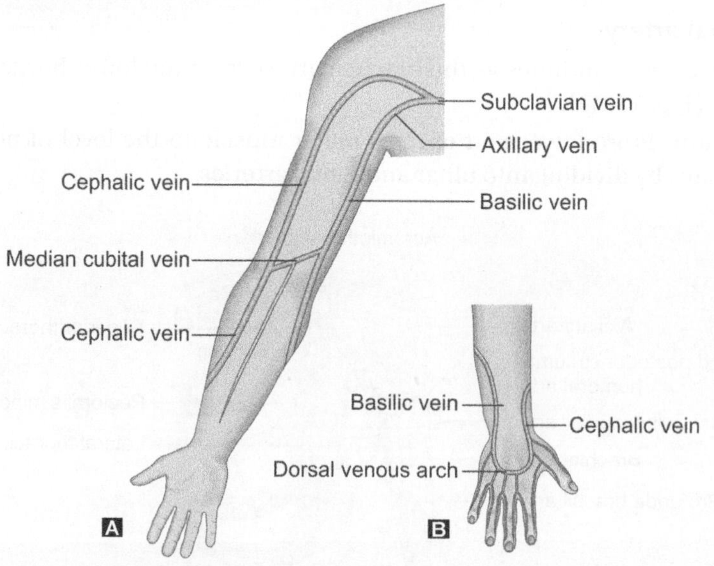

Figs. 11.21A and B: Veins of upper limb. (A) Palmar surface; (B) Dorsal surface.

22. Name the arteries of the lower limb.

Ans. The arteries of the lower limb are femoral artery, popliteal artery, anterior and posterior tibial artery and medial and lateral plantar artery **(Fig. 11.22)**.

- **Femoral artery** is the branch of external iliac artery. It continues as popliteal artery in the popliteal fossa behind the knee joint.
- **Popliteal artery** divides into anterior and posterior tibial arteries.
- **Anterior tibial artery**: It continues as dorsalis pedis artery in the dorsum of the foot.
- **Posterior tibial artery** divides into medial and lateral plantar arteries which enter the sole of the foot.
- **Lateral plantar artery** forms the plantar arch in the sole which supplies the toes.

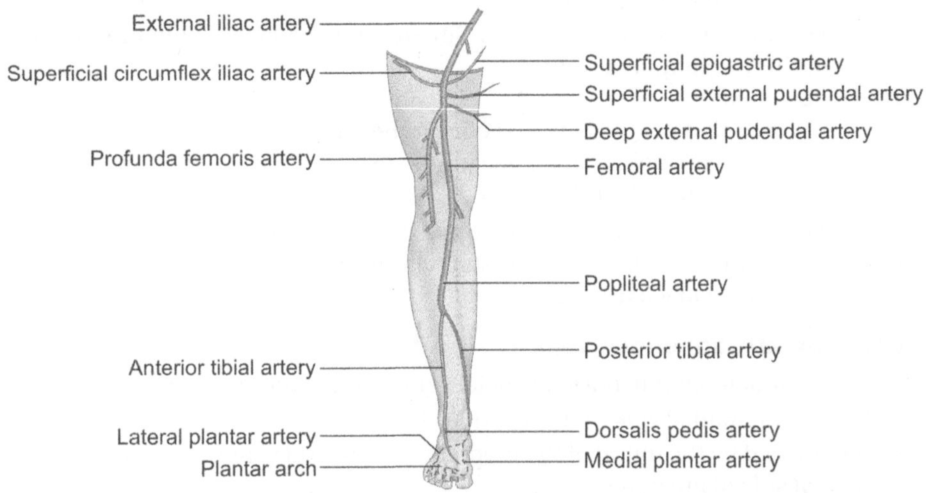

Fig. 11.22: Arteries of lower limb.

23. Femoral artery.

Ans.
- Femoral artery is the **continuation of external iliac artery**.
- It is the principal artery for the lower limb.
- It is situated in **femoral triangle** in the upper one-third of the anterior part of the thigh.
- It is enclosed in femoral sheath lateral to femoral vein and femoral canal.
- Femoral nerve is situated lateral to femoral artery. It is **not enclosed** within the femoral sheath.
- It **continues as popliteal artery** at the level of opening in the adductor magnus.

Branches (Fig. 11.22):
- Superficial external pudendal artery.
- Superficial epigastric artery.
- Superficial circumflex iliac artery.
- Deep external pudendal artery.
- Profunda femoris artery—it gives rise to medial and lateral circumflex femoral arteries and also perforating arteries.
- Descending genicular artery.
- Unnamed muscular branches.

Applied anatomy:
- Femoral pulse is felt below the midinguinal point.
- Femoral artery is used for catheterization in angiography.
- Artery can be compressed against the pubic bone in case of injury.

24. Name the veins of lower limb.

Ans. Lower limb is drained by superficial veins and deep veins. These veins have **valves** which direct the blood from superficial veins to deep veins and prevent the backflow (Since blood has to flow against gravity) **(Fig. 11.23).**

A. Superficial veins:
- Dorsal venous arch.
- Great (long) saphenous vein: Situated on the medial side of lower limb and drains into femoral vein.
- Short (small) saphenous vein: Situated on the lateral side of lower limb and drains into popliteal vein.

B. Deep veins:
- Anterior and posterior tibial veins in the leg.
- Popliteal vein behind the knee joint.
- Femoral vein in the thigh.

The superficial and deep veins are connected by **perforator veins** which also have valves. If the valves fail, blood can stagnate in the veins of lower limb leading to a condition called **varicose veins.**

25. Long (great) saphenous vein.

Ans.
- Great saphenous vein is a superficial vein which drains the lower limb **(Fig. 11.23).**
- Present on medial side of the lower limb.
- It is formed by the union of the medial end of dorsal venous arch and digital vein of medial side of great toe.
- It passes upwards in front of medial malleolus and behind the medial side of knee joint to the thigh.
- In the thigh it **terminates into the femoral vein by piercing the cribriform fascia.**
- Great saphenous vein has **5 perforator veins** which connect with the deep veins of lower limb.

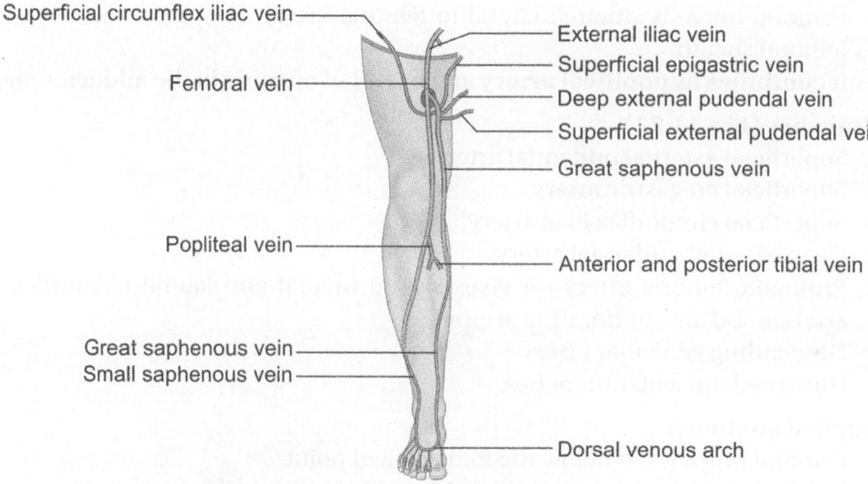

Fig. 11.23: Veins of lower limb.

Tributaries:

i. Medial marginal vein
ii. Communicating vein to short saphenous vein
iii. Anterior and posterior femoral cutaneous veins
iv. Superficial circumflex iliac vein
v. Superficial epigastric vein
vi. Superficial and deep external pudendal veins.

Applied anatomy:

- Dilatation of superficial veins is known as **varicose veins.**
- The veins of the lower limb have valves which direct the blood from superficial veins to deep veins.
- When the valves become incompetent, there is backflow of venous blood from deep veins to superficial veins. This results in tortuous dilated superficial veins in the lower limb.
- **Great saphenous vein:** It is used in **bypass grafting.** A segment of the vessel is taken, reversed and grafted at the site of coronary artery block.

26. Thoracic duct.

Ans.
- Thoracic duct is the main lymphatic channel which drains the chyle and lymph into blood.
- It is 45 cm long and begins at the level of 12th thoracic vertebra as a dilatation *called Cisterna chyli.*
- It enters the thoracic cavity through the aortic opening of the diaphragm.
- It crosses from right to left side at the level of 5th thoracic vertebra.
- At the root of the neck, it terminates into the junction of left subclavian and left internal jugular vein.

Thoracic duct **receives lymph from** the following regions:

- Left side of the head, neck and thorax
- Left upper limb
- Entire abdomen and pelvis
- Lower limbs.

Tributaries:

1. Intestinal trunks
2. Right and left lumbar lymph trunks
3. Left jugular lymph trunk
4. Left subclavian lymph trunk
5. Left brachiocephalic and mediastinal trunks.

27. Write a note on thymus and its function.

Ans.
- Thymus is a bilobed lymphoid organ situated in the superior mediastinum between the aorta and sternum.
- It is covered by capsule which sends in trabeculae dividing the gland into lobules.
- Each lobule consists of **outer cortex and inner medulla**. Cortex is composed of dense collection of T lymphocytes, few epithelial cells and macrophages.

- Medulla consists of less number of lymphocytes. The degenerated epithelial cells are flat and arranged in concentric layers with hyaline material in the center. These are called the thymic or Hassall's corpuscles.

Functions:

- It is a primary lymphoid organ and plays an important role in immune responses.
- Maturation, proliferation and selection of lymphocytes takes place in thymus.

28. Location, relations and functions of spleen.

Ans. Spleen is a lymphoid organ **(Fig. 11.24)**.

- Location: It is situated in the left hypochondrium, opposite 9th, 10th and 11th ribs, between the stomach and diaphragm.
- Surfaces: Visceral surface and diaphragmatic surface.
- Borders: Superior, inferior and intermediate borders.

Relations:

- Visceral surface: Stomach, left kidney, left colic flexure and tail of pancreas.
- Diaphragmatic surface: Diaphragm, left pleura, 9th, 10th and 11th ribs.
- Hilum—splenic blood vessels enter it.

Functions:

- Macrophages remove the defective and worn out blood cells and platelets.
- Storage of platelets.
- Production of red cells during fetal period.

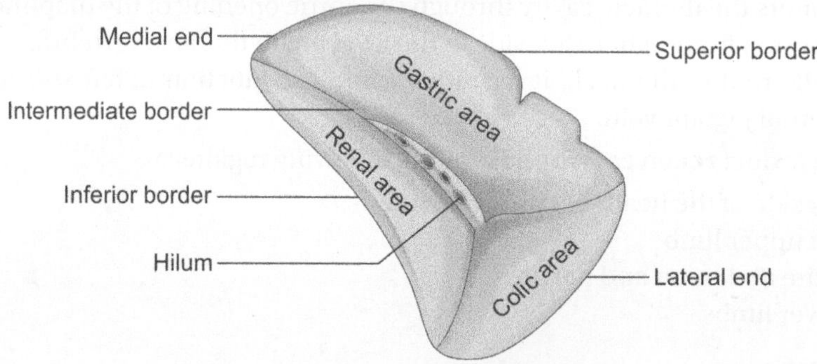

Fig. 11.24: Spleen—visceral surface.

29. Interior of right ventricle.

Ans. *Refer Q.No. 3, Long Essays.*

30. Interior of right atrium.

Ans. *Refer Q.No. 3, Long Essays.*

31. Right coronary artery.

Ans. *Refer Q.No. 2, Long Essays.*

32. Left coronary artery.

Ans. *Refer Q.No. 2, Long Essays.*

33. Venous drainage of heart.

Ans. *Refer Q.No. 2, Long Essays.*

SHORT ANSWERS 2 MARKS

34. Name the layers of a blood vessel.

Ans. *Refer* **Figures 11.11 and 11.12.**

- Tunica intima—inner layer. Lined by endothelium.
- Tunica media—middle layer. Contains connective tissue either smooth muscle fibers or elastic fibers.
- Tunica adventitia—outer layer. Made of connective tissue with nerves and blood vessels.

35. Give the formation and termination of superior vena cava.

Ans. **Formation:** By the union of right- and left brachiocephalic vein at the level of 1st right costal cartilage.

Termination: Into the right atrium at the level of the 3rd right costal cartilage **(Fig. 11.25).**

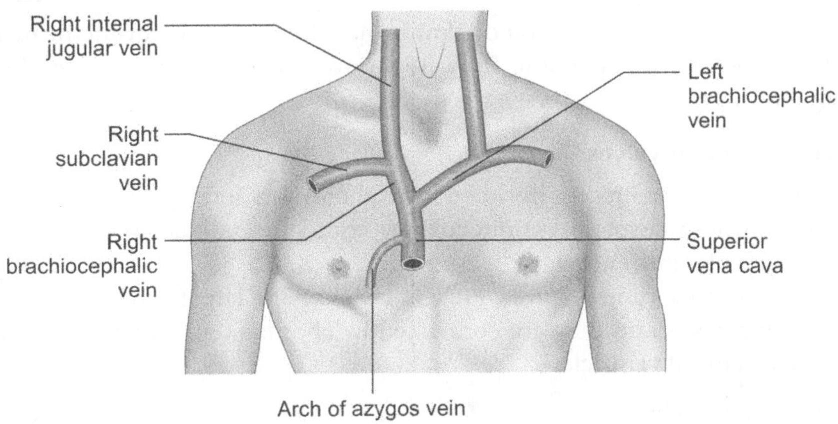

Fig. 11.25: Superior vena cava.

36. Name the branches of right coronary artery.

Ans.
- SA nodal artery
- Atrial branches
- Right marginal branch
- Posterior interventricular artery
- AV nodal artery.

37. Name the branches of left coronary artery.

Ans.
- Anterior interventricular artery [left anterior descending artery (LAD)]
- Circumflex branch
- Diagonal artery
- Atrial branches
- Ventricular branch
- SA nodal and AV nodal branch if not supplied by right coronary artery.

38. Name the veins opening into right atrium.

Ans.
- Superior vena cava
- Inferior vena cava
- Coronary sinus
- Venae cordis minimae (Thebesian veins)
- Anterior cardiac veins.

39. Structures present in the interventricular and atrioventricular sulci of heart.

Ans. *Refer* **Table 11.2 and Figure 11.7.**

Table 11.2: Structures present in the sulci of heart.

Structures present in the sulcus	Anterior interventricular sulcus	Posterior interventricular sulcus	Atrioventricular (coronary sulcus)
Arteries	Anterior interventricular artery	Posterior interventricular artery	Terminal parts of left and right coronary arteries
Veins	Great cardiac vein	Middle cardiac vein	Coronary sinus Small cardiac vein

40. Valves of the heart.

Ans. Valves of the heart direct the blood flow in one direction and prevent the regurgitation of blood in opposite direction. They are atrioventricular valves and semilunar valves **(Fig. 11.6)**.

Atrioventricular valves:

- Tricuspid valve: Present between the right atrium and right ventricle. It has three cusps. These cusps are connected by chordae tendinae to the three papillary muscles of right ventricle.
- Bicuspid valve (mitral valve): Present between the left atrium and left ventricle. It has two cusps and they are connected by chordae tendinae to the two papillary muscles of left ventricle.

Semilunar valves:

- These valves are present in the aorta and pulmonary artery. They are semilunar in shape and have three cusps.
- Aortic valve: It directs the blood from left ventricle to the ascending aorta.
- Pulmonary valve: It directs the blood from right ventricle to the pulmonary artery.

Applied anatomy:

- Stenosis—narrowing of the valve orifice, reducing blood flow.
- Regurgitation/incompetency/insufficiency—the valves cannot close completely leading to backflow of blood.

41. Median cubital vein.

Ans. Median cubital vein is a communication vein present in the cubital fossa of upper limb. It connects the cephalic vein and the basilic vein **(Fig. 11.26)**.

Applied anatomy: This vein is ideal for veni puncture and intravenous injections because it is supported by bicipital aponeurosis present beneath the vein.

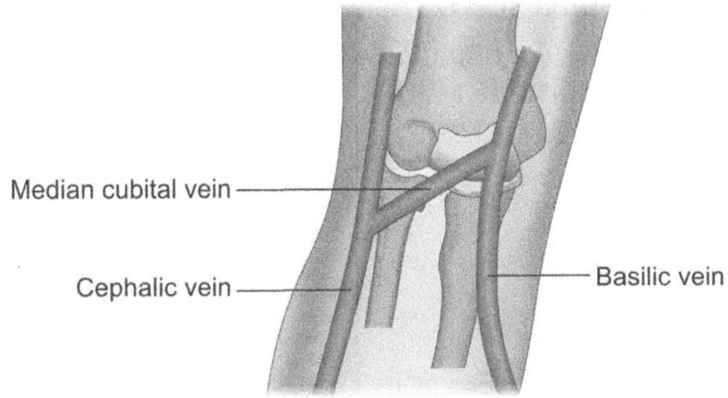

Fig. 11.26: Median cubital vein.

42. Nutrient artery.

Ans. Nutrient artery supplies the bone. It is a branch from the artery outside the periosteum and passes obliquely into the shaft of a bone through nutrient foramen. In the medullary cavity of bone, it divides into longitudinal branches and supplies the bone marrow, spongy bone and compact bone.

43. Superficial and deep palmar arch.

Ans.
- Arterial arches are present in the palm **(Fig. 11.27)**.
- These arches supply the hand.
- The superficial palmar arch is mainly formed by superficial branch of the ulnar artery. It anastomoses with the superficial branch of radial artery. It gives common digital branches to supply the fingers.
- The deep palmar arch is mainly formed by the deep branch of radial artery. It anastomoses with deep branch of ulnar artery. It gives palmar metacarpal and perforating digital arteries which supply the fingers.
- Princeps pollicis and radialis indicis arteries supply the thumb and index finger respectively.

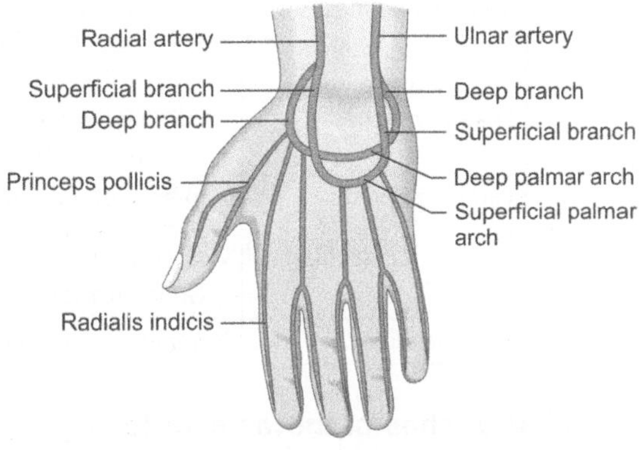

Fig. 11.27: Superficial and deep palmar arch.

44. Dorsalis pedis artery.

Ans.
- **Formation:** It is the continuation of the anterior tibial artery **(Fig. 11.22)**.
- It extends from the midpoint between the two malleoli on the dorsum of foot and passes downwards between the two heads of first dorsal interossei into the sole of foot.
- It joins the lateral plantar artery to complete the plantar arch.
- Arterial pulse can be felt in dorsum of foot in between the malleoli of tibia and fibula.

45. Branches of abdominal aorta.

Ans. Abdominal aorta is the continuation of thoracic aorta at the level of 12th thoracic vertebra **(Fig. 11.28 and Table 11.3).**

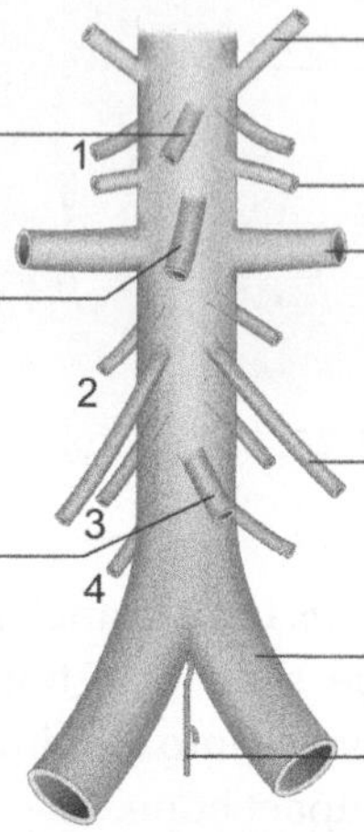

Fig. 11.28: Branches of abdominal aorta.

Table 11.3: Branches of abdominal aorta.

Ventral branches	• Celiac artery • Superior mesenteric artery • Inferior mesenteric artery
Dorsal branches	• Lumbar arteries • Median sacral artery
Lateral branches	• Inferior phrenic arteries • Middle suprarenal arteries • Renal arteries • Gonadal arteries (testicular artery in male and ovarian artery in female)
Terminal branches	Right and left common iliac arteries

46. Branches of thoracic aorta.

Ans. *Refer Q. No. 7, Short Essays*

47. Branches of popliteal artery.

Ans. **Formation:** It is the continuation of femoral artery.

Location: It is situated in the popliteal fossa behind the knee joint **(Fig. 11.22).**

Branches:

- Cutaneous branches
- Muscular branches
- Genicular branches
- Terminal branches are anterior and posterior tibial arteries.

48. Name the branches of axillary artery.

Ans. • **Formation:** It is the continuation of subclavian artery.

- It supplies upper limb and thoracic wall, breast.
- It has three parts divided by the pectoralis minor muscle **(Fig. 11.20)**.

Branches:

- First part: Superior thoracic artery
- Second part: Acromiothoracic and lateral thoracic artery
- Third part: Subscapular artery, anterior- and posterior circumflex humeral artery.

49. Radial artery.

Ans.
- Radial artery is a terminal branch of brachial artery.
- **Extension:** From the level of neck of radius in front of the forearm to the palm.
- **Termination:** Forms the deep palmar arch by anastomosing with deep branch of ulnar artery.
- **Branches:** Distribute to elbow, forearm and hand.
- **Radial pulse**—felt against lower end of radius.

50. Name the arteries where peripheral pulse is felt.

Ans. *Refer* **Table 11.4.**

Table 11.4: Site of peripheral pulsation.

	Artery	Location of pulse
Upper limb	• Radial artery • Brachial artery	• Lower end of radius • Front of elbow, medial to tendon of biceps brachii muscle
Neck and face	• Common carotid artery • Facial artery • Superficial temporal artery	• Lateral to the thyroid cartilage • Base of mandible in front of masseter muscle • In front of the ear
Lower limb	• Dorsalis pedis artery • Popliteal artery • Femoral artery	• In between the two malleoli of tibia and fibula • In the popliteal fossa • Just below the midinguinal point

51. Varicose veins.

Ans.
- Dilatation of superficial veins is known as varicose veins.
- The veins of the lower limb have valves which direct the blood from superficial veins to deep veins.
- When the valves become incompetent, there is backflow of venous blood from deep to superficial veins. This results in tortuous dilated superficial veins in the lower limb (great saphenous and small saphenous veins).
- Varicose ulcer develops in the leg as a complication of varicose veins.

52. Subclavian vein.

Ans.
- Subclavian vein drains the upper extremity **(Fig. 11.25)**.
- **Formation:** It is the continuation of axillary vein.
- **Termination:** Union of subclavian vein and the internal jugular vein form the brachiocephalic vein.
- **Applied anatomy**: Central venous catheterization is done for monitoring or to deliver medicine.

53. Name the tributaries of coronary sinus.

Ans. Coronary sinus is situated in the coronary sulcus. It terminates into the right atrium after receiving the following tributaries.

Tributaries are: Great cardiac vein, middle cardiac vein, small cardiac veins, oblique vein of left atrium (oblique vein of Marshall) and posterior vein of the left ventricle.

54. Formation and termination of portal vein.

Ans.
- **Formation:** Union of superior mesenteric vein and splenic vein **(Fig. 11.3)**.
- **Termination:** Divides into right and left branch in the liver.
- Portal vein receives venous blood from spleen, pancreas, gallbladder, stomach and intestines.

55. Portocaval anastomosis.

Ans. It is the anastomosis between the portal and systemic veins. In case of portal vein obstruction, the veins at the following sites are distended.
- Lower end of esophagus: Causes esophageal varices.
- Lower end of rectum and anal canal: Causes hemorrhoids or piles.
- Umbilicus: Distension of veins around umbilicus causes caput medusae.
- Bare area of liver.
- Posterior abdominal wall.

56. Azygos system of veins.

Ans. Azygos vein drains the lumbar region and thoracic wall. It connects the superior vena cava and inferior vena cava **(Fig. 11.29)**.

Formation: It is formed by the right subcostal vein, ascending lumbar vein and a vein from inferior vena cava.

Termination: It passes through the aortic opening of the diaphragm into the thorax. It receives accessory hemiazygos vein and hemiazygos vein from the left side. Then it terminates into the superior vena cava.

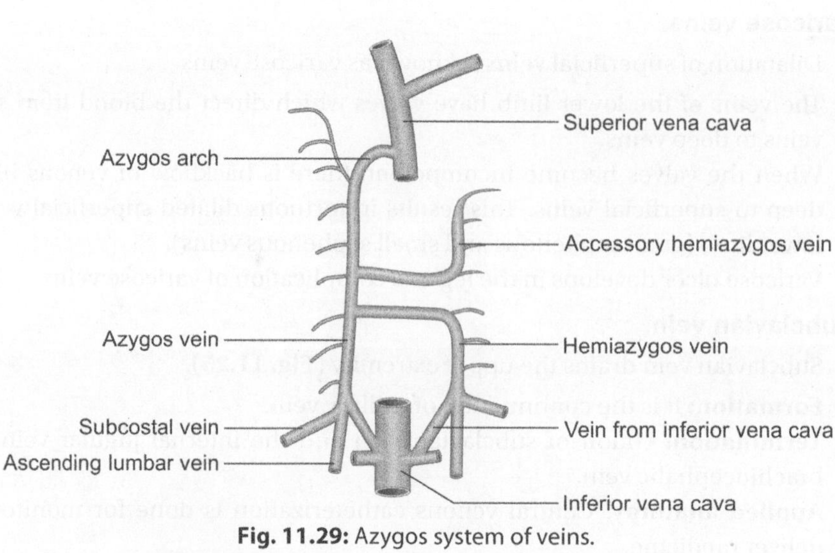

Fig. 11.29: Azygos system of veins.

Applied anatomy: In case of superior vena caval obstruction, azygos and hemiazygos veins form the collateral channel with the inferior vena cava.

57. Name the arteries supplying cerebrum.

Ans. Main arterial supply for cerebrum is from internal carotid and basilar arteries **(Figs. 11.15 and 11.30)**.

- Anterior cerebral artery—branch of internal carotid artery.
- Middle cerebral artery—branch of internal carotid artery.
- Posterior cerebral artery—branch of basilar artery.

Area of distribution:

- Superolateral surface—by middle cerebral artery, and partly by anterior cerebral.
- Medial surface—by anterior cerebral artery, partly by posterior cerebral.
- Inferior surface—by posterior cerebral artery, partly by anterior cerebral.

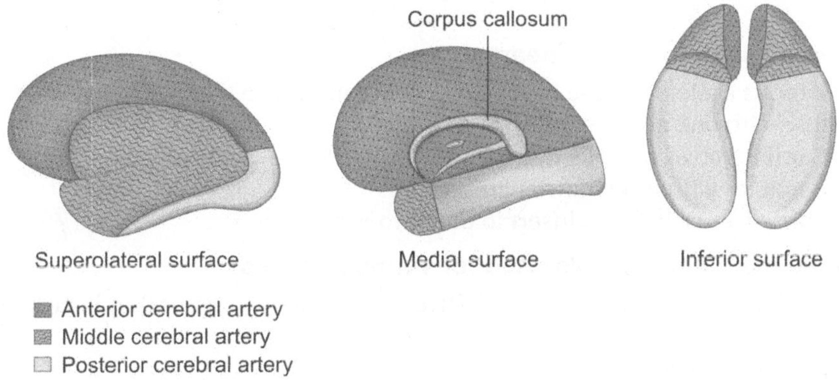

Fig. 11.30: Arterial supply of cerebrum and area of distribution.

58. Conducting system of heart.

Ans. Conducting system of heart consists of sinoatrial node, atrial muscle fibers, atrioventricular node, atrioventricular bundle of His, right and left bundle branches and the Purkinje fibers **(Fig. 11.31)**.

- **Sinoatrial node (SA node)** is situated in the right atrial wall to the right of the superior vena caval opening.
- The **atrioventricular node (AV node)** is located anterior to the opening of coronary sinus.
- **Atrioventricular bundle (of His)** begins at the AV node and passes through the interventricular septum. It gives off right and left bundle branches.
- **Purkinje fibers** form the subendocardial plexus.

59. Name the lymphoid organs of the body.

Ans.
- Primary lymphoid organs are bone marrow and thymus.
- Secondary lymphoid organs are lymph node, spleen and palatine tonsil. These organs are covered by capsule.
- Mucosa-associated lymphatic tissue (MALT): Lymphatic nodules (follicles) which are not covered by capsule is present in the mucosa of gastrointestinal, urinary, reproductive and respiratory systems. They are seen in the lamina propria of the mucosa.

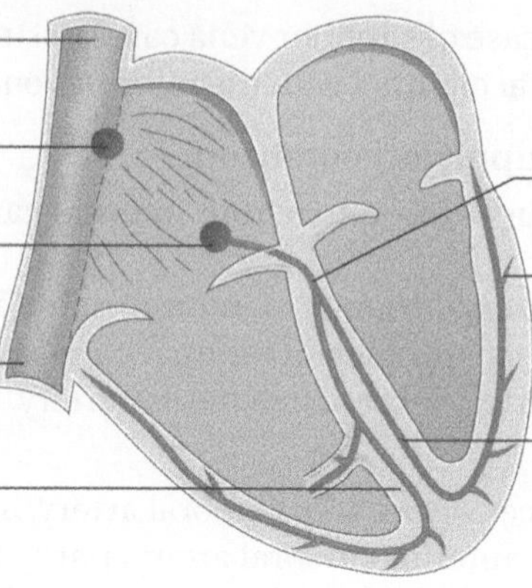

Fig. 11.31: Conducting system of heart.

60. Fibrous skeleton of the heart.

Ans.
- Fibrous skeleton of the heart consists of four dense connective tissue rings, which fuse with one another.
- Cardiac valves are attached to it.
- It merges with interventricular septum.
- Cardiac muscle fibers insert to the fibrous skeleton.

61. Name the blood vessels used for venous access.

Ans. The following blood vessels are preferred for venous access, as they have larger lumen:
- Internal jugular vein
- Subclavian vein
- Axillary vein
- Femoral vein.

62. Differentiate capillaries and sinusoids.

Ans. **Capillaries:** These are minute blood vessels with a single layer of endothelial cells lining. They allow for exchange of substances (nutrition, O_2, waste products).

Sinusoids: It is a type of capillary, but are irregular, have large pores between the cells. They connect arterioles with venules, e.g., liver, spleen, bone marrow, etc.

Notes:
- Heart is the first organ to start functioning in a fetus.
- Cardiology—scientific study of heart and associated diseases.
- Inflammation can affect any of the layers of heart—pericarditis, myocarditis or endocarditis.
- Wall of the left ventricle is thick since it has to pump blood to whole body.
- Coronary artery disease (CAD)—occurs due to deposition of atherosclerotic plaques in the coronary blood vessels.
- Artificial pacemaker—it is a mechanical device inserted in the body which helps to regulate the beating of heart if SA node is damaged/diseased.
- Valve replacement—can be done in severe cases of valvular stenosis/insufficiency.

12
CHAPTER

Respiratory System

LONG ESSAYS — 10 MARKS

1. Enumerate the parts of respiratory system and write in detail about the lung.

Ans. Parts of respiratory system **(Fig. 12.1).**

Respiratory system is divided into upper and lower respiratory tracts.

The **upper respiratory tract** includes the external nose, nasal cavity, pharynx and larynx.

The **lower respiratory tract** includes the trachea, bronchial tree and lungs.

(*Note:* Larynx belongs to both upper- and lower respiratory passages. Above vocal folds it is upper respiratory tract and, below it is lower respiratory tract).

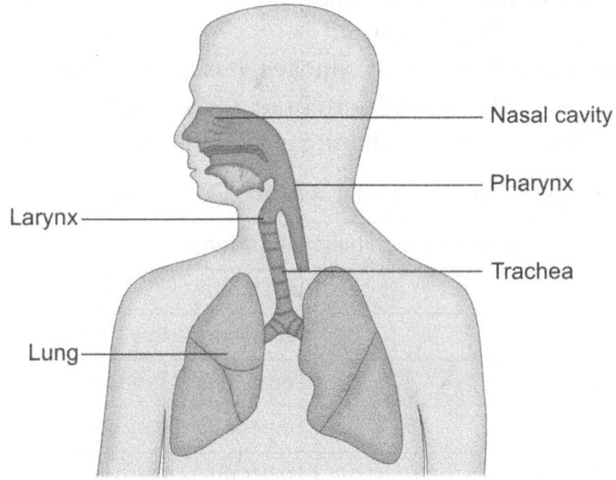

Fig. 12.1: Organs of respiration.

Lungs:

Lungs are the principal organs of respiration situated in the thoracic cavity. Each lung has:

- An apex that extends 2.5 cm above the clavicle.
- A base which rests on the diaphragm.
- Lobes: Right lung has three lobes and left lung has two lobes.
- Three surfaces: Costal, medial, and inferior surfaces.
- Three borders: Anterior, posterior and inferior borders.

Fissures of the lung: *Refer* **Figure 12.2**

- Right lung is divided into three lobes by two fissures: Horizontal and oblique.
- Left lung is divided into two lobes by an oblique fissure.

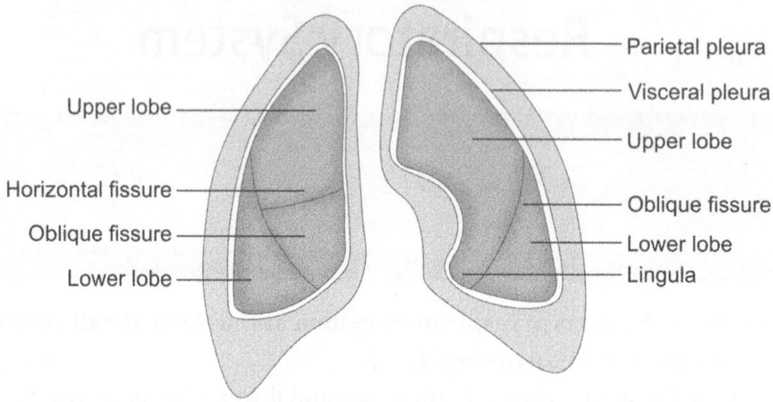

Fig. 12.2: Pleura and lung.

Relations of the lung: *Refer* **Figures 12.3 and 12.4**

- Costal surface: It is related to the costal pleura which covers the thoracic wall. The posterior part of the costal surface is related to thoracic vertebrae.
- Inferior surface or the diaphragmatic surface is concave and forms the base of the lung. It rests on the diaphragm.
- Medial surface (mediastinal) is concave. It is related to the heart and pericardium. Posteriorly, it is related to the vertebrae. Right lung is also related to the superior vena cava and azygos arch. Left lung is related to the arch of aorta.

Hilum of the lungs: *Refer* Table 12.1, Figures 12.3 and 12.4

Table 12.1: Structures passing through hilum of the lungs.

Right lung	Left lung
Eparterial bronchus	Pulmonary artery
Pulmonary artery	Left principal bronchus
Hyparterial bronchus	Upper pulmonary vein
Upper pulmonary vein	Lower pulmonary vein
Lower pulmonary vein	Bronchial arteries
Bronchial arteries	Pulmomary plexus of nerves
Pulmonary plexus of nerves	

Blood supply:

- Pulmonary artery: It carries deoxygenated blood from right ventricle to lung for oxygenation.
- Pulmonary veins: Two veins arise from each lung which carries oxygenated blood from lung to left atrium.

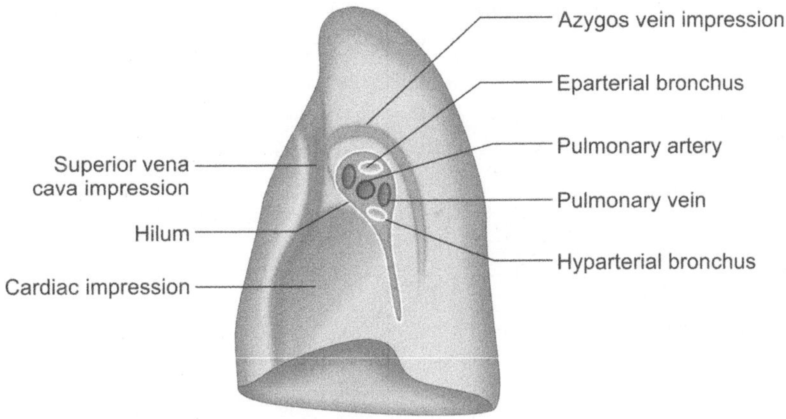

Fig. 12.3: Medial surface of right lung.

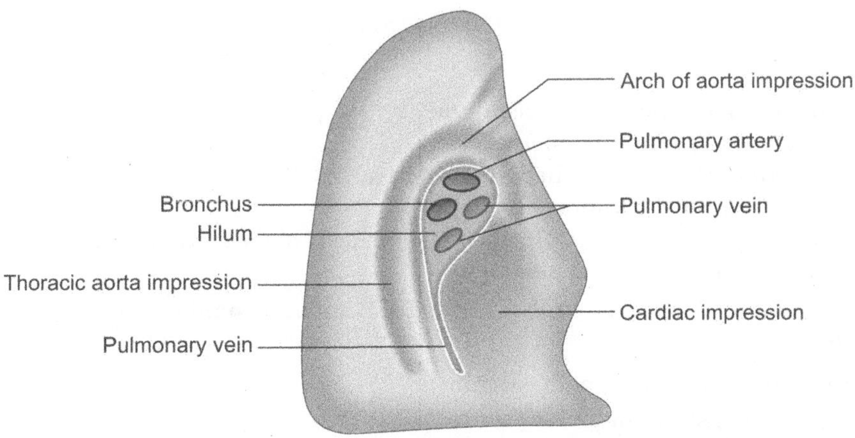

Fig. 12.4: Medial surface of right lung.

- Bronchial artery and vein: Bronchial arteries arise from descending thoracic aorta. Bronchial veins drain into azygos vein on the right side and hemiazygos vein on the left side.

Nerve supply:

- Sympathetic innervation is from second to fifth thoracic spinal segments.
- Parasympathetic innervation is from vagus nerves.

SHORT ESSAYS 5 MARKS

2. Boundaries and subdivisions of mediastinum.

Ans. *Refer* **Figure 12.5**.

The space between the right and left pleural sacs is called the mediastinum.

Subdivisions:

Superior mediastinum and inferior mediastinum by an imaginary line drawn at the level of the sternal angle. The line passes through the 4th thoracic vertebra.

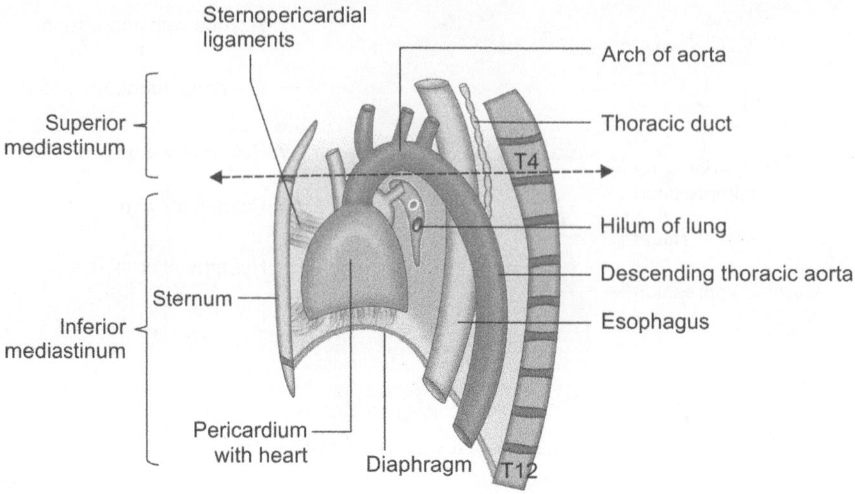

Fig. 12.5: Mediastinum.

Boundaries of superior mediastinum:

- *Anteriorly:* Manubrium sterni
- *Posteriorly:* Upper four thoracic vertebrae
- *Superiorly:* Inlet of thorax
- *Inferiorly:* An imaginary line drawn at the level of the sternal angle
- *Laterally:* Right and left pleural sacs

Inferior mediastinum is further divided into anterior, middle and posterior mediastinum.

Boundaries of inferior mediastinum:

- *Anteriorly:* Sternum
- *Posteriorly:* Lower eight thoracic vertebrae
- *Superiorly:* An imaginary line drawn at the level of the sternal angle
- *Inferiorly:* Diaphragm
- *Laterally:* Right and left pleural sacs

Anterior mediastinum

Boundaries:

- *Anteriorly:* Sternum
- *Posteriorly:* Middle mediastinum
- *Superiorly:* Superior mediastinum
- *Inferiorly:* Diaphragm
- *Laterally:* Right and left pleural sacs

Contents: Sternopericardial ligaments, few lymph nodes and branches of internal thoracic artery

Middle mediastinum: *Refer Q. No. 3, Short Essays*
Posterior mediastinum: *Refer Q. No. 4, Short Essays*

3. Boundaries and contents of middle mediastinum.

Ans. *Refer* **Figure 12.5.**

Boundaries:

- *Anteriorly:* Anterior mediastinum
- *Posteriorly:* Posterior mediastinum
- *Superiorly:* Superior mediastinum
- *Inferiorly:* Diaphragm
- *Laterally:* Right and left pleural sacs

Contents:

- Heart and pericardium
- Ascending aorta
- Bifurcation of trachea
- Pulmonary trunk and pulmonary veins

4. Boundaries and contents of posterior mediastinum.

Ans. *Refer* **Figure 12.5**

Boundaries:

- *Anteriorly:* Middle mediastinum
- *Posteriorly:* Lower eight thoracic vertebrae
- *Superiorly:* superior mediastinum
- *Inferiorly:* Diaphragm
- *Laterally:* Right and left pleural sacs

Contents:

- Esophagus
- Thoracic duct
- Descending thoracic aorta
- Azygos and hemiazygos veins

5. Boundaries and contents of superior mediastinum.

Ans. *Refer* **Figure 12.5**

Boundaries:

- *Anteriorly:* Manubrium sterni
- *Posteriorly:* Upper four thoracic vertebrae
- *Superiorly:* Inlet of thorax
- *Inferiorly:* An imaginary line drawn at the level of the sternal angle
- *Laterally:* Right and left pleural sacs

Contents:

- Trachea
- Esophagus
- Thymus
- Arch of aorta and its branches: Brachiocephalic, left subclavian and left common carotid arteries.

6. Pleura.

Ans. *Refer* **Figure 12.6**

Pleura is a *closed serous sac* formed by two layers.

1. The **outer parietal layer** lines the wall of thoracic cavity. It is further divided into:
   a. Diaphragmatic pleura
   b. Costal pleura

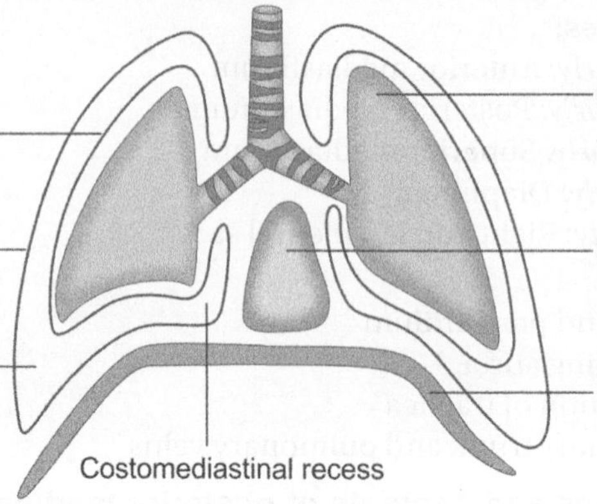

Fig. 12.6: Pleural recesses.

c. Mediastinal pleura
d. Cervical pleura

- The **inner visceral layer** lines the lung.
- Pleural cavity is a *potential space* between the two layers and is filled with thin layer of lymph-like fluid. This fluid lubricates and reduces friction during the movements of respiration.

Blood supply and nerve supply of pleura: *Refer* **Table 12.2.**

Table 12.2: Blood and nerve supply of pleura.

	Arterial supply	Venous drainage	Nerve supply
Parietal pleura	• Intercostal arteries • Internal thoracic arteries • Musculophrenic arteries	• Intercostal veins • Internal thoracic veins • Musculophrenic veins • Azygos vein	• Intercostal nerves • Phrenic nerves – Sensitive to pain
Visceral pleura	Bronchial arteries	Bronchial veins	Autonomic nerves • Insensitive to pain

Applied anatomy:

- Pleuritis—inflammation of pleura.
- Pleural effusion—collection of fluid in the pleural cavity.
- Pneumothorax—collection of air in pleural cavity.
- Hemothorax—collection of blood in pleural cavity.
- Hydropneumothorax—collection of fluid and air in the pleural cavity.
- Paracentesis thoracis: Aspiration of fluid from the pleural cavity which is usually done in the 6th intercostal space in the midaxillary line to avoid injury to the lung.

7. Pleural recesses.

Ans. *Refer* **Figure 12.6.**

Pleural recesses are spaces present in the pleural cavity. These recesses act a reserve space for the lung to expand during respiration. The two pleural recesses are costodiaphragmatic and costomediastinal recesses.

- Costodiaphragmatic recess is situated between the costal and diaphragmatic pleurae inferiorly along the midaxillary line. It extends from 8th to 10th ribs.

- Costomediastinal recess lies posterior to sternum and costal cartilages between the costal and mediastinal pleurae.

Applied anatomy: Paracentesis thoracis—aspiration of fluid from the pleural cavity which is usually done in the 6th intercostal space in the midaxillary line to avoid injury to the lung.

8. Bronchopulmonary segments.

Ans. *Refer* **Table 12.3 and Figures 12. 7 to 12.10.**

Bronchus and its divisions are accompanied by the pulmonary artery and its branches.

Each bronchus divides continuously into primary, secondary and tertiary (or segmental) bronchi. Each division of bronchi is accompanied by divisions of pulmonary artery.

Definition: Each segmental bronchus along with a branch of pulmonary artery supplies a definite segment of the lung and is called as *bronchopulmonary segment.*

- The segments are pyramidal in shape
- It has a segmental bronchus and segmental artery
- The pulmonary veins are intersegmental
- Each lung has 10 bronchopulmonary segments.

Applied anatomy:

- Infections are confined to the segments. In tuberculosis and malignancy, it can spread to other segments.
- Segmental resection: In lung disease, a segment could be resected by surgery (segmentectomy).

Table 12.3: Bronchopulmonary segments of right and left lungs.

Right lung		Left lung	
Upper lobe	• Apical • Anterior • posterior	**Upper lobe**	• Apical • Anterior • Posterior
Middle lobe	• Medial • Lateral	**Lingula**	• Superior lingular • Inferior lingular
Lower lobe	• Apical • Anterior basal • Posterior basal • Medial basal • Lateral basal	**Lower lobe**	• Apical • Anterior basal • Posterior basal • Medial basal • Lateral basal

9. Paranasal sinuses.

Ans. *Refer* **Figures 12.11 and 12.12.**

Paranasal air sinuses are air-filled cavities in the skull bones. There are four air sinuses:

1. Frontal air sinus
2. Ethmoidal air sinus
3. Sphenoidal air sinus
4. Maxillary air sinus.

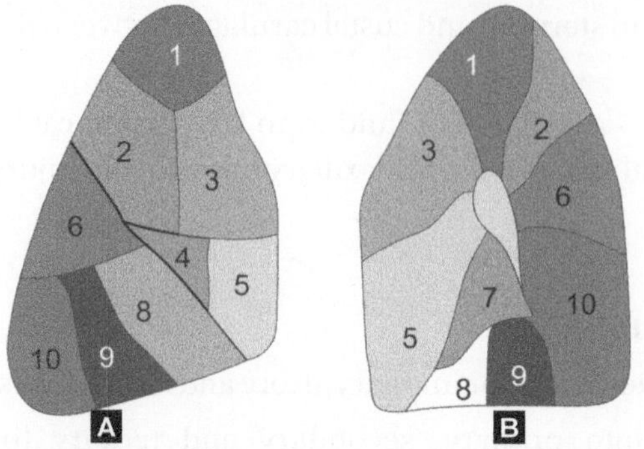

Figs. 12.7A and B: Bronchopulmonary segments—right lung. (A) Costal surface; (B) Mediastinal surface.

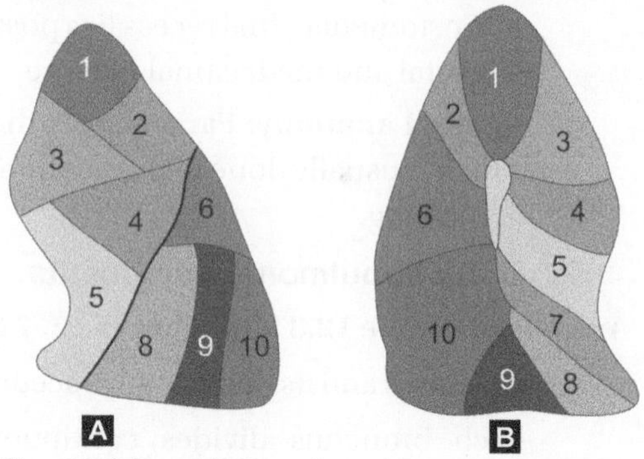

Figs. 12.8A and B: Bronchopulmonary segments—left lung. (A) Costal surface; (B) Mediastinal surface.

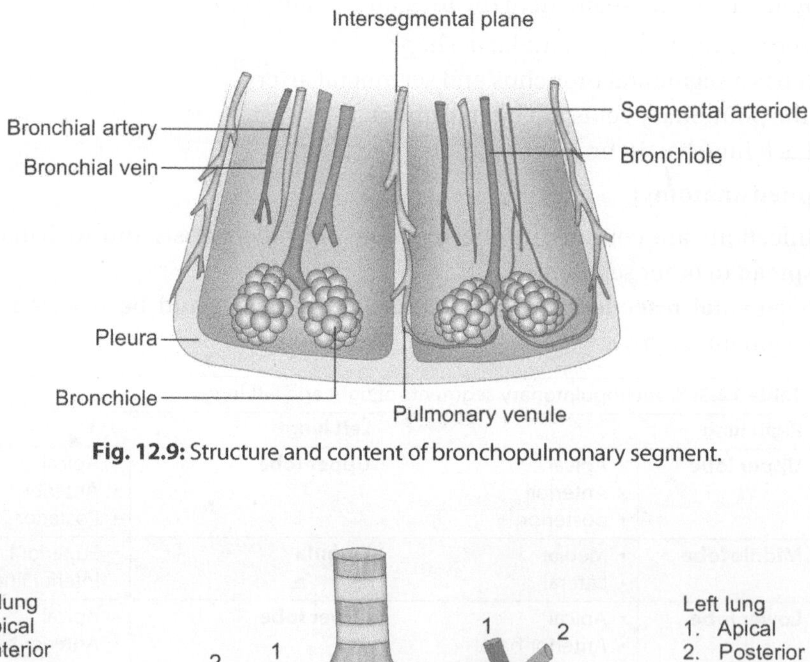

Fig. 12.9: Structure and content of bronchopulmonary segment.

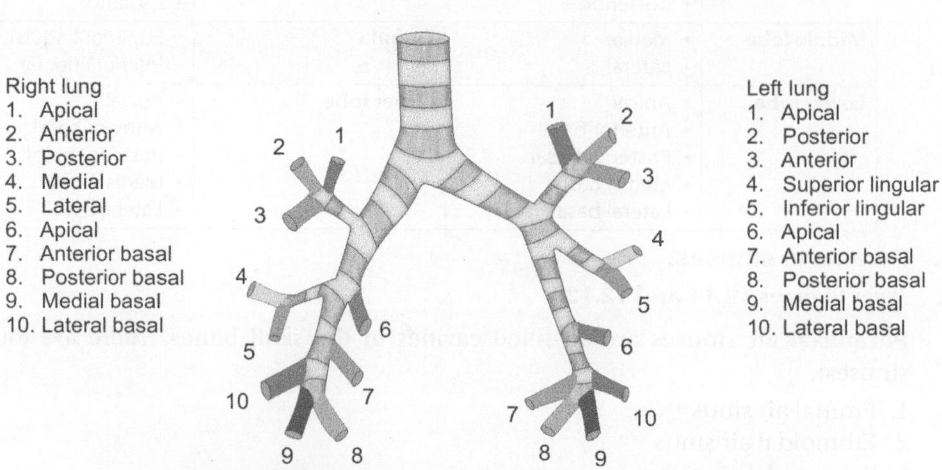

Fig. 12.10: Tracheobronchial tree supplying the bronchopulmonary segments.

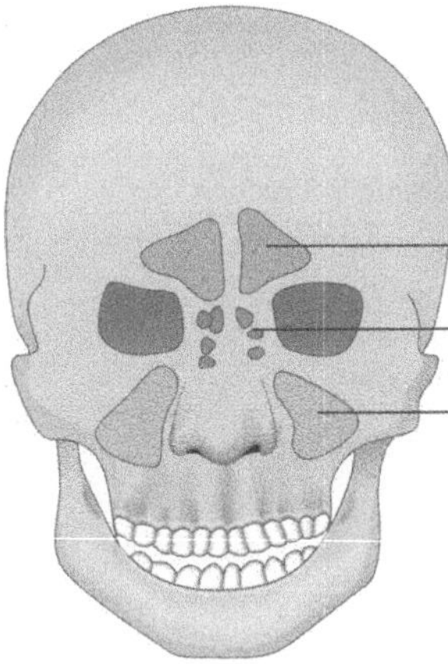

Fig. 12.11: Paranasal sinuses—frontal view.

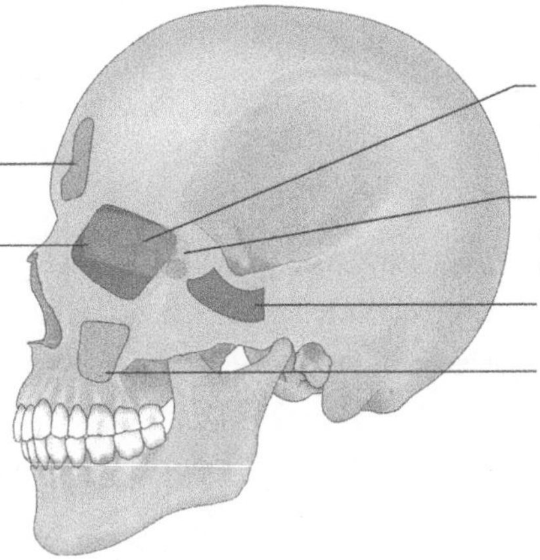

Fig. 12.12: Paranasal sinuses—lateral view.

The air sinuses are lined by mucous membrane. They drain into the lateral wall of nasal cavities which are as follows **(Fig. 12.13)**.

- Superior meatus—posterior ethmoidal air sinus.
- Middle meatus—frontal air sinus, maxillary sinus, anterior and middle ethmoidal air sinuses.
- Sphenoethmoidal recess—sphenoidal air sinus.

Functions of air sinuses:

- To add resonance to the voice
- To lighten the weight of the skull
- Convert the inspired air to optimum temperature and humidity for respiration.

Applied anatomy: Sinusitis—inflammation of sinuses is sinusitis. It leads to pain over the sinus and headache.

10. Lateral wall of nasal cavity.

Ans. Lateral wall of nasal cavity is divided into three parts **(Figs. 12.13 and 12.14):**

- Vestibule: Dilated anterior part which is lined by skin with hair follicles
- Respiratory part: Lower 2/3rd of the nasal cavity
- Olfactory part: Upper 1/3rd of the nasal cavity.

Lateral wall consists of three shelf-like projections called concha. The space below each concha is called meatus.

- Superior, middle and inferior conchae
- Sphenoethmoidal recess: Present above the superior concha. Sphenoidal air sinus opens into it.
- Superior meatus:
  - Between the superior and middle concha.
  - Posterior ethmoidal air sinus opens into it.
- Middle meatus:
  - Space between the middle and inferior conchae.
  - Bulla ethmoidalis: It is a spherical bulge into which middle ethmoidal sinus opens.

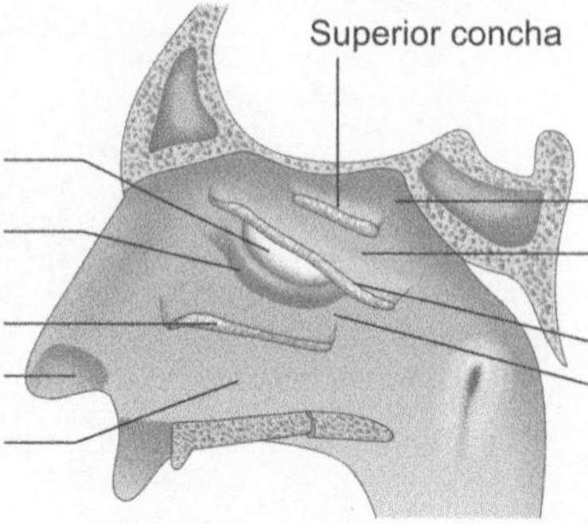

Fig. 12.13: Lateral wall of nasal cavity.

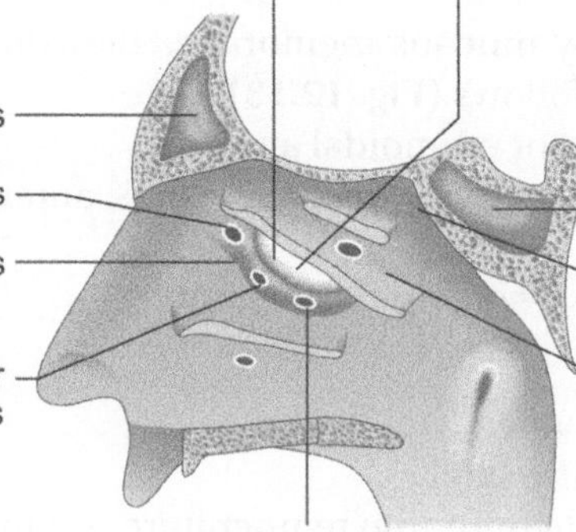

Fig. 12.14: Structures opening into lateral wall of nasal cavity.

- Hiatus semilunaris: Cleft present below the bulla ethmoidalis. Frontal air sinus, anterior ethmoidal air sinus and maxillary air sinus opens here.

- Inferior meatus:
  - Space below the inferior concha
  - Nasolacrimal duct opens into it

11. Blood supply and nerve supply of lateral wall of nasal cavity.

Ans. *Refer* **Table 12.4** and **Figures 12.15 and 12.16.**

Table 12.4: Lateral wall of nasal cavity: Blood supply and nerve supply.

Arterial supply	Venous drainage	Nerve supply
• Sphenopalatine artery • Greater palatine artery • Anterior ethmoidal artery • Lateral nasal branch of facial artery	• Facial vein • Pterygoid venous plexus • Pharyngeal venous plexus	• Anterior ethmoidal branch (ophthalmic nerve) • Anterior superior alveolar nerve (infraorbital nerve) • Posterior superior and inferior lateral nasal nerves • Internal nasal branch of infraorbital nerve

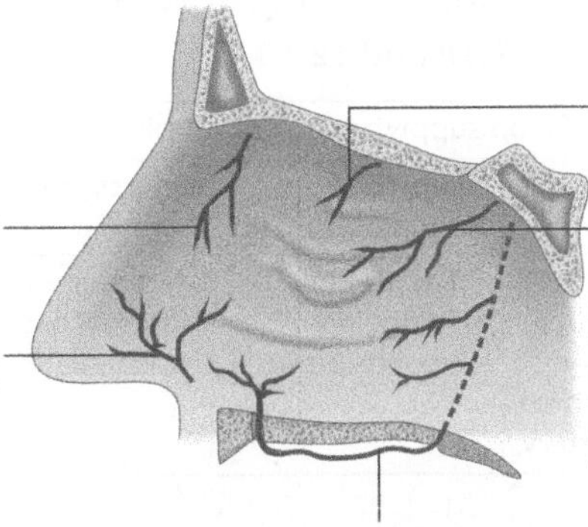

Fig. 12.15: Lateral wall of nasal cavity—arterial supply.

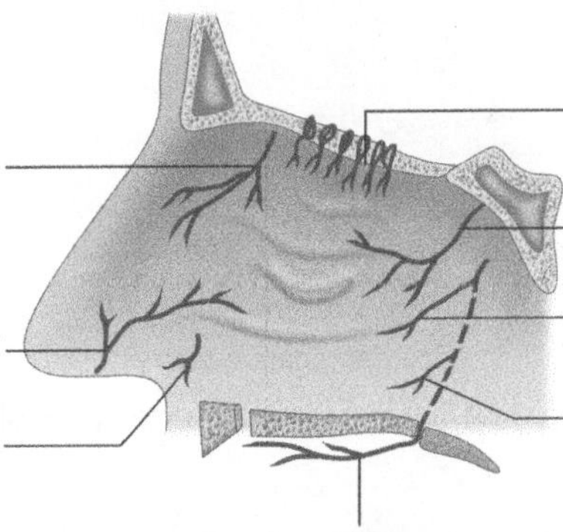

Fig. 12.16: Lateral wall of nasal cavity—nerve supply.

12. Nasal septum (medial wall of nasal cavity).

Ans. *Refer* **Figure 12.17**

- Nasal septum is formed by bone and cartilage.
- Bony part: Posterior part formed by ethmoid bone and vomer.
- Cartilaginous part is formed by septal cartilage, greater alar cartilage and lesser alar cartilages.
- In the anteroinferior part of nasal septum the branches from sphenopalatine, greater palatine, facial and anterior ethmoidal arteries form arterial plexus called Kiesselbach's plexus. This area is called the Little's area and is a common site of bleeding from nose/ epistaxis.

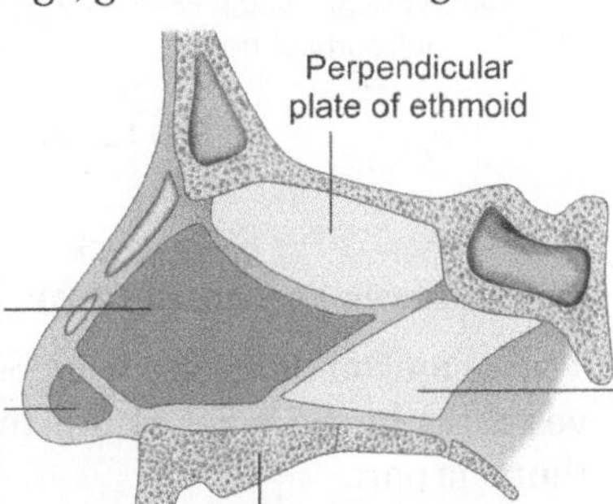

Fig. 12.17: Nasal septum (medial wall of nasal cavity).

13. Blood supply and nerve supply of nasal septum.

Ans. *Refer* **Table 12.5, Figures 12.18 and 12.19.**

Table 12.5: Nasal septum: Blood supply and nerve supply.

Arterial supply	Venous drainage	Nerve supply
• Sphenopalatine artery • Greater palatine artery • Anterior ethmoidal artery • Superior labial branch of septal branch of facial artery	• Facial vein • Pterygoid venous plexus	• Anterior ethmoidal branch (ophthalmic nerve) • Internal nasal branch of intraorbital nerve • Nasopalatine nerve

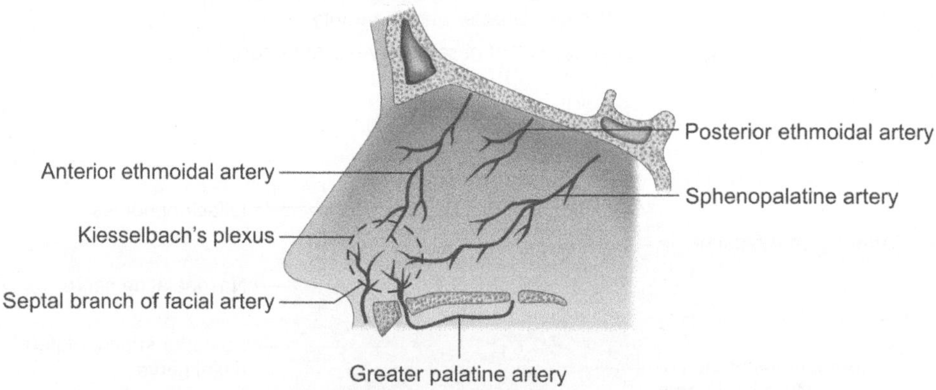

Fig. 12.18: Nasal septum—arterial supply.

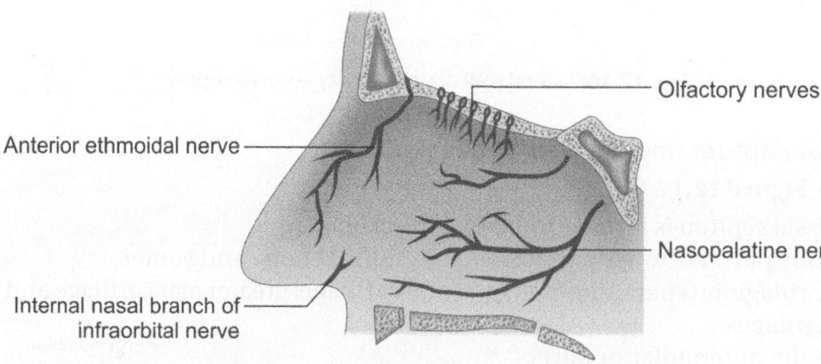

Fig. 12.19: Nasal septum—nerve supply.

14. Trachea.

Ans. *Refer* **Figures 12.20 and 12.21.**

Trachea extends from lower border of cricoid cartilage (at the level of 6th cervical vertebra) to the level of 5th thoracic vertebra. It is divided into cervical part and thoracic part.

- Length of the trachea is about 12 cm.

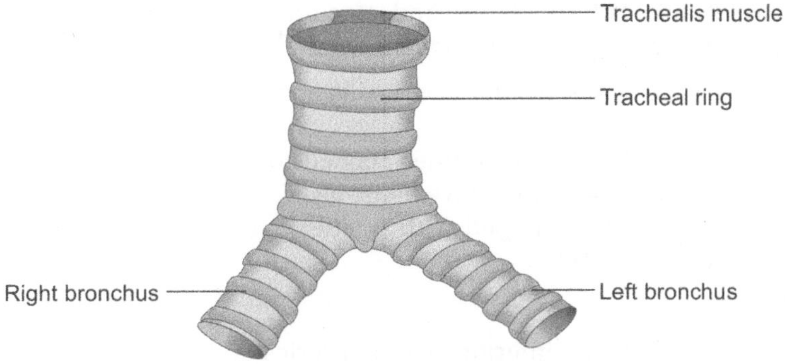

Fig. 12.20: Trachea.

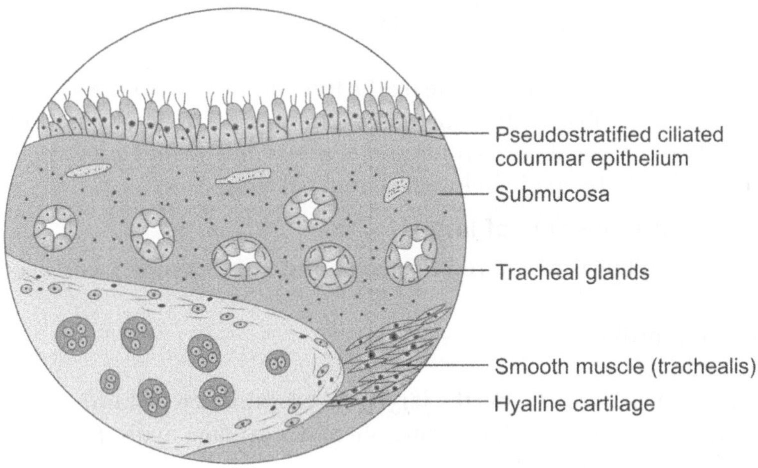

Fig. 12.21: Histology of trachea.

- It divides into left and right primary bronchi.
  - Right primary bronchi divide into three secondary bronchi for the three lobes.
  - Left primary bronchi divide into two secondary bronchi for its two lobes.
- The secondary bronchi divide further into 10 segmental bronchi or the tertiary bronchi on either side.

Relations:

Cervical part:

- Anterior: Isthmus of thyroid gland on 2nd, 3rd and 4th tracheal rings, brachiocephalic artery
- Posterior: Esophagus
- Laterally: Lobes of thyroid gland and common carotid arteries.

Thoracic part:

- Anterior: Sternum, thymus, arch of aorta
- Posterior: Esophagus

- On the left side: Left subclavian and left common carotid arteries.
- On the right side: Arch of azygos vein.

Histology: Trachea consists of mucosa, submucosa, cartilage rings and outer fibrous layer.

- Mucosa is lined by pseudostratified ciliated columnar epithelium with goblet cells.
- Submucosa is a loose connective tissue layer.
- Cartilage rings are C-shaped with trachealis muscles between two ends of the cartilage **(Fig. 12.21)**.

Blood supply:

Arterial supply is by the inferior thyroid arteries and the venous drainage is by the inferior thyroid veins.

Applied anatomy:

- Foreign bodies usually get lodged in right bronchus because it is wider and straight in line with trachea.
- Tracheostomy: Incision is made on the trachea and a tracheostomy tube is inserted to relieve any obstruction to the respiratory tract. Strap muscles of the neck (sternohyoid and sternothyroid) and isthmus of thyroid gland are divided and the incision should be made below 2nd tracheal ring.

15. Cartilages and muscles of larynx.

Ans. Larynx is formed by three paired cartilages and three unpaired cartilages **(Figs. 12.22 and 12.23)**.

- Unpaired cartilages:
  - Epiglottis
  - Thyroid cartilage forms the laryngeal prominence (Adam's apple).
  - Cricoid cartilage: Signet ring-shaped cartilage with posterior lamina and anterior narrow arch.

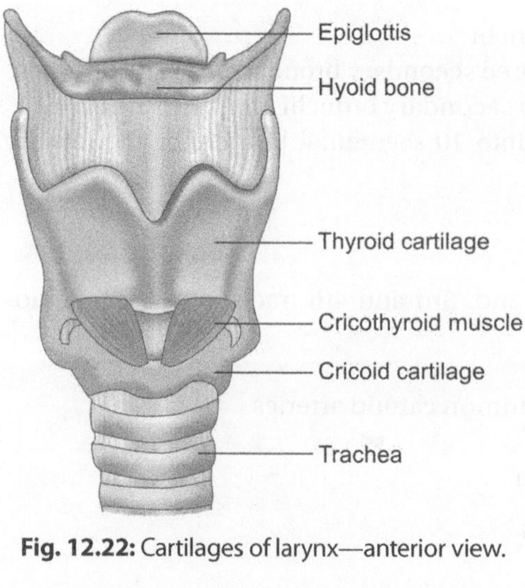

Fig. 12.22: Cartilages of larynx—anterior view.

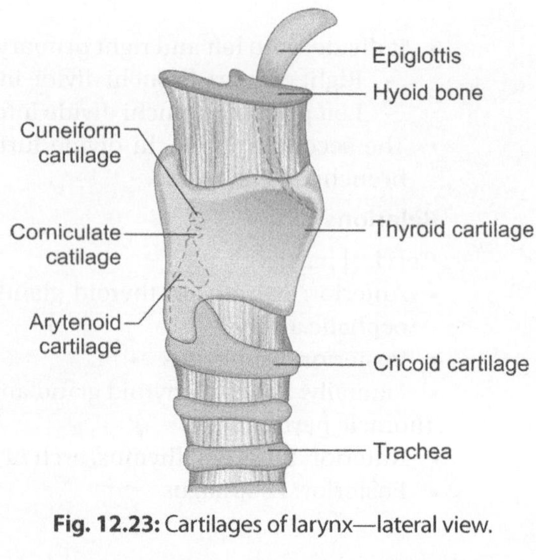

Fig. 12.23: Cartilages of larynx—lateral view.

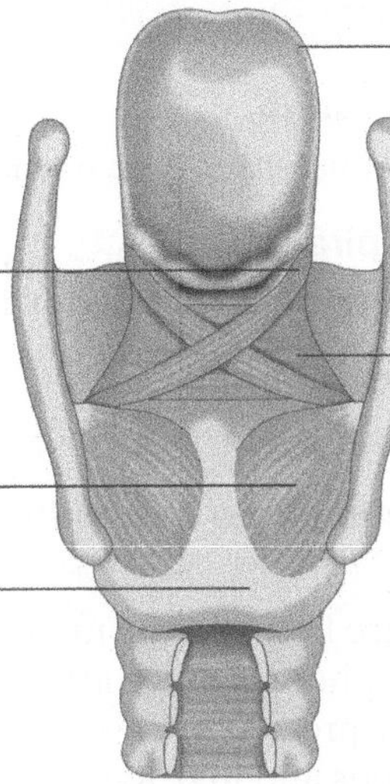

Fig. 12.24: Muscles of larynx—posterior view.

- Paired cartilages:
  - Arytenoid, corniculate and cuneiform.

Based on the type of cartilage, they are as follows:

- Elastic cartilages: Epiglottis, arytenoid, corniculate and cuneiform.
- Hyaline cartilage: Thyroid, cricoid.

Muscle of the larynx: *Refer* **Table 12.6 and Figures 12.22 and 12.24.**

Nerve supply to muscles: It is by external and recurrent laryngeal nerves.

Applied anatomy:

Vocal cord paralysis: Injury to recurrent laryngeal nerve results in paralysis of muscles of larynx. This results in hoarseness of voice. If both vocal cords involved, it leads to breathing difficulty.

Table 12.6: Muscles of larynx.

Intrinsic muscles of larynx	Action	Nerve supply
Cricothyroid	Tensor of vocal cord	Cricothyroid by external laryngeal nerve. All the other muscles are supplied recurrent laryngeal nerve
Thyroarytenoid	Relaxes of vocal cord	
Posterior cricoarytenoid	Abduction of vocal cord	
Lateral cricoarytenoid	Adduction of vocal cord	
Transverse arytenoid	Brings the arytenoids cartilage closer	
Oblique arytenoid	Brings the arytenoids cartilage closer	
Aryepiglotticus	Closes the inlet of larynx	
Thyroepiglotticus	Opens the inlet of larynx	
Vocalis	Differential tension of vocal cord	
Posterior cricoarytenoid is the safety muscle of the larynx, as it is the only abductor of larynx.		

SHORT ANSWERS 2 MARKS

16. Name the organs of respiration.

Ans. Nasal cavity, nasopharynx, oropharynx, larynx, trachea, bronchial tree and lungs (**Fig. 12.1**).

17. Name the muscles of respiration.

Ans. Diaphragm, external intercostal muscles, internal intercostal muscles, scalene muscles.

18. Contents of superior mediastinum.

Ans. *Refer Q. No. 5, Short Essays*

19. Name the structures opening into the middle meatus.

Ans. *Refer* **Figure 12.14.**

- Middle meatus is the space between the middle and inferior conchae.
- Bulla ethmoidalis: It is a spherical bulge into which middle ethmoidal sinus opens.
- Hiatus semilunaris: Cleft present below the bulla ethmoidalis. Frontal air sinus, anterior ethmoidal air sinus and maxillary air sinus opens here.

20. Name the structures present in the hilum of the right lung.

Ans. *Refer* **Figure 12.3.**

- Eparterial and hyparterial bronchi are situated posteriorly.
- Pulmonary artery is present in front and between the two bronchi.
- Upper pulmonary vein is seen anteriorly and lower pulmonary vein is seen inferiorly.
- Bronchial arteries are situated posterior to the bronchi.

21. Interior of larynx.

Ans. *Refer* **Figure 12.25.**

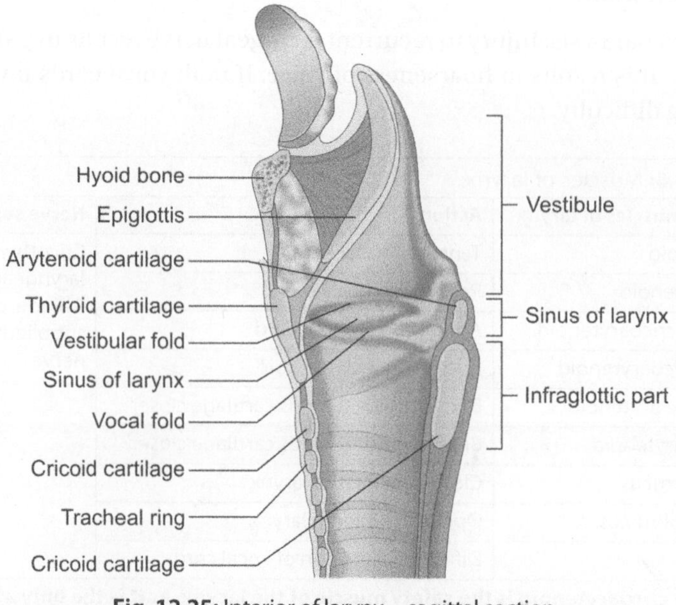

Fig. 12.25: Interior of larynx—sagittal section.

The cavity of larynx extends from laryngeal inlet to trachea. It has three parts.

1. **Vestibule:** Between the laryngeal inlet and vestibular folds.
2. **Sinus of larynx**: Between the vestibular and vocal folds. It has a saccule with mucous secreting glands which lubricates the vocal cords during speech.
3. **Infraglottic part:** Below the vocal folds. It is continuous with the trachea.

22. Vocal cords/folds.

Ans. *Refer* **Figure 12.25**.

- Cricovocal membrane or conus elasticus is a membrane present in the larynx. The lower border of the membrane is attached to the cricoid cartilage.
- The upper border is free and stretches between the arytenoid and thyroid cartilage. The **free border** is **thickened to form vocal ligament**. It is covered by mucous membrane to form the vocal folds.
- Vocal fold is lined by stratified squamous epithelium and is lubricated by mucus glands in the saccule of larynx.
- The space between the vocal folds is Rima glottidis.
- Vocal fold is responsible for sound production. It vibrates as expired air passes through narrowed glottis.

23. Name the paranasal air sinuses.

Ans. The paranasal air sinuses are:

- Frontal air sinus
- Maxillary sinus
- Ethmoidal air sinuses
- Sphenoidal sinus

24. Name the parts of pharynx.

Ans. The pharynx consists of three parts:

1. Nasopharynx.
2. Oropharynx.
3. Laryngopharynx

25. Name the cartilages of larynx.

Ans.

- Unpaired cartilages:
  - Epiglottis
  - Thyroid cartilage
  - Cricoid cartilage
- Paired cartilages: Arytenoid, corniculate and cuneiform

26. Name the lobes and fissures of lungs.

Ans. *Refer* **Table 12.7**.

Table 12.7: Lobes and fissures of lungs.

	Right lung	Left lung
Fissures	• Oblique fissure • Horizontal fissure	Oblique fissure
Lobes	• Upper lobe • Middle lobe • Lower lobe	• Upper lobe • Lower lobe

27. Name the functional zones of the respiratory passages.

Ans. Functionally respiratory passage is divided into conducting and respiratory zone.

Conducting zone: It extends from larynx till terminal bronchiole. It filters, warms and moistens the inspired air.

Respiratory zone: Extends below the respiratory bronchiole till alveoli. These are involved in air exchange.

28. Alveoli of lungs.

Ans.
- Alveoli are the terminal air passages. They are enlarged sacs filled with air. It is lined by simple squamous epithelium and within this two types of cells have been identified.
- Type I pneumocyte—they are the principal cells responsible for air exchange.
- Type II pneumocyte—they secrete surfactant which consists of protein-lipid mixture. It maintains the surface tension within the alveoli and prevent their collapse during expiration.

Notes:
- The respiratory membrane or the air-blood barrier is 0.5 microns thick. It consists of endothelium and its basement membrane, plus type I pneumocyte with its basement membrane.
- Lungs have dual blood supply—from bronchial and pulmonary arteries.
- Medulla has the respiratory and cardiovascular center.
- Respiratory epithelium is nothing but pseudostratified ciliated columnar epithelium with goblet cells.

13
CHAPTER

Digestive System

LONG ESSAYS — 10 MARKS

1. Enumerate the organs of digestion including accessory organs of digestion. Describe in detail about stomach under the following: (a) Situation, (b) Parts, (c) Relation, (d) Blood supply, (e) Nerve supply, (f) Applied anatomy.

Ans.
- Organs of digestion: Mouth, pharynx, esophagus, stomach, small intestine and large intestine **(Fig. 13.1)**.
- Accessory organs of digestion: Salivary glands, tongue, gallbladder, liver and pancreas.

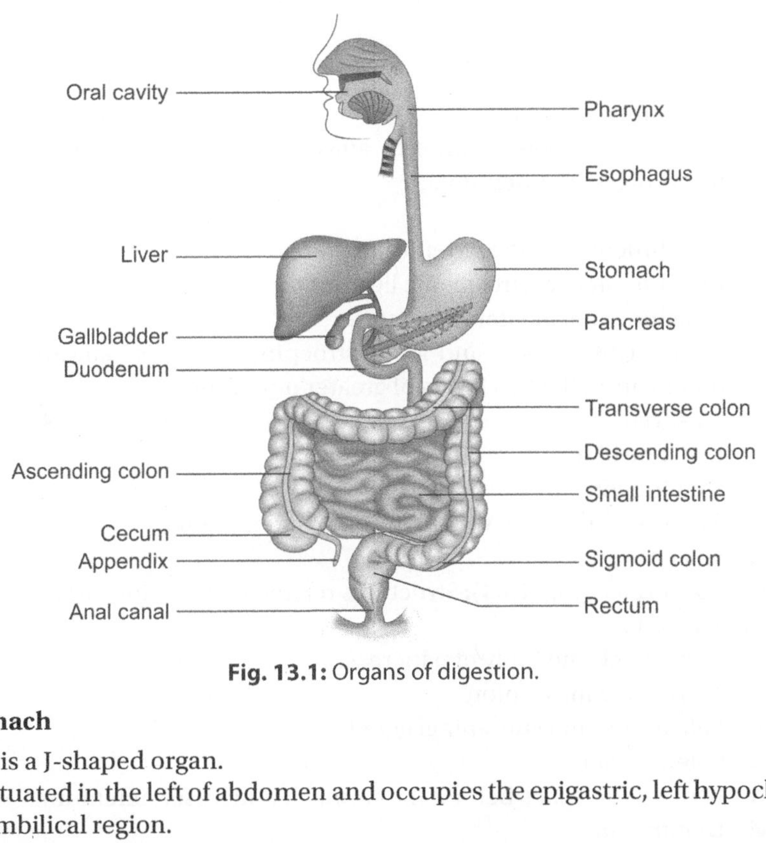

Fig. 13.1: Organs of digestion.

Stomach

- It is a J-shaped organ.
- Situated in the left of abdomen and occupies the epigastric, left hypochondriac and umbilical region.

Anatomical Parts (Fig. 13.2):

- **Fundus**: Portion above the cardiac notch.
- **Body**
- **Pylorus:** It is divided into pyloric antrum and pyloric canal.
- **Two sphincters** are cardiac and pyloric sphincters.
- **Surfaces:** Anterosuperior and posteroinferior surface.
- **Curvatures:** Lesser and greater curvature.

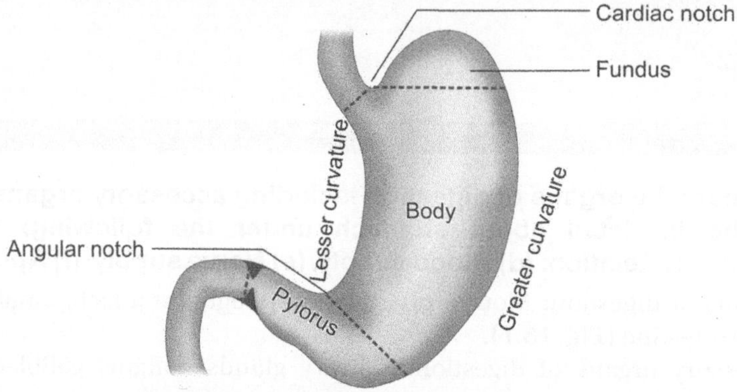

Fig. 13.2: Parts of stomach.

Relations:

- Lesser curvature:
  i. Attachment of lesser omentum.
  ii. Right and left gastric arteries anastomose with each other within the two layers of lesser omentum.
- Greater curvature:
  i. Attachment of gastrophrenic ligament.
  ii. Attachment of gastrosplenic ligament.
  iii. Attachment of greater omentum.
  iv. Right gastroepiploic and left gastroepiploic arteries anastomose with each other within the two layers of greater omentum.
- Anterior surface:
  i. Left lobe of liver.
  ii. Diaphragm.
  iii. Anterior abdominal wall between costal margins.
  iv. Spleen.
- Posterior surface **(Fig. 13.3):** Structures related to posterior surface is also called as 'stomach bed':
  i. Head, neck and body of pancreas.
  ii. Transverse mesocolon.
  iii. Left kidney and suprarenal gland.
  iv. Splenic artery
  v. Lesser sac—space behind the stomach and lesser omentum
  vi. Diaphragm

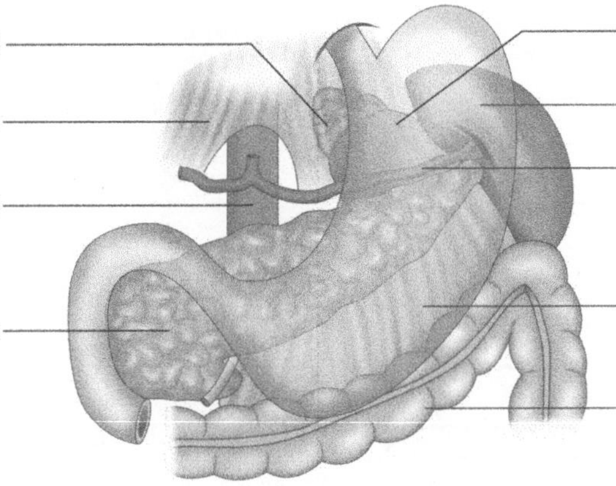

Fig. 13.3: Stomach—posterior relations (stomach bed).

Arterial supply (Fig. 13.4):

It is contributed by branches of celiac trunk: Hepatic artery, splenic artery, left gastric artery.

- Left gastric artery—branch of celiac artery
- Right gastric artery—branch of hepatic artery
- Left gastroepiploic artery—branch of splenic artery
- Right gastroepiploic artery—branch of gastroduodenal artery
- Short gastric arteries—branches of splenic artery.

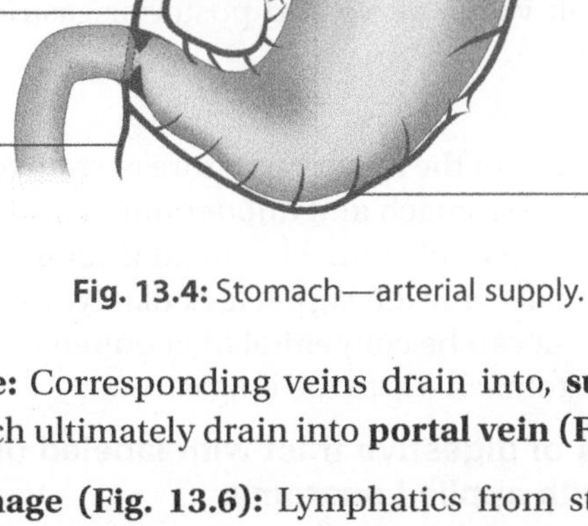

Fig. 13.4: Stomach—arterial supply.

Venous drainage: Corresponding veins drain into, **superior mesenteric vein** and **splenic vein** which ultimately drain into **portal vein (Fig. 13.5).**

Lymphatic drainage (Fig. 13.6): Lymphatics from stomach drain into left gastric nodes, pancreaticosplenic nodes, right gastroepiploic nodes, subpyloric nodes, hepatic nodes and celiac nodes.

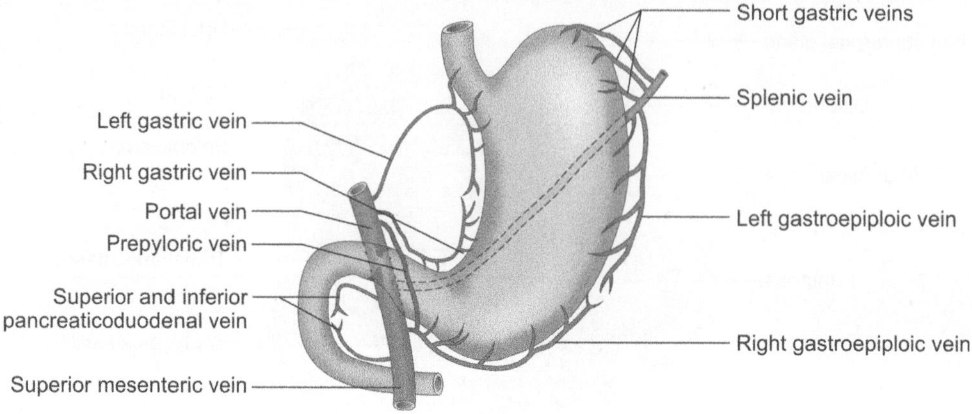

Fig. 13.5: Stomach—venous drainage.

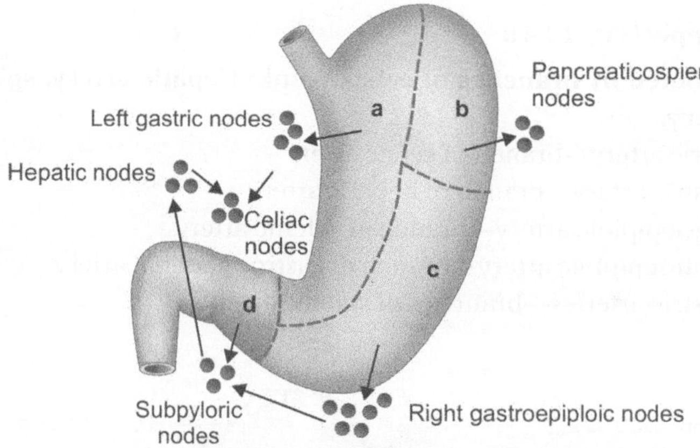

Fig. 13.6: Stomach—lymphatic drainage.

Nerve supply:
- Sympathetic nerves from T6 to T10 spinal cord segments.
- Parasympathetic innervation: Right and left vagus nerves. The anterior gastric nerves arise from left vagus nerve and posterior gastric nerves from right vagus nerve.

Applied anatomy:
- Gastric ulcer—common in the lesser curvature of stomach.
- Peptic ulcer—affect the stomach and duodenum.
- Gastric carcinoma—cancer of stomach spread through lymphatics which reaches the thoracic duct and also the left supraclavicular lymph node.
- Pyloric obstruction—it can be congenital or acquired.
- Referred pain from stomach—is to the epigastrium.

2. Enumerate the parts of digestive tract with labeled diagram. Describe about pancreas in detail with applied anatomy.

Ans. For parts of gastrointestinal tract (GIT)—*Refer Q.No. 1, Long Essays* **(Organs of Digestion and Figure 13.1).**

Pancreas

Pancreas is a *retroperitoneal organ* situated on the posterior abdominal wall in the epigastric and umbilical regions.

It extends from the C-shaped concavity of duodenum to the hilum of the spleen, horizontally across in front of the vertebral column.

Parts of the pancreas: Head, neck, body and tail **(Fig. 13.7)**.

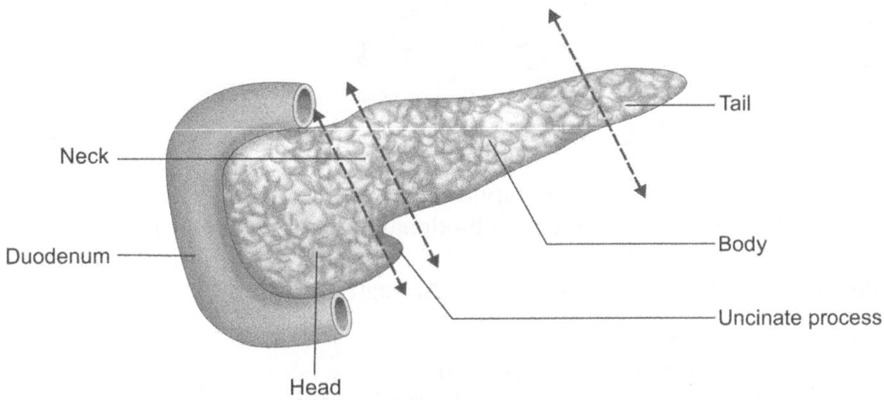

Fig. 13.7: Parts of pancreas.

Relations:

A. **Head of pancreas:**
   - Anterior surface—it is covered with peritoneum, transverse mesocolon, first part of duodenum and small intestine.
   - Posterior surface—right renal vein. inferior vena cava and the common bile duct.

B. **Neck of pancreas:**
   - Anterior surface—lesser sac.
   - Posterior surface—portal vein.

C. **Body of pancreas:**
   - Anterior surface—greater omentum, coils of small intestine.
   - Posterior surface—abdominal aorta, left kidney, left renal vein, left suprarenal gland and splenic vein.

D. **Tail of pancreas:** It is situated within the lienorenal ligament which extends between the kidney and hilum of spleen.

Ducts of pancreas (Fig. 13.8):

- Main pancreatic duct or the duct of Wirsung: It unites with common bile duct to form hepatopancreatic of **ampulla of Vater** and *opens into the second part of duodenum.*
- Accessory pancreatic duct opens 2 cm above the main duct into the duodenum.

Blood supply:

Arterial supply

- Branches of superior pancreaticoduodenal and inferior pancreaticoduodenal arteries supplies the head
- Branches from the splenic artery supplies the body and tail of pancreas.

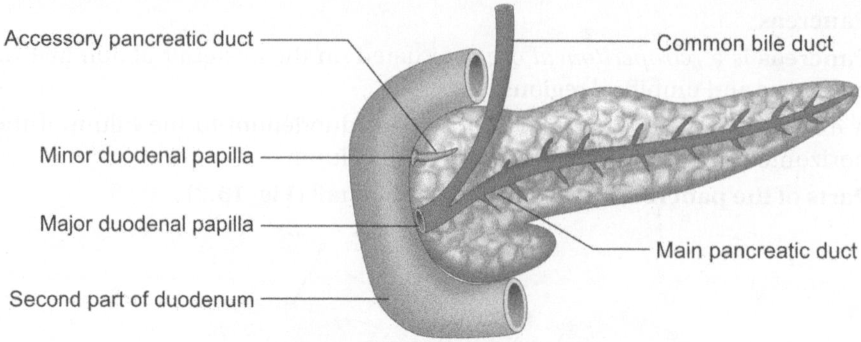

Fig. 13.8: Pancreatic ducts.

Venous drainage is by the corresponding veins.
Lymphatic drainage: Pancreaticoduodenal nodes and splenic nodes.
Nerve supply: Sympathetic innervation—from the lower thoracic spinal segments
Parasympathetic innervation: From the vagus nerves.

Applied anatomy:
- Pancreatitis: Inflammation of pancreas.
- Carcinoma of head of pancreas: The tumor may compress the common bile duct and splenic vein leading to jaundice and ascites.
- Pancreatic pain is referred to the back.

3. Describe the anatomy of the pharynx under the following headings: Subdivisions, muscles, nerve supply.

Ans. Pharynx is a muscular tube and acts as a passage for air as well as food.
Extension: Base of the skull to the level of C6 vertebra where it continues as esophagus.
It *communicates* with oral cavity, nasal cavity and larynx.

Subdivisions: Nasopharynx, oropharynx and laryngopharynx **(Fig. 13.9)**.

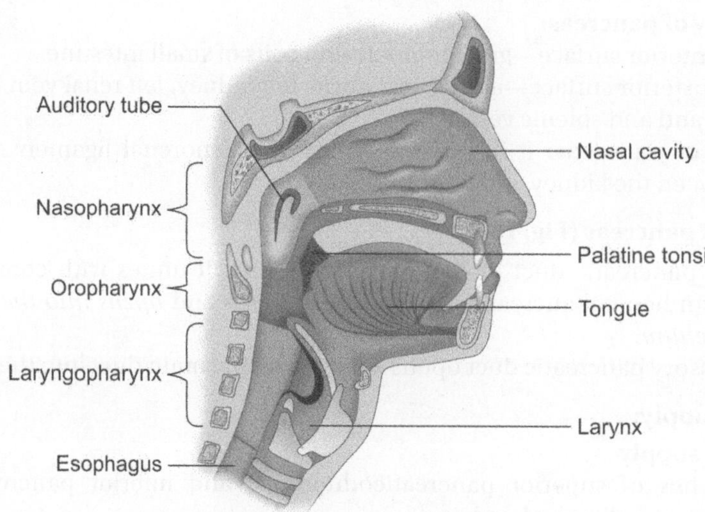

Fig. 13.9: Interior of pharynx.

Nasopharynx:

- Situated posterior to nasal cavity up to the level of soft palate.
- Communications:
  - Anteriorly with nasal cavity.
  - Inferiorly with oropharynx.

Features in interior of nasopharynx

- Lateral wall:
  - **Tubal opening of auditory tube**
  - **Tubal elevation**—by cartilaginous part of auditory tube
  - **Tubal tonsils**—seen around the tubal opening.

  Behind tubal elevation—depression called pharyngeal isthmus (fossa of Rosenmuller) is present.
- Roof and posterior wall—**pharyngeal tonsils** are present. When enlarged they are called **adenoids.**

Oropharynx:

- Extension: From soft palate to upper border of epiglottis.
- *Communications*:
  - Superiorly with nasal cavity.
  - Anteriorly with oral cavity.
  - Inferiorly with laryngopharynx.
- Lateral walls: **Palatine tonsils** are present.

Laryngopharynx:

- Extension: From upper border of epiglottis to lower border of cricoid cartilage.
- *Communications*:
  - Superiorly with oropharynx and inferiorly with esophagus
  - Anteriorly, laryngeal inlet is present.
- *Piriform fossa*: Present on either side of laryngeal inlet. Foreign bodies like fish bone get lodged in the fossa. The internal laryngeal nerve is present beneath the mucosa. Therefore care should be taken to avoid any injury to nerve while removing foreign bodies.

Muscles of the pharynx:

- Outer circular muscles:
  - Superior constrictor
  - Middle constrictor
  - Inferior constrictor
- Inner longitudinal muscles:
  - Stylopharyngeus
  - Salphingopharyngeus
  - Palatopharyngeus

Nerve supply:

Motor innervation:

- All the constrictor muscles, salphingopharyngeus and palatopharyngeus are supplied by **cranial accessory** nerve through vagus nerve.
- Stylopharyngeus is supplied by glossopharyngeal nerve.

Sensory innervation:
- Glossopharyngeal nerve
- Vagus nerve

Blood supply:

Arterial supply: Ascending pharyngeal artery, branches from facial artery, lingual artery and maxillary artery.

Venous drainage: By pharyngeal plexus of veins which drains into facial vein and internal jugular vein.

Lymphatic drainage: Upper deep cervical nodes and retropharyngeal nodes.

Function: Passage of food and air. During swallowing, the food passage is closed by sphincter. Soft palate is very important for this.

Applied anatomy:
- Paralysis of soft palate muscles leads to regurgitation of food into nasal cavity.
- Tonsillitis and adenoids are common condition which affect children.
- Forms an air passage, important in sound production.

4. Describe the salivary glands of the body.

Ans. The salivary glands secrete saliva which helps in mixing and digestion of food.

They are classified as major and minor:
- *Major salivary glands* are parotid, submandibular and sublingual glands **(Fig. 13.10)**.
- *Minor salivary glands* are present in the beneath the mucosa of the oral cavity, floor of the mouth and soft palate.

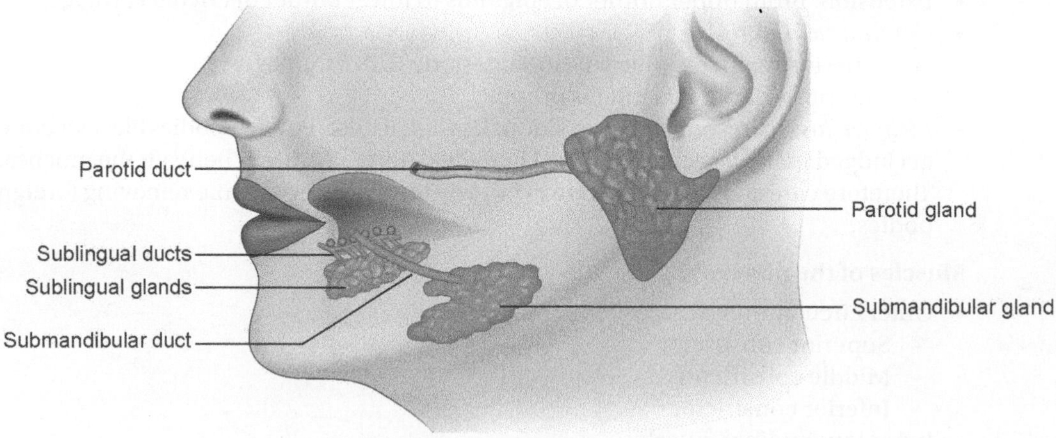

Fig. 13.10: Major salivary glands.

Salivary glands are of three types based on structure: Serous, mucus and mixed glands.

Parotid Salivary Gland
- It is predominantly a serous salivary gland and the largest of the three glands. Pyramidal in shape, lobulated and yellowish-brown in color.
- Location: Front of ear, below the zygomatic arch, superficial to infratemporal fossa.
- Capsule: Gland is covered by deep cervical fascia.

- Structures passing through the gland:
  - External carotid artery
  - Superficial temporal artery
  - Maxillary artery
  - Retromandibular vein
  - Facial nerve.
- Parotid duct or Stenson's duct:
  - Length of the duct is 5 cm
  - Duct opens opposite to the upper second molar tooth into the vestibule of the oral cavity.

Submandibular Salivary Gland

- It is a mixed salivary gland with serous and mucous acini.
- Location: In the submandibular triangle.
- Parts: Divided into superficial and deep parts by the mylohyoid muscle.
- Important relations: Facial artery, hypoglossal nerve.
- Mucous acini have serous demilunes.
- Submandibular duct or Wharton's duct:
  - Length is 5 cm
  - Opens into sublingual papilla in the floor of mouth.

Sublingual Salivary Gland

- It is predominantly a mucus salivary gland.
- Situated underneath the mucosa of floor of the mouth.
- Duct:
  - 15–20 ducts
  - Open into the sublingual fold in the floor of mouth.
  - Some ducts may open into the Wharton's duct.

Nerve supply:

- *Sympathetic fibers* from superior cervical ganglion reach the salivary glands via the nerve plexus around external carotid artery.
- *Parasympathetic fibers for parotid gland*: Inferior salivatory nucleus in medulla oblongata → **glossopharyngeal nerve** → tympanic branch → tympanic plexus in middle ear → lesser superficial petrosal nerve → relay in **Otic ganglion** → postganglionic fibers reach the gland through **auriculotemporal nerve.**
- *Parasympathetic fibers for submandibular and sublingual gland*: Parasympathetic fibers—superior salivatory nucleus in pons → nervus intermedius → chorda tympani branch of facial nerve—through **lingual nerve** → relay in **submandibular ganglion** → postganglionic fibers reach the submandibular and sublingual gland.

Applied anatomy:

- Mumps parotitis: Viral infection of parotid gland leads to painful swelling.
- Facial nerve is in danger during surgery on parotid gland.
- Tumors can involve the glands.
- Salivary gland ducts can get affected with stones, leads to painful swelling. The stone requires surgical removal.

SHORT ESSAYS **5 MARKS**

5. Regions and quadrants of the abdomen.

Ans. **Regions:** There are nine regions for the description of the abdominal contents divided by three imaginary lines.

1. Midclavicular line: Vertical line drawn downwards from the midpoint of clavicle on the right and left side.
2. Transpyloric plane: Horizontal line drawn on the midpoint between the suprasternal notch and pubic symphysis. It passes through the tip of 9th costal cartilage.
3. Transtubercular plane: Horizontal line passes through the L5 vertebra between the iliac tubercle of the right and left hip bone.

Nine regions are (Fig. 13.11A):

- Right hypochondrium, epigastrium, left hypochondrium.
- Right lumbar region, umbilical region, left lumbar region.
- Right iliac fossa, hypogastrium, left iliac fossa.

Quadrants: Abdomen is also divided into **four quadrants** by two lines **(Fig. 13.11B)**. A vertical and horizontal line intersecting at the umbilicus.

The quadrants are:

1. Upper right quadrant
2. Upper left quadrant
3. Lower right quadrant
4. Lower left quadrant

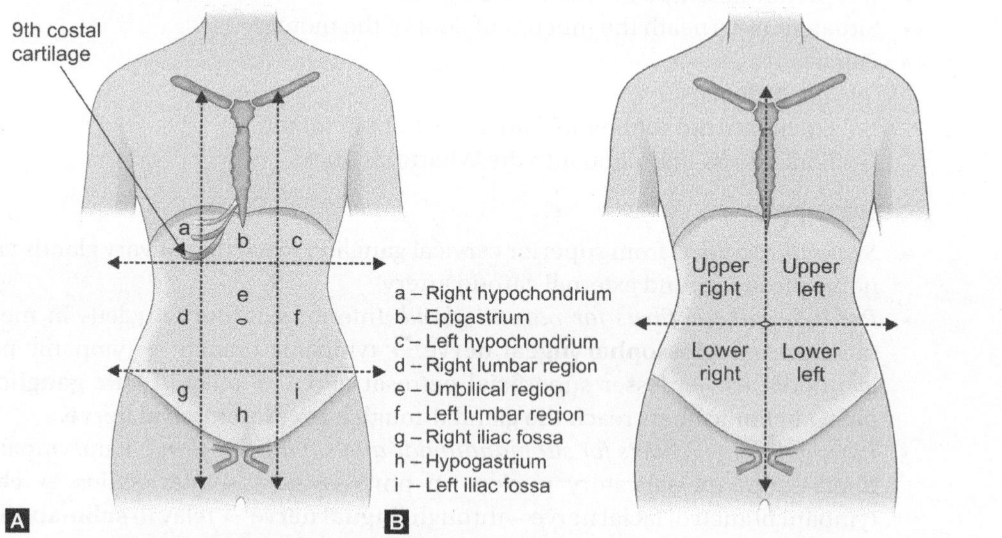

Figs. 13.11A and B: Areas in the abdomen. (A) Regions of the abdomen; (B) Quadrants of the abdomen.

6. Peritoneum.

Ans.

- Peritoneum is a serous membrane lined by simple squamous epithelium.
- It is made of two layers: (1) parietal and (2) visceral.
- **Parietal peritoneum** lines the abdominal wall, whereas the **visceral peritoneum** lines the abdominal organs.

- Space between the parietal and visceral layers is called the peritoneal cavity. It contains the serous peritoneal fluid.
- *Retroperitoneal organs*: Some organs are situated in the posterior abdominal wall. Only the anterior surface of those organs are covered with peritoneum. They are pancreas, kidneys, duodenum, ascending and descending colons.

Peritoneal folds (Figs. 13.12 and 13.13):

- **Greater omentum**:
  - Attached to the greater curvature of the stomach.
  - It extends downwards and covers the transverse colon and coils of small intestine.
  - In any infection, it tries to limit the spread. Hence called the **Policeman of abdomen.**

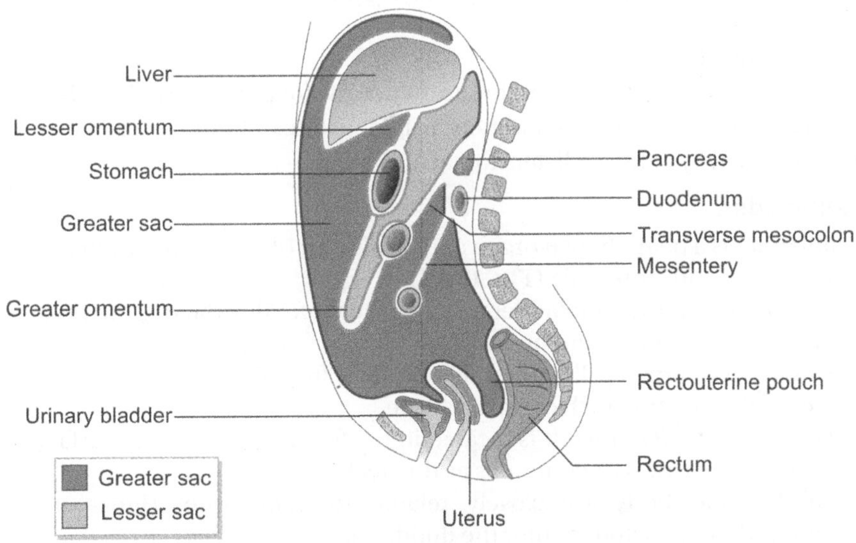

Fig. 13.12: Peritoneum—longitudinal section.

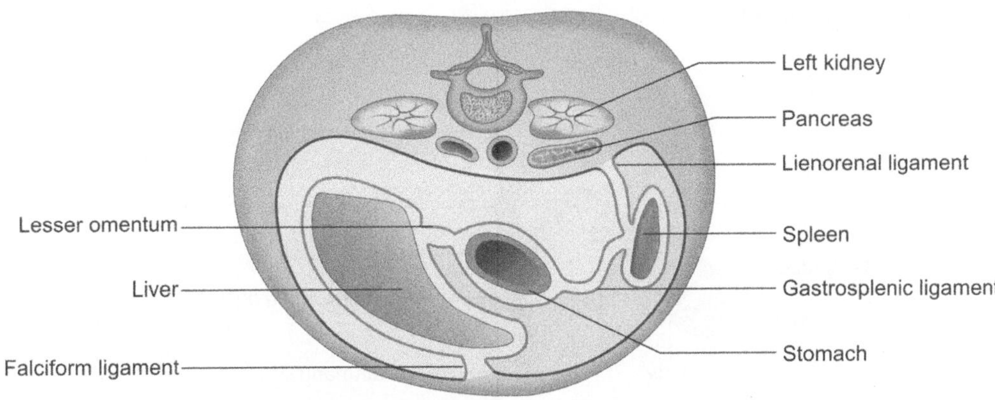

Fig. 13.13: Peritoneum—cross-section.

- **Lesser omentum:** Attached to the lesser curvature of stomach and the hilum of liver.
- **Falciform ligament**: It is attached to the liver and connects the anterior abdominal wall and diaphragm to the liver.
- **Mesentery:** It attaches the jejunum and ileum of small intestine to the posterior abdominal wall. It contains superior mesenteric artery and its branches, corresponding veins, lymph nodes.
- **Mesocolon:**
  - *Transverse mesocolon*: It connects the transverse colon to the posterior abdominal wall.
  - *Sigmoid mesocolon*: It connects the sigmoid colon to the posterior abdominal wall.

Functions of peritoneum:
- The folds of peritoneum suspend the organs so that they are freely mobile.
- Gives passage to vessels, nerves and lymphatics.
- Storehouse of fat.
- Fights infection.
- Acts as semipermeable membrane, hence useful in *peritoneal dialysis.*

Applied anatomy: In a condition called **ascites,** fluid accumulates inside the peritoneal cavity causing distension of abdomen.

7. Gallbladder.

Ans. Gallbladder is a pear-shaped organ and forms part of extrahepatic biliary apparatus. It concentrates and stores bile **(Fig. 13.14)**.
- It is situated in the gallbladder fossa, in the visceral surface of the liver.
- **Parts:** Fundus, body and neck.
- *Fundus*: It is part of gallbladder that projects from the inferior margin of the liver at the level of the tip of 9th costal cartilage.
- *Body of the gallbladder*: It is located in the fossa in the visceral surface of the liver. Its upper narrow part continues as the neck.
  Fundus and body are closely related to duodenum. Hence in gallbladder perforations, gallstones enter the duodenum.
- *Neck*: It is the funnel-shaped upper narrow end of the gallbladder. Hartmann's pouch is the dilated right wall of the neck. It is the common site where gallstones may get lodged.

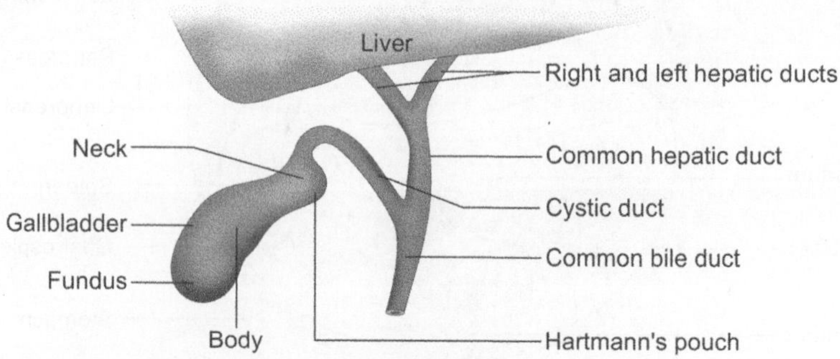

Fig. 13.14: Parts of gallbladder.

Cystic duct: It extends from the neck of gallbladder. It is spirally curved. It joins the common hepatic duct and forms the *common bile duct.*

Blood supply:

Arterial supply:

- **Cystic artery is** the main artery of supply.
- Right hepatic artery also supplies it.

Venous drainage:

- Cystic vein
- Hepatic veins
- Portal vein

Lymphatic drainage: Hepatic nodes, cystic node and pancreaticosplenic nodes.

Applied anatomy:

- Cholelithiasis—stones in gallbladder.
- Cholecystitis—inflammation of gallbladder.
- Cholecystectomy—surgical removal of gallbladder.

8. Describe stomach under following headings: Location, parts, blood supply, nerve supply, applied anatomy.

Ans. *Refer Q. No. 1, Longs Essays (Stomach)*

Refer **Figures 13.2, 13.4 and 13.5.**

9. Vermiform appendix.

Ans. *Location:* In the *right iliac fossa.* It is attached to the posteromedial wall of the cecum. Its length ranges from 2 to 20 cm.

Base of the appendix: The part attached to the cecum.

Tip of the appendix: It may point towards any direction.

Positions of appendix: The tip of the appendix can point to any of the following directions **(Fig. 13.15)**.

- Retrocecal: 12 o'clock position behind the cecum.
- Preileal and postileal: 2 o'clock position, upwards to the right.
- Promontoric: 3 o'clock position towards the sacral promontory.
- Pelvic: 4 o' clock position towards the pelvic cavity.
- Subcecal: 6 o' clock position points downwards to the inguinal ligament.

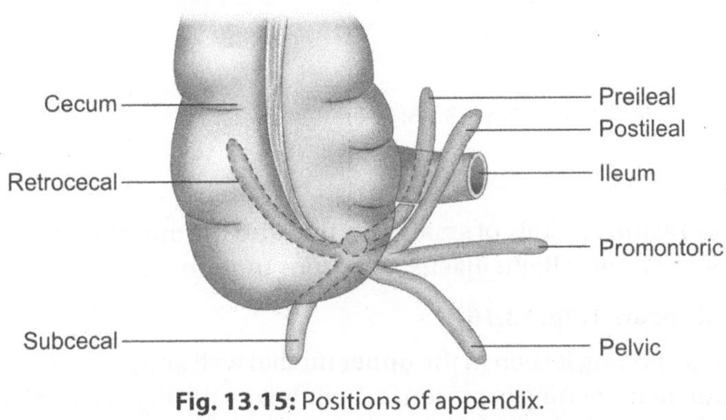

Fig. 13.15: Positions of appendix.

Arterial supply:

Appendicular artery: It is a branch of ileocolic artery.
Venous drainage: By appendicular vein which drains into ileocolic vein.
Lymphatic drainage: Into the ileocolic lymph nodes.

Nerve supply:

- Sympathetic innervation: From T9 and T10 spinal cord segments.
- Parasympathetic innervation: Vagus nerves.

Applied anatomy:

- **Appendicitis:** Inflammation of appendix.
- **McBurney's point**: At this site, there is maximum tenderness in case of appendicitis. It is the point at the junction of lateral one-third and medial two-third of the line joining the umbilicus and anterior superior iliac spine.
- **Appendectomy**: Removal of the appendix by surgery.

10. Cecum.

Ans.
- Cecum is the most proximal part of large intestine which continues as the ascending colon
- Ileum opens into the cecum
- Situated in the right iliac fossa
- It has a blind end inferiorly
- It is completely covered with peritoneum.

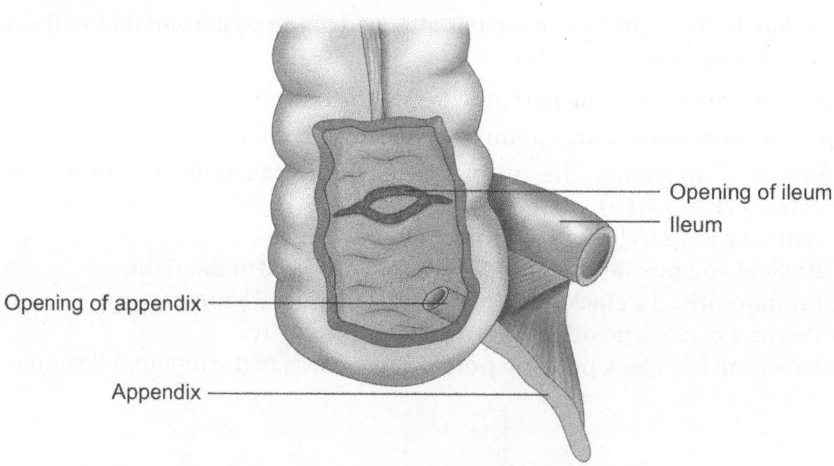

Fig. 13.16: Interior of cecum.

Relations:

- *Anterior relations:* Coils of small intestine and the anterior abdominal wall.
- *Posterior relations:* Right iliacus and psoas muscle.

Interior of cecum (Fig. 13.16):

- Ileocecal opening is seen in the upper medial wall and is guarded by ileocecal valve.
- Appendicular opening is present 2.5 cm below the ileocecal valve.

Types of cecum: Shape of cecum varies

- Conical type (fetal type): cecum is conical in shape with appendix attached to the apex.
- Quadrate type (infantile): Right and left wall are equal in length.
- Asymmetrical type (normal): Right wall of cecum bulges more than the left wall and the appendix opens into the posteromedial part of cecum.
- Exaggerated asymmetrical type: Right wall grows more and left wall atrophies.

Blood supply:

- **Arterial supply**: Anterior cecal artery, posterior cecal artery, branches of ileocolic artery.
- **Venous drainage**: By the corresponding veins which finally drains into portal vein.
- **Lymphatic drainage**: Ileocolic nodes present around the ileocolic artery.

Nerve supply:

Sympathetic innervations: From T10–T11 spinal segments.

Parasympathetic innervations: From the vagus nerves.

11. Rectum.

Ans.
- Rectum is the distal end of large intestine and a reservoir of feces.
- Rectum is situated between the sigmoid colon and anal canal **(Fig. 13.17)**.
- Extent: Rectosigmoid junction at 3rd sacral vertebra to anorectal junction just below and anterior to the tip of coccyx.
- 12 cm long and the widest part is called ampulla.
- Does not have appendices epiploicae, sacculations or Taenia coli.

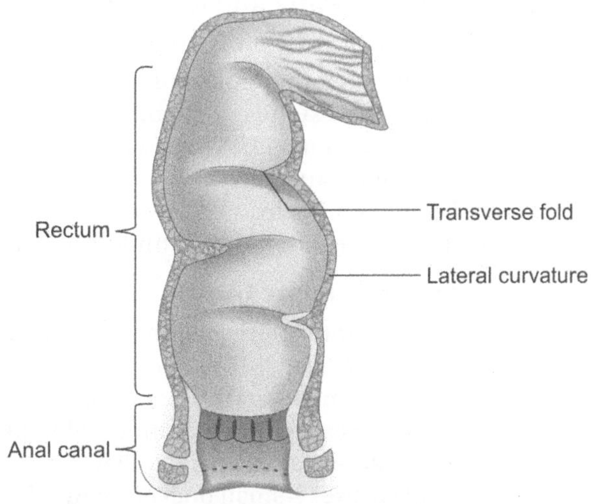

Fig. 13.17: Interior of rectum.

- Two anteroposterior curvatures and three lateral curvatures.
- Internal features: **Houston's valves**—permanent transverse folds. Largest fold is called Nelaton's valve.
- Peritoneal covering:
  - Upper 1/3rd of rectum is covered on the anterior and lateral sides
  - Middle 1/3rd of rectum is covered only anteriorly.
  - Lower 1/3rd is devoid of peritoneum.
- Anorectal junction is pulled anteriorly by puborectal sling.

Anterior relations:

- In female—rectouterine pouch (space between rectum and uterus).
- In male—rectovesical pouch and rectovesical fascia or Denonvillier's fascia. It separates the urinary bladder and prostate from rectum.

Posterior relations: Lower three sacral vertebrae, piriformis muscle.

Blood supply:

Arterial supply:
- Superior rectal artery: Branch of inferior mesenteric artery.
- Middle rectal artery: Branch of internal iliac artery.
- Inferior rectal artery: Branch of internal pudendal artery.
- Median sacral artery: From abdominal aorta.

Venous drainage:
- Superior rectal vein: It drains into the inferior mesenteric vein.
- Middle and inferior rectal veins: These veins drain into internal iliac veins.

Lymphatic drainage:
- Upper part: Preaortic and para aortic lymph nodes.
- Lower part: Internal iliac nodes.

Applied anatomy:
- Rectum and anal canal are site of portocaval anastomosis.
- Per rectum (PR) examination—is a part of examination. Prostate, seminal vesicles in male, cervix in females can be palpated by PR examination.

12. Anal canal: Parts and features.

Ans.
- Anal canal is the most terminal part of GIT.
- It plays important role in defecation and maintaining fetal continence.
- Anal canal extends from anorectal junction to the anal opening. Anal opening exits to the exterior within the anal triangle of perineum.
- Location—true pelvis.
- Length is 3.75 cm.
- It has three parts: Upper, middle and lower parts (**Fig. 13.18**).

Upper zone (upper 1/3rd)
- Extends from anorectal junction to pectinate line.
- Length—1.5 cm.
- **Anal columns**—vertical mucosal folds.
- **Anal valves**—horizontal mucosal folds connecting the anal columns. Each valve has nodules called anal papillae.
- **Anal sinuses**—small pockets above the anal sinuses.

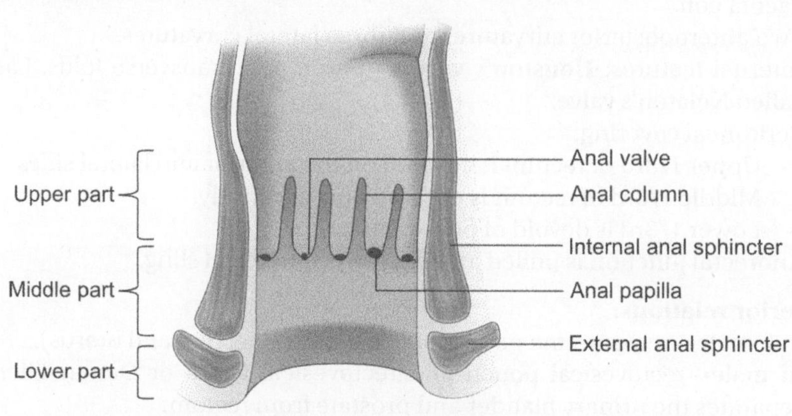

Fig. 13.18: Interior of anal canal.

- **Pectinate line (dentate line)**—line connecting all the anal valves.
- Lined by simple columnar epithelium.

Middle zone (middle 1/3rd)

- Extends between pectinate and Hilton's line.
- Length—1.5 cm.
- Lined by stratified columnar epithelium.
- No anal columns or valves.
- No sebaceous glands or sweat glands.
- Hilton's line (White line of Hilton) is a demarcation between true skin and mucosa. It also demarcates junction between internal and external anal sphincter.

Lower zone (lower 1/3rd)

- Length—0.75 cm.
- Lined by true skin.
- Hair follicles, sebaceous glands and sweat glands are present.

Applied anatomy:

- Rectum and anal canal are the sites of portocaval anastomosis.
- Hemorrhoids or piles can affect the anal canal leading to bleeding. Here the rectal veins enlarge and filled with blood. It occurs due to portal hypertension or prolonged constipation.

13. Importance of pectinate line of anal canal.

Ans. *Refer* **Table 13.1**.

Table 13.1: Comparison of features of anal canal in relation to above and below pectinate line.

Features	Above the pectinate line	Below the pectinate line
Development	Endoderm	Ectoderm (proctodeum)
Lining epithelium	Simple columnar epithelium	Stratified squamous epithelium
Arterial supply	Superior rectal artery	Inferior rectal artery
Venous drainage	Superior rectal veins	Inferior rectal veins
Lymphatic drainage	Internal iliac nodes	Superficial inguinal nodes
Nerve supply	Autonomic nerves: • Sympathetic—inferior hypogastric plexus • Parasympathetic: – Pelvic splanchnic nerves – Insensitive to pain	Somatic nerves: • Inferior rectal nerves • Sensitive to pain
Hemorrhoids	Internal hemorrhoids • Painless	External hemorrhoids • Painful

14. Extrahepatic biliary apparatus.

Ans. The biliary tree consists of series of ducts that collect and store bile synthesized by liver. The bile is synthesized by hepatocytes and carried via the bile canaliculi which unite and terminate in hepatic ducts.

Components of extrahepatic biliary apparatus (Fig. 13.19):

- Right and left hepatic ducts
- Common hepatic duct

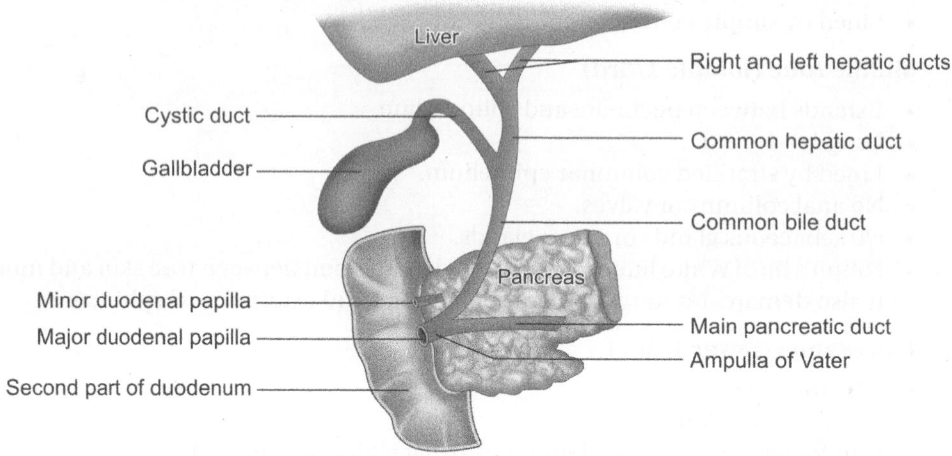

Fig. 13.19: Extrahepatic biliary apparatus.

- Gallbladder
- Cystic duct
- Common bile duct

A. **Hepatic duct**: The right and left hepatic ducts arise from the right and left lobe of the liver. They unite to form the common hepatic duct at the hilum (porta hepatis) of liver.

B. **Gallbladder**: Gallbladder is a pear-shaped structure which stores bile. It has fundus, body and neck. The neck is the upper narrow end of the gallbladder which continues as cystic duct. The cystic duct is 3–4 cm long. It joins the common hepatic duct to form the common bile duct.

C. **Cystic duct**: It extends from the neck of gallbladder. It is spirally curved. It joins the common hepatic duct and forms *the common bile duct.*

D. **Common bile duct**: It is about 8 cm long. It passes posterior to first part of the duodenum and unites with the main pancreatic duct. The hepatopancreatic ampulla or ampulla of Vater opens into the second part of the duodenum at the major duodenal papilla.

Blood supply: Cystic artery is the chief artery. It also receives blood from the superior pancreaticoduodenal and right hepatic arteries.

Venous drainage—is by the cystic vein, hepatic veins and portal vein.

Lymphatics: From the biliary apparatus drain into cystic node, hepatic nodes and pancreaticosplenic nodes.

Nerve supply:

Parasympathetic nerves: Cystic plexus of nerves.
Sympathetic nerves arise from the T7 to T9 spinal cord segments.

Applied anatomy:

- Cholecystitis: Inflammation of the gallbladder.
- Cholelithiasis: Formation of stones in gallbladder.
- Cholecystectomy: Removal of gallbladder by surgery.

- Biliary obstruction: Bile duct can be obstructed by gallstones or by cancer of head of pancreas leading to jaundice.

15. Gross anatomy of spleen.

Ans. Spleen is a lymphoid organ. It is situated in the left hypochondrium opposite 9th, 10th and 11th ribs.

Parts (Fig. 13.20): It has 2 ends—medial and lateral, 2 borders—superior and inferior border and 2 surfaces—anterior (visceral) and posterior (diaphragmatic). It is intraperitoneal.

- **Visceral surface**: Related to stomach, left kidney, tail of pancreas and left colic flexure.
- **Diaphragmatic surface**: Related to diaphragm, left pleura, 9th, 10th and 11th ribs.
- **Hilum** of the spleen: Splenic vessels, nerves and lymphatics enter or leave the spleen.
- **Hilum also** gives attachment to gastrosplenic and lienorenal ligaments.

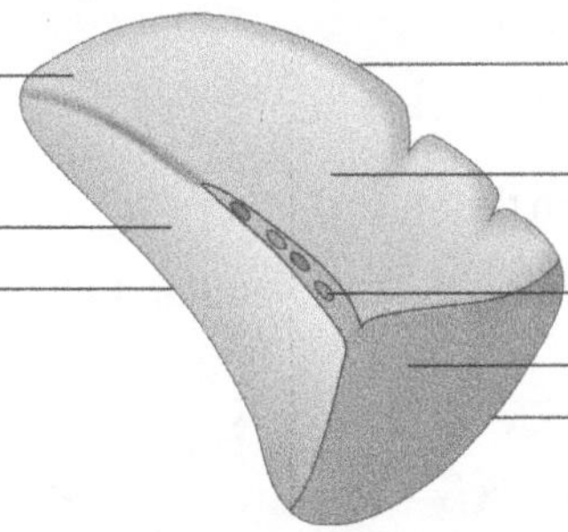

Fig. 13.20: Spleen—visceral surface.

Ligaments related to spleen:

- Gastrosplenic ligament attached to hilum.
- Lienorenal ligaments are attached to the hilum.
- Phrenicocolic ligament supports the lateral end of the spleen. It extends from left colic flexure to the diaphragm and is not attached to the spleen.

Blood supply:

Arterial supply: Splenic artery which is a branch of celiac artery.

Venous drainage: By splenic vein. It forms the portal vein by uniting with the superior mesenteric vein.

Lymphatic drainage: Pancreaticosplenic nodes.

Functions:

- Lymphoid organ—defense against blood-borne antigens.
- Removes dead RBCs.
- Hematopoiesis in fetal life.

Applied anatomy:

- It is prone to rupture leading to massive hemorrhage inside the abdomen.

- Enlargement of spleen is called **splenomegaly**. Spleen enlarges towards the umbilicus and not downwards because of the presence of phrenicocolic ligament at the lateral end.
- **Splenectomy**—removal of spleen.

16. Liver.

Ans. Liver is situated in the right hypochondrium, epigastrium and may extend into the left hypochondrium.

Parts:

- **Surfaces of liver (Figs. 13.21 to 13.23):**
  - Anterior surface
  - Superior surface
  - Posterior surface
  - Inferior surface
  - Right surface
- **Anatomical lobes:** Divided into right and left lobes by the attachment of ligaments on the liver.
  - Falciform ligament on the anterosuperior surface

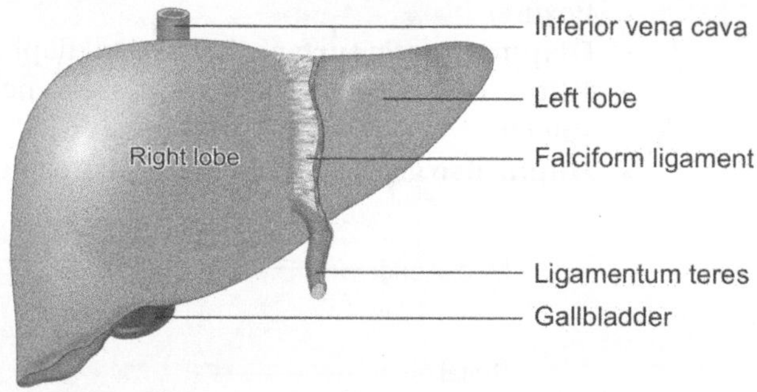

Fig. 13.21: Liver—anterior surface.

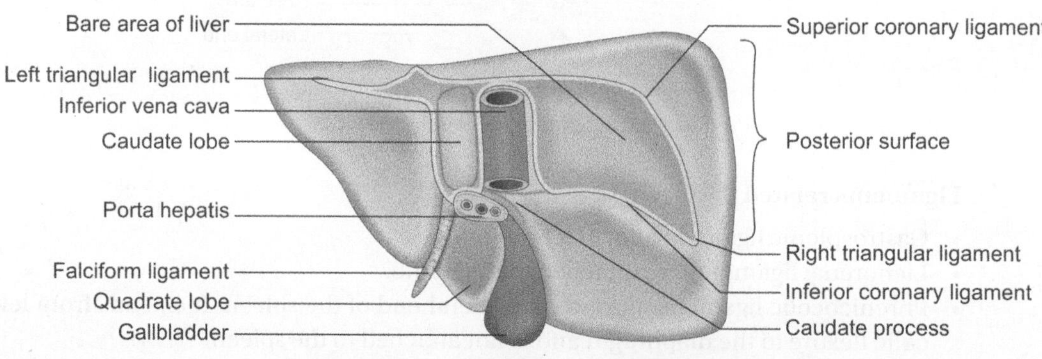

Fig. 13.22: Liver—posterior and inferior surface.

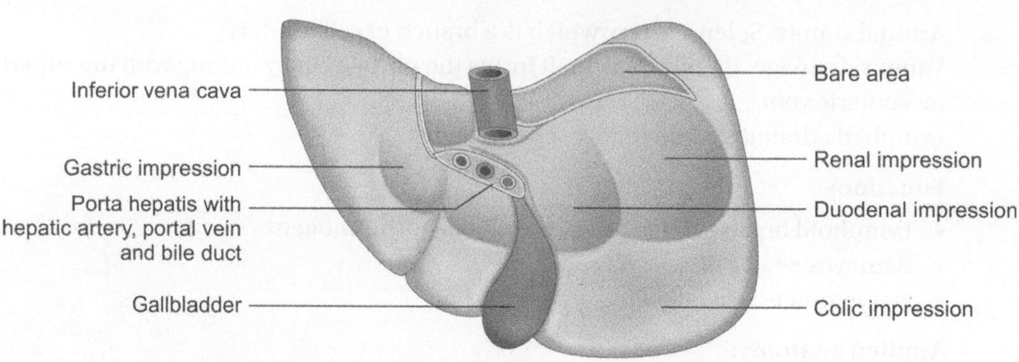

Fig. 13.23: Liver—relations of Inferior surface.

  - By the fissures for ligamentum teres and ligamentum venosum on the postero-inferior surface.
- *The quadrate and caudate lobes* belongs to the left lobe.
- **Functional lobes:** Divided functionally into right and left lobes by the intrahepatic distribution of the portal vein, hepatic artery and bile duct.

Relations:
- *Anterior surface*: Anterior abdominal wall and diaphragm.
- *Posterior surface*:
  - Esophagus.
  - Bare area of liver: Not covered by peritoneum. It is related to right suprarenal gland.
- *Superior surface*: Above the diaphragm, it is related to the pericardium with heart, and pleura with lung on both sides.
- *Inferior surface*:
  - Stomach, lesser omentum, pylorus, duodenum and colon.
  - Gallbladder and right kidney.
  - Fissure for ligamentum teres and ligamentum venosum.

Blood supply:

Arterial supply:
- Hepatic artery: 20% of blood supply
- Portal vein: 80% of blood supply

Venous drainage:
- Hepatic veins: Drains into inferior vena cava.

Lymphatic drainage: Hepatic nodes, caval nodes, celiac nodes and paracardial nodes.

Function:
- Bile synthesis
- Glycogen synthesis
- Clotting factors production
- Metabolic functions
- Detoxification.

Applied anatomy:
- Liver biopsy—care should be taken to do biopsy without injuring the pleura.
- Liver transplantation—can be carried out since liver can regenerate.
- Hepatomegaly—enlarged liver can occur due to various causes.

17. Esophagus.

Ans. Esophagus is a muscular tube for the passage of food.
- It is 25 cm long.
- Parts: Cervical part, thoracic part and abdominal part.
- It is a content of posterior mediastinum.
- Connects the pharynx and stomach.
- Extent—from lower border of cricoid cartilage (C6 vertebral level) to cardiac orifice of stomach (T11 vertebral level).
- It is closely related to trachea, abdominal aorta, azygos system, thoracic duct.
- Wall of the esophagus has four layers. The inner epithelium is nonkeratinized stratified squamous epithelium.

- The muscles in wall is a mixture of smooth and skeletal. But still the action is involuntary.
- It passes through the esophageal opening of the diaphragm.
- Sphincters of esophagus
  a. Upper esophageal sphincter—formed by the cricopharyngeus muscle. It prevents the passage of air into esophagus.
  b. Lower esophageal sphincter—at the gastroesophageal (GE) junction.

Constrictions of esophagus:

- 15 cm from incisor teeth—at the junction of esophagus and pharynx.
- 22.5 cm from incisor teeth—it is crossed by aortic arch.
- 27.5 cm from incisor teeth—it is crossed by left bronchus.
- 37.5 from incisor teeth—as it pierces the diaphragm.

Blood supply: ***Refer*** **Table 13.2**

Table 13.2: Blood supply and lymphatic drainage of esophagus.

Parts	Arterial supply	Venous drainage	Lymphatic drainage
Cervical	Inferior thyroid arteries	Brachiocephalic veins	Deep cervical nodes
Thoracic	Esophageal branches from aorta	Azygos veins	Posterior mediastinal nodes
Abdominal	Left gastric artery	Left gastric and hemiazygos veins	Left gastric nodes

Applied anatomy:

- Esophageal varices: Veins at lower end of esophagus are dilated in portal hypertension. Rupture of these veins cause hematemesis.
- Esophagoscopy: Constrictions of esophagus should be kept in mind while doing the procedure.
- It can get inflamed due to regurgitation of acidic food contents from cardiac end of stomach—esophagitis. It leads to pain behind the sternum.
- Dysphagia is the difficulty in swallowing.

18. Tooth.

Ans.
- Tooth is an accessory organ of alimentary tract.
- Located in the alveolar sockets.
- Gums cover the alveolar processes, and attached by periodontal ligament.
- Three regions: Crown, neck, root.
- Dentin: Covers pulp cavity, harder than bone. It has more calcium. It is synthesized by odontoblasts.
- Enamel is the outermost covering on the crown of tooth. It consists of calcium phosphate and carbonate. It protects from wear and tear. If enamel is damaged, it cannot be replaced.
- Cementum—bone like substance covering the root. It attaches root to the socket by periodontal ligament.
- Two set of dentitions is observed in a man's life
  a. Primary/milk/deciduous—appears around 6 months of life and persists till 6 years.
  b. Secondary/permanent—appears around 6 years and continues till adulthood.

Note:
Endodontics: Study of diseases of pulp, root, ligament and alveolar bone.
Orthodontics: Prevention and correction of abnormally aligned teeth.
Periodontics: Study and treatment of tissues around teeth.

SHORT ANSWERS 2 MARKS

19. Name the components of extrahepatic biliary apparatus.

Ans.
- Right and left hepatic ducts
- Common hepatic duct
- Gallbladder
- Cystic duct
- Bile duct

20. What are the anatomical lobes of the liver?

Ans. **Anatomical lobes:** Divided into right and left lobes by the attachment of ligaments on the liver.
- Falciform ligament on the anterosuperior surface
- By the fissures for ligamentum teres and ligamentum venosum on the postero-inferior surface.
- The quadrate and caudate lobes belong to the left lobe.

21. Name the subdivisions of small and large intestine.

Ans. *Refer* **Table 13.3**

Table 13.3: Parts of small and large intestine.

Small intestine	Large intestine
• Duodenum • Jejunum • Ileum	• Cecum, appendix • Ascending colon • Transverse colon • Descending colon • Sigmoid colon

22. Parts of the duodenum and its blood supply.

Ans. Duodenum is the C-shaped fixed part of small intestine. It has four parts: I, II, III and IV **(Fig. 13.24)**:
- First part: It is 5 cm in length. It extends from pyloric end of stomach to superior duodenal flexure.
- Second part: It is 7.5 cm in length. It passes vertically downwards from superior duodenal flexure to inferior duodenal flexure.
- Third part: It is the longest and horizontal part, about 10 cm in length.
- Fourth part: It is 2.5 cm in length and becomes continuous with jejunum at duodenojejunal flexure.

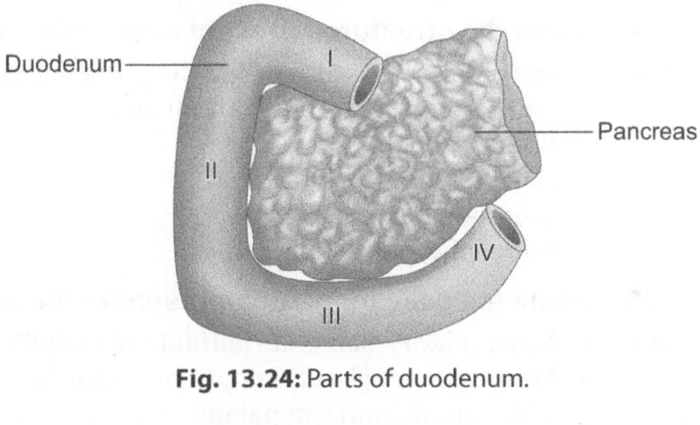

Fig. 13.24: Parts of duodenum.

Blood supply:

Arterial supply: Superior pancreaticoduodenal artery—branch of gastroduodenal artery.

Inferior pancreaticoduodenal artery—branch of superior mesenteric artery.

Venous drainage:
- Superior pancreaticoduodenal vein drains into portal vein.
- Inferior pancreaticoduodenal vein drains into superior mesenteric vein.

Lymphatic drainage: Pancreaticosplenic nodes and pyloric nodes.

23. Differences between small intestine and large intestine.

Ans. *Refer* **Table 13.4 and Figures 13.25A and B.**

Table 13.4: Differences between small and large intestine.

Features	Small intestine	Large intestine
Sacculations	Absent	Present
Appendices epiploicae	Absent	Present
Taenia coli	Absent	present
Peyer's patches—large lymphatic aggregations	Present	Absent
Fixation to posterior abdominal wall	Mobile	Fixed except transverse colon and sigmoid colon

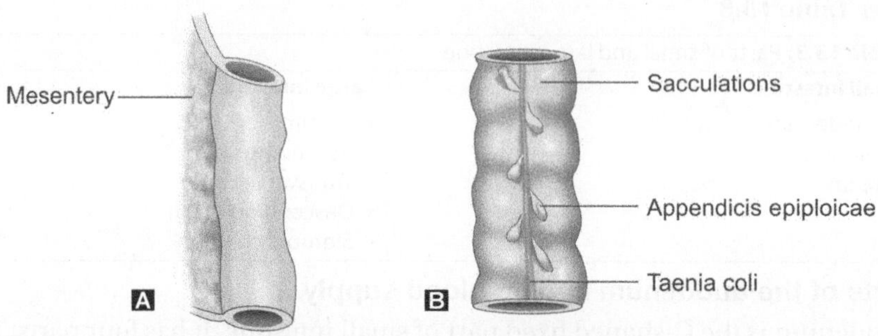

Figs. 13.25A and B: Difference between small and large intestines.

24. Name the structures present at the hilum of liver.

Ans. Hilum of the liver is also called the porta hepatis.

Structures passing through hilum are:
- Portal vein
- Hepatic artery
- Common hepatic duct
- Nerve plexus and lymphatics.

25. Name the salivary glands present in the body.

Ans.
- Major salivary glands are parotid, submandibular and sublingual glands **(Fig. 13.10)**.
- Minor salivary glands are present in the beneath the mucosa of the oral cavity, floor of the mouth and soft palate.

26. Name the arteries supplying the stomach.

Ans. Stomach is supplied by the following arteries **(Fig. 13.4)**:
- Left gastric artery—a branch of celiac artery.
- Right gastric artery—a branch of hepatic artery.
- Left gastroepiploic artery—a branch of splenic artery.
- Right gastroepiploic artery—a branch of gastroduodenal artery.
- Short gastric arteries—branches of splenic artery.

27. Name the muscle of soft palate and their nerve supply.

Ans. Muscles of soft palate are as follows:
- Musculus uvulae
- Tensor palatini
- Levator palatini
- Palatopharyngeus
- Palatoglossus

Innervations:
- All the muscles except palatoglossus: By pharyngeal plexus (cranial accessory through vagus nerve)
- Palatoglossus: By mandibular nerve.

28. What are hemorrhoids?

Ans. Hemorrhoids (piles) are caused by dilatations of rectal venous plexuses. There are two types: (1) External and (2) internal hemorrhoids **(Fig. 13.26)**.

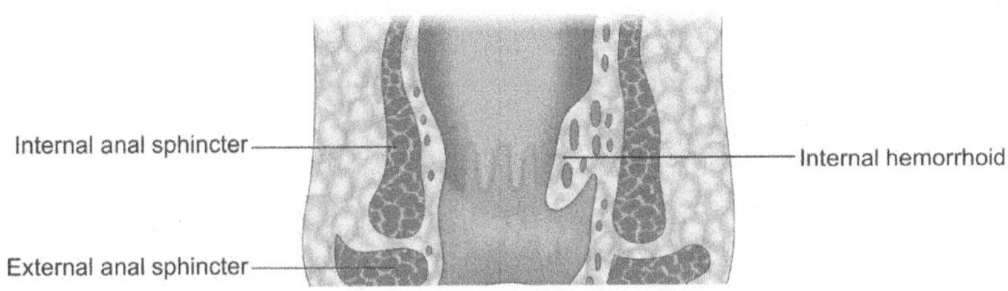

Fig. 13.26: Hemorrhoids in anal canal.

Internal hemorrhoids:
- Above the pectinate line
- Dilatations of superior rectal venous plexuses
- Painless

External hemorrhoids:
- Below the pectinate line
- Dilatations of inferior rectal venous plexuses
- Painful

14
CHAPTER

Urinary System

LONG ESSAYS — 10 MARKS

1. Mention the parts of urinary system. Describe the gross anatomy of kidneys.

Ans. Parts of urinary system (Fig. 14.1):

- Two kidneys
- Two ureters
- Urinary bladder
- Urethra

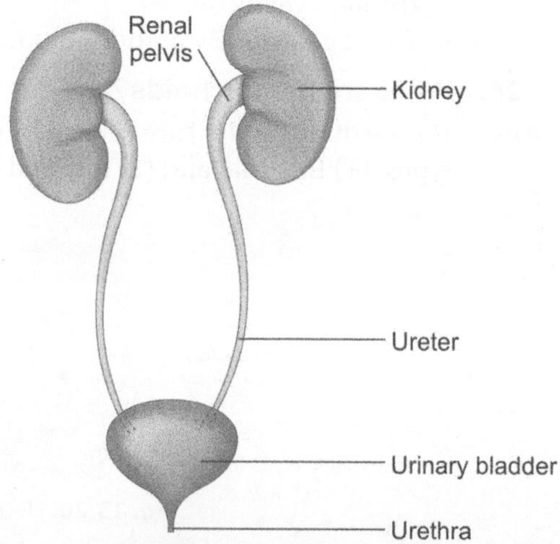

Fig. 14.1: Parts of urinary system.

Kidney:

- **Gross anatomy:** Paired, main organs of urinary system.
- **Function:**
  - Removes metabolic waste products by producing urine.
  - Regulates fluid balance of body.
  - Secretes renin and erythropoietin.
- **Location/position:**
  - On posterior abdominal wall.
  - Retroperitoneal.
  - Extent: From T12 to L3 vertebrae.
  - Right kidney lower than left (due to presence of liver on right).
- **Shape and size:**
  - Bean-shaped
  - 10 × 5 × 2.5 cm
- **Coverings (*refer* Fig. 14.19):**
  - Two—inner fibrous capsule and outer renal fascia.
  - Fibrous capsule:
    - ¤ Dense sheet of connective tissue.
    - ¤ Can be stripped off in healthy kidney.
    - ¤ Protects and maintains shape of kidney.
  - Renal fascia—thin layer between kidney and surrounding structures.
  - Perinephric fat—between capsule and renal fascia.
  - Peritoneum covers the anterior aspect.

External features (Fig. 14.2):

- Two poles, two surfaces and two borders.
- **Poles**: Upper and lower.
- **Surfaces**:
  - Anterior and posterior.
  - Anterior surface—convex, related to viscera.
  - Posterior surface—flat and rests on the posterior abdominal wall.
- **Borders**:
  - Lateral and medial.
  - Lateral border is convex.
  - Hilum—depression on the medial aspect.
  - **Structures passing through hilum** (from anterior to posterior): Renal vein, renal artery and pelvis of ureter **(Fig. 14.2)**.

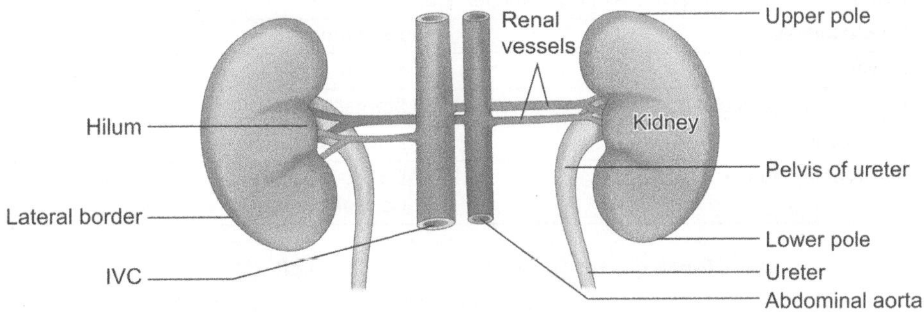

Fig. 14.2: Right and left kidneys—parts and blood vessels. (IVC: inferior vena cava)

Internal features (Fig. 14.3)

- Outer region is **cortex** and inner part is **medulla**.
- Medulla: Consists of conical **renal pyramids** (8-18).
- Cortex: Parts—cortical arches and columns.
- **Renal papilla**—narrow part of renal pyramid towards hilum.
- Renal papillae open into minor calyces.

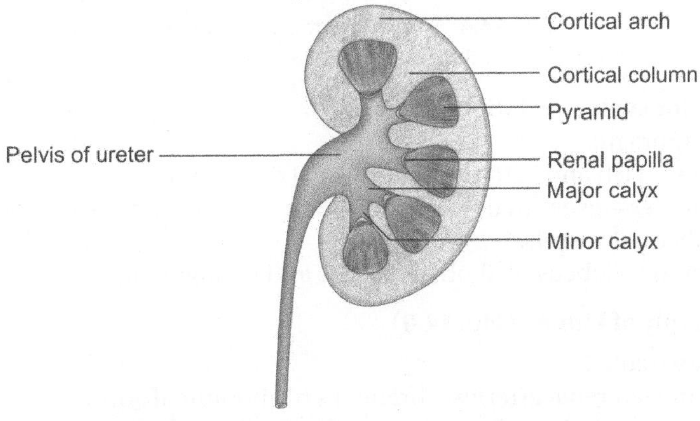

Fig. 14.3: Internal features of kidney in a coronal section.

- Minor calyces—join to form major calyces which open into pelvis of ureter.
- **Renal lobe**—consists of a renal pyramid with cortex around it.
- **Nephron**:
  - Functional unit of kidney.
  - Parts—renal corpuscle and renal tubule.
- Collecting tubules:
  - Receive tubules from nephron.
  - Form ducts of Bellini.
- Ducts of Bellini open in renal papilla.

Relations:

- **Upper pole:** Suprarenal gland.
- **Anterior surface**—*Refer* **Table 14.1 and Figure 14.4.**

Table 14.1: Anterior relations of right and left kidney.

Right kidney	Left kidney
Liver	Spleen
Duodenum (2nd part)	Stomach
Right colic flexure	Pancreas (body)
Coils of jejunum	Left colic flexure Coils of jejunum

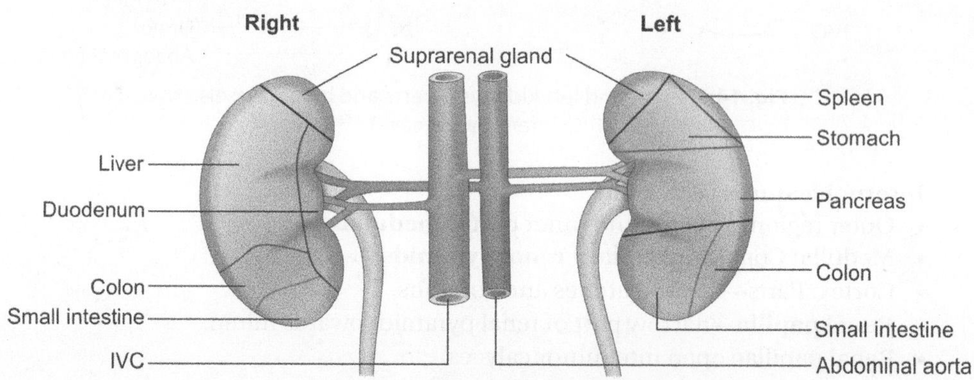

Fig. 14.4: Anterior relations of kidney.
(IVC: inferior vena cava)

- **Posterior surface relations (Fig. 14.5):**
  - Diaphragm.
  - Ribs—11th and 12th (left side), 12th (right side).
  - Muscles—psoas major, quadratus lumborum and transversus abdominis.
  - Subcostal vessels.
  - Nerves—subcostal, iliohypogastric and ilioinguinal.

Blood supply of kidney (Fig. 14.6)

- Highly vascular.
- Right and left renal arteries—branches of abdominal aorta.
- Renal veins—drain into inferior vena cava.

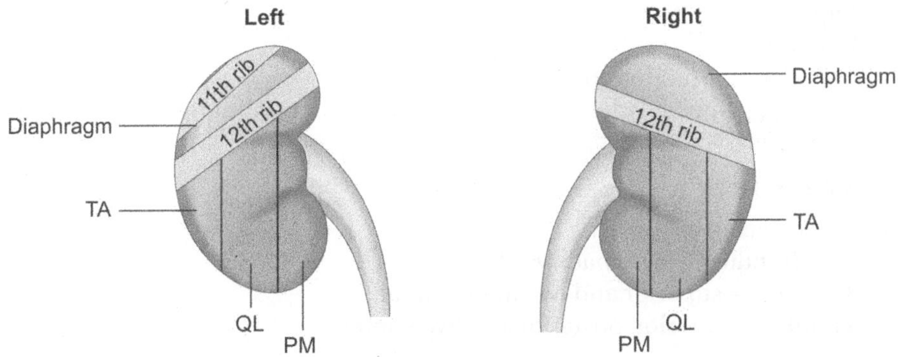

Fig. 14.5: Posterior relations of kidney.
(PM: psoas major; QL: quadratus lumborum; TA: transversus abdominis).

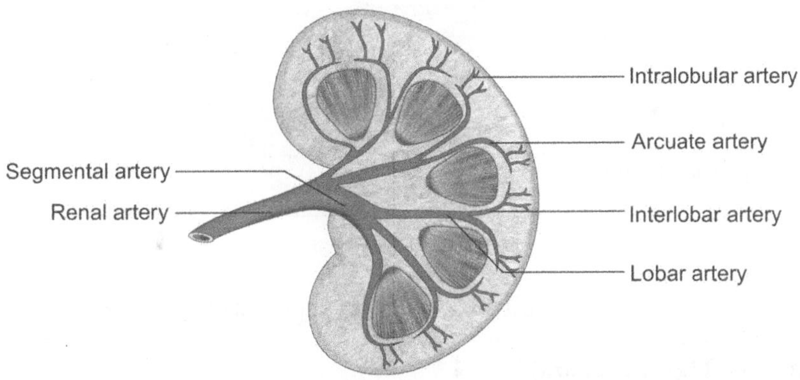

Fig. 14.6: Blood supply of kidney.

- Renal artery → segmental artery → lobar artery → interlobar artery → arcuate artery → interlobular artery → afferent arteriole → glomerulus → efferent arteriole → peritubular capillaries → interlobular vein → arcuate vein → interlobar vein → lobar vein → renal vein
- Lymphatic drainage: Lateral aortic lymph nodes.
- **Nerve supply**—renal ganglion and renal plexus.

Applied anatomy:
- Nephrectomy—surgical removal of kidney.
- Renal pain—dull pain in lumbar region.
- Pyelonephritis presents as—inflammation of kidney.

2. Draw a neat labeled diagram of urinary system. Explain in detail about urinary bladder.

Ans. *Refer* **Figure 14.1**.

Urinary bladder:
- Hollow, muscular viscera
- **Shape**:
  - Empty bladder—tetrahedral
  - Filled bladder—ovoid.

- **Capacity**: 120–320 mL
- **Position**:
  - Children—abdominopelvic
  - Adults—pelvic when empty and becomes abdominopelvic when filled with urine.

Parts (Fig. 14.7)

- Apex—facing forwards
- Base (fundus)—faces backwards
- 3 surfaces—superior and two inferolateral.
- 4 borders—anterior, posterior and two lateral.

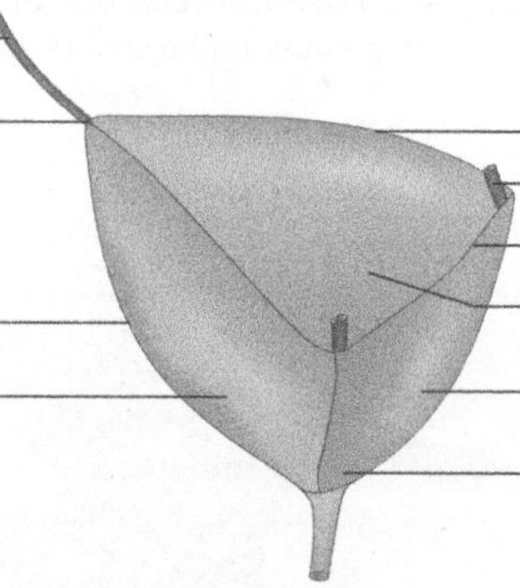

Fig. 14.7: External features of urinary bladder.

Relations (Figs. 14.8A and B)

- **Apex**—attached to median umbilical ligament.
- **Base**:
  - *In male:*
    - ¤ Upper part—rectovesical pouch between bladder and ampulla of rectum.
    - ¤ Lower part—seminal vesicles, ampulla of vas deferens and rectovesical fascia.
  - *In female:* Related to vagina and supravaginal part of cervix.
- **Superior surface:**
  - Related to sigmoid colon, coils of small intestine.
  - In females, rectouterine pouch is present between bladder and uterus.
- **Inferolateral surface**
  - Related to body of pubis, symphysis pubis, levator ani and obturator internus.
  - Space of Retzius—between bladder and pubis bone. Contains fat and vesical plexus of veins.
- **Anterior border**—separates two inferolateral surfaces.
- **Posterior border**—seen between two ureters. Separates superior surface and base.
- **Lateral border**—between ureter and apex. Separates superior and Inferolateral surfaces.
- **Neck of bladder:**
  - Lowest and most fixed part.
  - Seen 3–4 cm behind lower margin of symphysis pubis.
  - Related to prostate in males and to urogenital diaphragm in females.

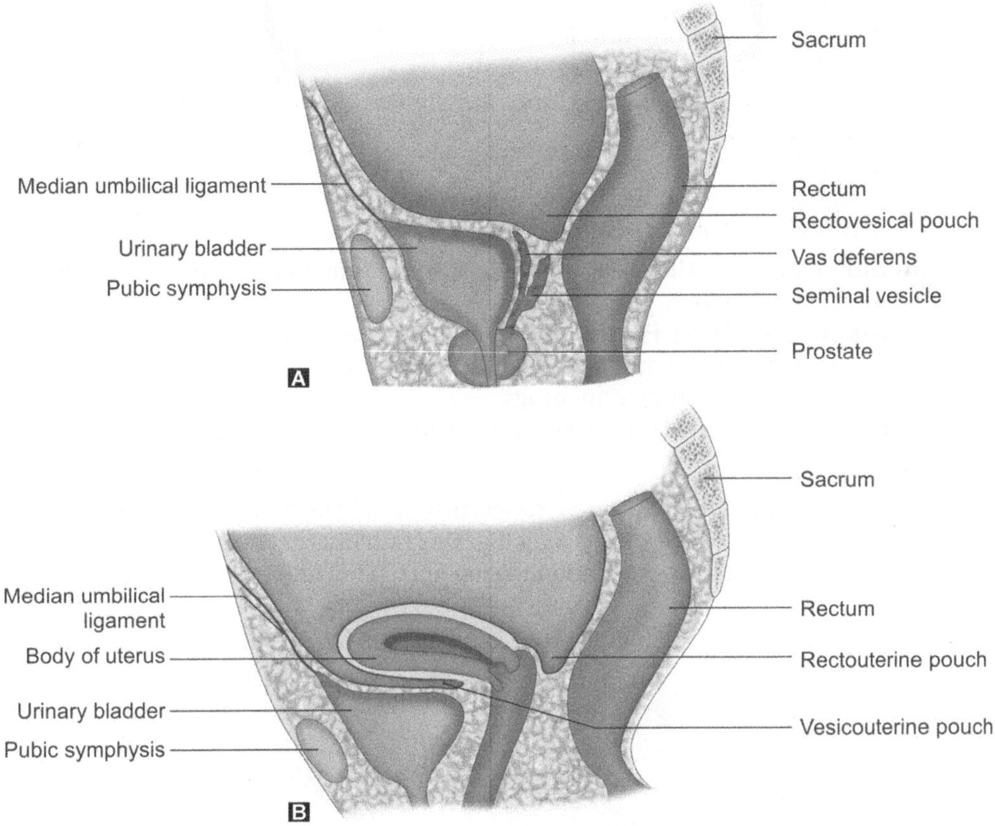

Figs. 14.8A and B: Relations of urinary bladder. (A) Male; (B) Female.

Ligaments of the urinary bladder:

True ligaments:

- Median umbilical ligament
- Puboprostatic or pubovesical ligaments
- Lateral ligaments
- Posterior ligaments

False ligaments: Peritoneal folds

- Median umbilical fold
- Medial umbilical fold
- Sacrogenital folds

Layers of urinary bladder (Fig. 14.9):

1. *Mucosa*:
   - Transitional epithelium
   - Surface cells are called as umbrella cells
2. *Lamina propria*:
   - Loose connective tissue
   - Absent in trigone

3. *Muscle layer:*
   - Consists of smooth muscle
   - Called as *detrusor* muscle
   - Arranged in three layers: Inner longitudinal, middle circular and outer longitudinal.
4. *Serosa:*
   - Lined by peritoneum (mesothelium and connective tissue)
   - Partially covers the bladder.

Interior of bladder: Mucosa is thrown into temporary folds or rugae. They disappear on filling of the bladder.

Internal trigone (*refer* Figure 14.10): It is a smooth area seen inside the urinary bladder. It is triangular with the following boundaries:

- Base: Between two ureter openings.
- Apex: Downwards, at internal urethral orifice.

Blood supply:

- Arterial—superior and inferior vesical arteries (branch of internal iliac artery)
- Veins—vesical venous plexus which drains into internal iliac vein
- Lymph drainage—external and internal iliac group of lymph nodes.

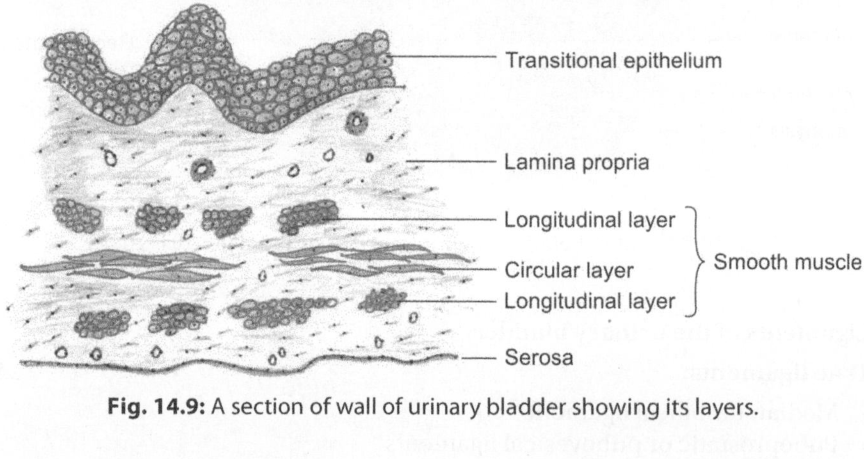

Fig. 14.9: A section of wall of urinary bladder showing its layers.

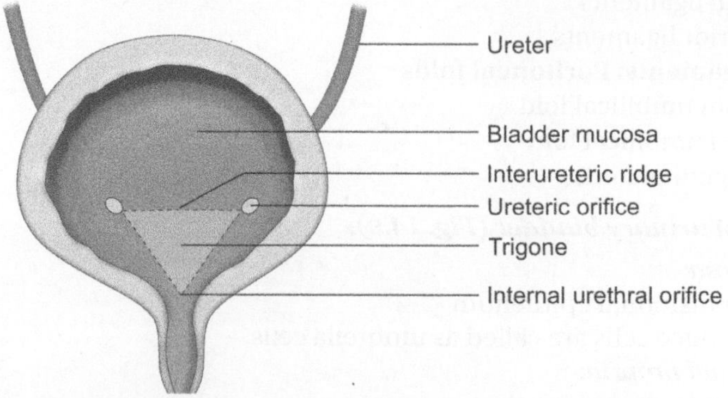

Fig. 14.10: Interior of bladder showing internal trigone.

Nerve supply:

A. Parasympathetic:
   - S2-S4 segments via pelvic splanchnic nerves.
   - Stimulates detrusor.
   - Causes emptying of bladder.

B. Sympathetic:
   - T10-L2 segments of the spinal cord via hypogastric plexus.
   - Inhibits detrusor and stimulates sphincter vesicae.
   - Prevents emptying of bladder.

Function of urinary bladder:

- To store urine till its excretion through urethra.
- To release urine by contraction of detrusor muscle.

Applied anatomy:

- Ectopia vesicae—congenital anomaly wherein urinary bladder is open to outside. The anterior wall of bladder and lower part of anterior abdominal wall are absent.
- Cystoscopy—an endoscopic instrument is passed into urinary bladder to examine its interior.
- Suprapubic cystostomy—a procedure to relieve distension of urinary bladder by puncturing it above pubic symphysis.

SHORT ESSAYS — 5 MARKS

3. Internal structure of kidney.

Ans. *Refer* **Figure 14.3.**

Coronal section:

Parts—inner medulla and outer cortex.

A. Cortex
   - Outer portion and granular in appearance.
   - Contains renal corpuscles, renal tubules except loop of Henle, and collecting ducts.

Parts

- Cortical arches—over the pyramids. Have medullary rays in between cortical tissue.
- Renal columns—in between the pyramids. Contain nephrons.
- Renal lobe—one renal pyramid with cortical tissue around it.

B. Medulla
   - Inner portion and striated in appearance.
   - Consists of renal pyramids.
   - Contains loop of Henle and collecting tubules.

Renal pyramids:

- Pale, conical.
- Base—outwards, towards cortex.
- Apex—round, forms renal papilla, inwards towards hilum.

Renal sinus is a space in kidney near the hilum.

Contents of renal sinus:
- Minor calyces—7 to 13 in numbers, cup-shaped and receive renal papillae
- Major calyces—2 to 3, formed by union of minor calyces
- Pelvis of ureter—funnel shaped and formed by union of major calyces
- Renal blood vessels
- Renal nerves and lymphatics
- Fat

4. Location and parts of urinary bladder.

Ans. Location:
- In children: It is abdominopelvic (since pelvis is small).
- In adults: When bladder is empty, it is situated within pelvis. The full bladder extends into abdomen.

Parts (Fig. 14.7):

In an empty bladder: Bladder is tetrahedral.

It has an apex, base, superior surface, two inferolateral surfaces, four borders and neck.

A. Apex—faces forwards, median umbilical ligament (urachus) is attached to it.
B. Borders—anterior, posterior and two lateral.
C. Base—located posteriorly.
D. Superior surface—covered with peritoneum.
E. Inferolateral surface—related to vesical plexus of veins.
F. Neck—lowest and most fixed. At the level of lower border of symphysis pubis.

5. Ureter.

Ans.
- Thick tube.
- Connects kidney to the urinary bladder.
- **Function**: Transfers urine from kidney to bladder by peristaltic contraction of ureter muscle.
- **Length**: 25 cm.

Parts (Fig. 14.11):
- Three parts—renal pelvis, abdominal and pelvic parts.
- *Pelvis of ureter*:
  - Upper dilated part
  - Formed by union of major calyces.
  - Continuous with abdominal part at lower end of kidney.
- *Abdominal part*:
  - On posterior abdominal wall.
  - Related to psoas major and transverse processes of lumbar vertebrae.
  - Becomes pelvic part after crossing pelvic brim.

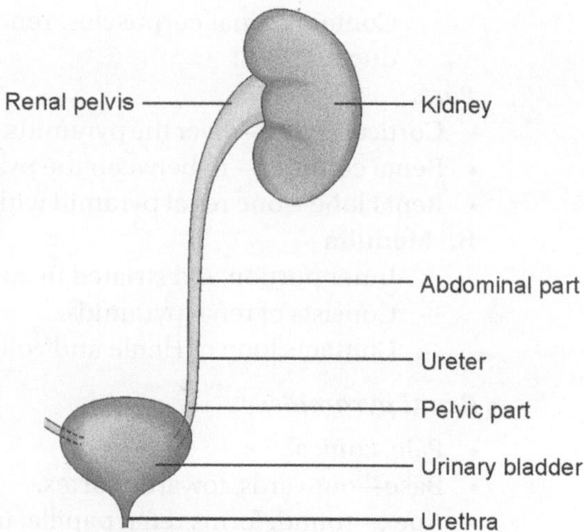

Fig. 14.11: Left ureter—parts.

- *Pelvic part*:
  - Opens inside bladder (at the trigone).
  - Lower end passes through bladder wall.
  - In females, it is related to cervix and uterine artery before entry into bladder and can be injured during surgery on uterus.

Constrictions:

Three constrictions.

- **First**—at the junction of renal pelvis and ureter.
- **Second**—at the pelvic brim.
- **Third**—just before entry into bladder.
- Importance—renal stones get lodged at constrictions.

Layers of ureter: The lumen is star shaped **(Fig. 14.12).**

- Mucosa (with transitional epithelium), muscle layer and adventitia.

Arterial supply: Branches from common iliac, internal iliac and ovarian arteries.

6. Male urethra.

Ans.

- Extends from internal urethral orifice to external urethral orifice.
- **Length**: 18–20 cm.
- **Parts**: Prostatic, membranous and spongy (**Fig. 14.13**).

A. Prostatic part (Fig. 14.14)

- Widest part, passes through the prostate gland.
- Length—3 cm.
- Features in the posterior wall:
  - Urethral crest—median, long mucous fold
  - Colliculus seminalis—an elevation in the middle of urethral crest which receives 3 openings: Prostatic utricle and two ejaculatory ducts
  - Prostatic sinuses—has openings of ducts of prostate.

B. Membranous part (Fig. 14.13)

- 5 mm in length
- Narrowest part
- Passes through urogenital diaphragm
- Sphincter urethrae muscle is present around it.

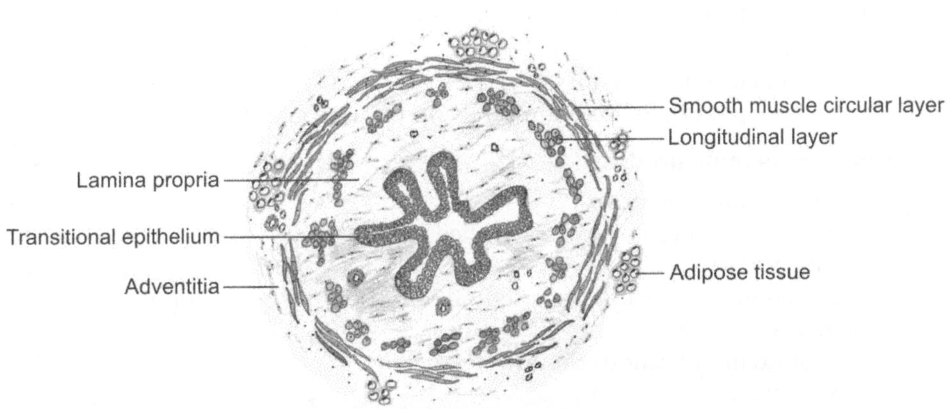

Fig. 14.12: Layers of ureter.

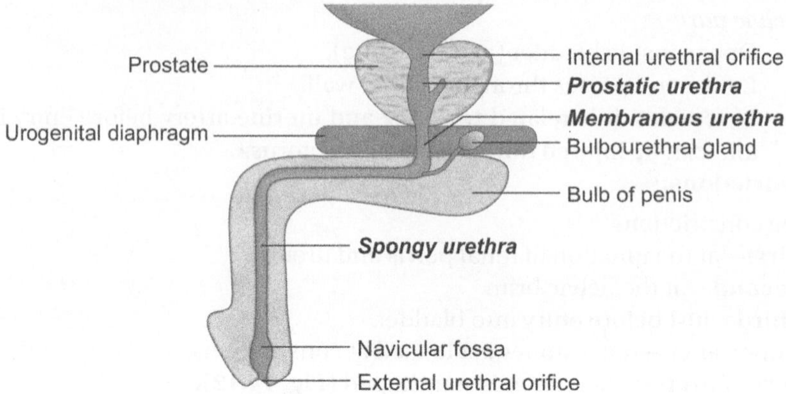

Fig. 14.13: Parts of male urethra.

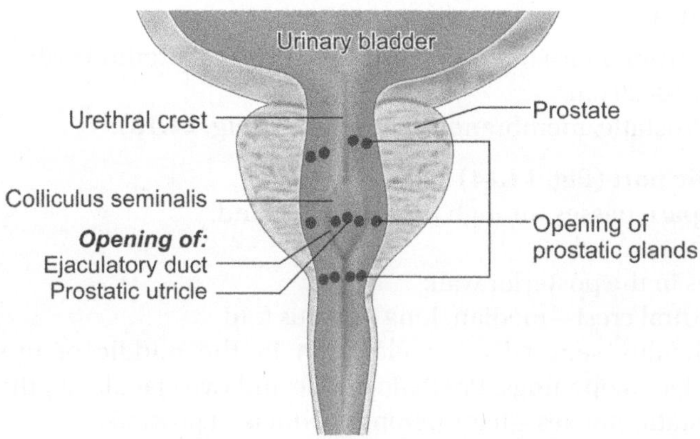

Fig. 14.14: Features of prostatic urethra.

C. Spongy part (Fig. 14.13)

- Length—15 cm, longest part of urethra
- Passes through bulb, body and glans of penis
- Shows two dilatations:
  - Intrabulbar fossa.
  - Navicular (terminal) fossa.
- It receives openings of bulbourethral and urethral glands.

Sphincters of male urethra:

- *Internal sphincter vesicae:*
  - Around the internal urethral orifice
  - Involuntary
  - Function—closes internal urethral orifice during ejaculation.
- *External sphincter:*
  - Around membranous urethra
  - Voluntary
  - Formed by sphincter urethrae muscle.

Anomalies:
- Hypospadias—urethra opening on undersurface of penis
- Epispadias—urethra opening on dorsal surface of penis.

7. Draw a neat labeled diagram of nephron and describe its parts.

Ans.
- Nephron is the functional unit of kidney.
- *Refer* **Figure 14.15** for diagram.
- Two types: Cortical and juxtamedullary.
- Cortical nephrons constitute 85% of total number of nephrons in kidney.
- Two parts: Renal corpuscle and renal tubule.

Renal corpuscle (*refer* Fig. 14.17):
- Consists of glomerulus and Bowman's capsule.
- Seen in renal cortex.
- *Glomerulus contains*: It is a capillary network within the Bowman's capsule. The afferent arteriole brings blood to the glomerular network and efferent arteriole takes blood away from it. The mesangial cells are present between capillaries.
- *Bowman's capsule:*
  - A double layer, cup-shaped structure around the glomerulus.
  - Layers: Outer parietal and inner visceral.
    i. Parietal layer—made of simple squamous epithelium.
    ii. Visceral layer:
      ¤ Close to glomerulus.
      ¤ Consists of podocytes.
  - **Capsular space**—between parietal and visceral layers.
  - The fluid filtered from the glomerulus enters the **capsular space** between two layers.

Renal tubules (Fig. 14.15)
- Consists of proximal convoluted tubule (PCT), nephron loop and distal convoluted tubule (DCT).
- Convoluted tubules are seen in cortex and nephron loop is seen in medulla.
- Proximal convoluted tubule:
  - Simple cuboidal epithelium with brush border.

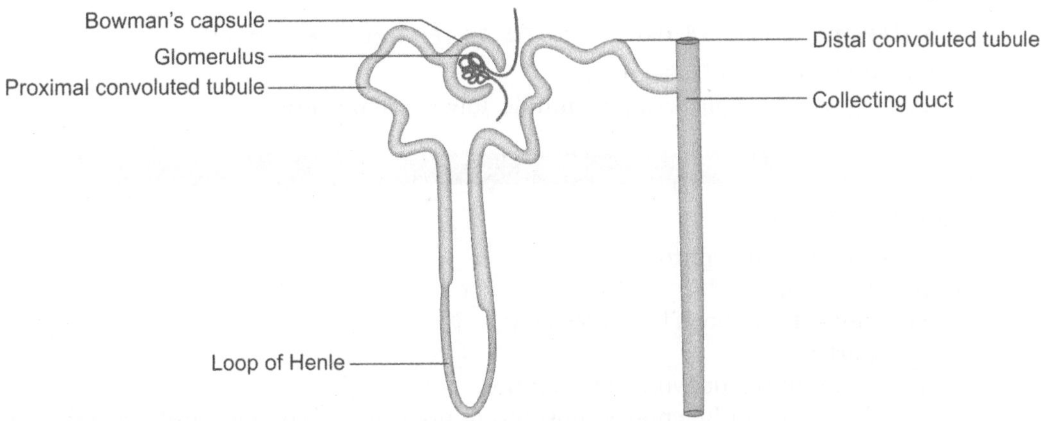

Fig. 14.15: Parts of nephron.

   - Lined by function—absorption of glucose, amino acids, sodium, chloride, phosphate and bicarbonate.
- Nephron loop:
   - U-shaped.
   - Parts—descending limb, loop of Henle and ascending limb.
- Distal convoluted tubule:
   - Extends from nephron loop to collecting tubule.
   - Cuboidal epithelium.
   - Lined by function—active absorption of water.

8. Blood supply of kidney.

Ans. **Arterial supply (Fig. 14.6):**

- Right and left renal arteries—branch from abdominal aorta.
- Right renal artery—longer than the left renal artery.
- Branching pattern of renal artery is given in **Flowchart 14.1**.

Flowchart 14.1: Branches of renal artery.

Segmental artery five in number → Lobar artery → Interlobar artery between renal pyramids → Arcuate artery over base of pyramid → Interlobular artery → Afferent arteriole → Glomerular plexus → Efferent arteriole → Peritubular plexus

Venous drainage:

- Renal veins—drain into inferior vena cava.
- Left renal vein—longer than the right renal vein.
- Tributaries:
   - Interlobular veins
   - Arcuate
   - Interlobar
   - Lobar

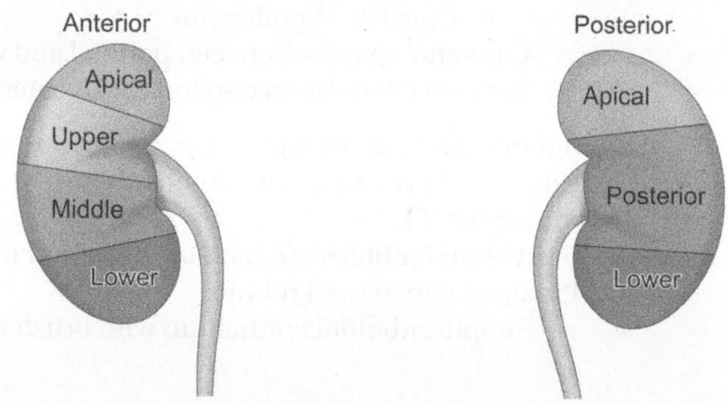

Fig. 14.16: Vascular segments of right kidney.

Renal segments (Fig. 14.16):

- Independent vascular segments.
- Five segments—apical, upper, middle, lower and posterior.

SHORT ANSWERS — 2 MARKS

9. Renal corpuscle.

Ans.
- Proximal part of nephron.
- Size: 0.2 mm.
- Function—filtration of blood plasma.
- Two parts:
   1. Glomerulus—network of capillaries.
   2. Glomerular or Bowman's capsule—double layered (parietal and visceral), cup-shaped and lined by epithelium **(Fig. 14.17)**.

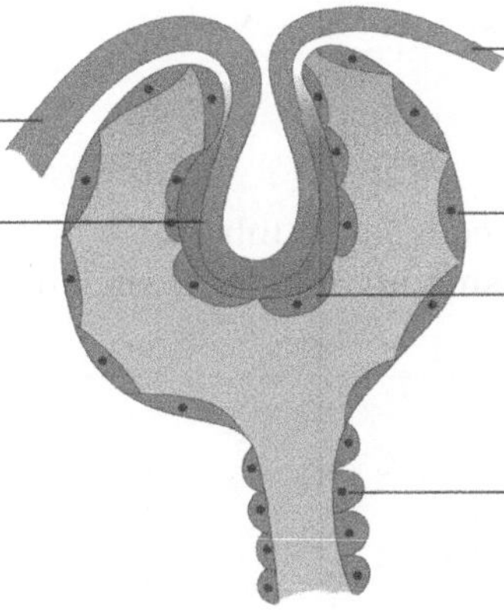

Fig. 14.17: A renal corpuscle.

10. Uriniferous tubule.

Ans.
- Two parts—secretory and collecting part.
  1. Secretory part—nephron.
  2. Collecting part—collecting tubule and duct.
- Function—to convert filtrate from glomerulus into urine.

11. Obstructive urinary disorders.

Ans.
- Normal flow of urine is affected.
- Hydronephrosis—swelling in kidney due to obstruction in flow of urine.
- Causes—kidney stones, stricture, bladder disorders and renal tumors.

12. Name the parts of ureter and the sites of its constrictions.

Ans. Three parts (*refer* **Fig. 14.11**)
1. Pelvis of ureter
2. Abdominal part
3. Pelvic part

Three constrictions:
1. At the pelvi-ureteric junction
2. At the pelvic brim and
3. At entry into bladder wall

13. Parts of a nephron.

Ans.
- Functional unit of kidney **(Fig. 14.15)**.
- Two parts—renal corpuscle and renal tubule.
  1. Renal corpuscle—consists of glomerulus and Bowman's capsule
  2. Renal tubule—made of:
     a. Proximal convoluted tubule (PCT).
     b. Loop of Henle.
     c. Distal convoluted tubule (DCT).

14. Name the structures at the hilum of kidney.

Ans. *Refer* **Figure 14.2**
- From anterior to posterior—renal vein, renal artery and renal pelvis.
- These structures are present in a space called as renal sinus.
- Renal pelvis—upper expanded part of the ureter.

15. Juxtaglomerular apparatus.

Ans.
- Situated near glomerulus.
- Function—produces renin.
- Formed by **(Fig. 14.18)**:
  - Macula densa of distal convoluted tubule.
  - Juxtaglomerular cells (smooth muscle) of afferent arteriole.

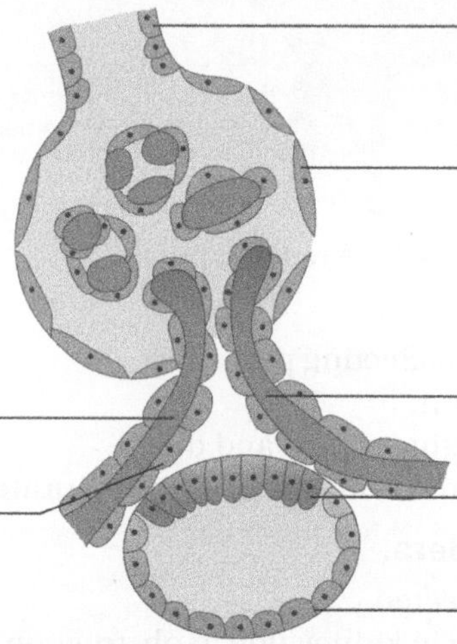

Fig. 14.18: Juxtaglomerular apparatus.

16. Internal trigone of urinary bladder.

Ans.
- It is a triangular, smooth area of the mucosa (*refer* **Fig. 14.10**)
- Seen inside the urinary bladder.
- It is present on the posterior wall.
- Boundaries:
  - Base—upwards, between openings of ureters.
  - Apex—downwards, at urethra opening (internal urethral orifice).

17. Name the parts of urinary/excretory system.

Ans. Two kidneys, two ureters, one urinary bladder and one urethra.

18. Functions of parts of urinary system.

Ans.
- Kidney
  - Removes metabolic waste products by producing urine.
  - Regulates fluid balance of body.
  - Secretes renin and erythropoietin.
- Ureter— brings urine from kidney to urinary bladder.
- Urinary bladder:
  - Stores the urine till its excretion.
  - Expels urine from the body through the urethra.

19. Differences between urethra in male and female urethra.

Ans. *Refer* **Table 14.2.**

Table 14.2: Comparison between male and female urethra.

Feature	Male urethra	Female urethra
Length	20 cm	4 cm
Function	Passage for urine and semen	Passage for urine
Course	Passes through prostate, urogenital diaphragm and penis	Passes through urogenital diaphragm, close to anterior vaginal wall
Parts	Prostatic, membranous and spongy	None
Openings	Glands, prostatic utricle and ejaculatory duct	Glands
Fossae	Intrabulbar and navicular	None
Glands related	Prostatic, bulbourethral and urethral	Urethral, paraurethral and greater vestibular
Urethral artery	Branch from internal pudendal artery	Branch from vaginal artery
Infections	Less common	More common due to short length

20. Renal capsule.

Ans.
- Inner fibrous capsule **(Fig. 14.19)**.
- Covers kidney.
- It is made of dense connective tissue.
- Can be easily stripped off in a healthy kidney.
- Function:
  - Gives protection from injury.
  - Maintains shape of kidney.

21. Name the layers of ureter.

Ans. Three layers **(*refer* Figure 14.12):**
- Mucosa: Transitional epithelium and lamina propria.
- Muscle layer: Made of inner longitudinal and outer circular smooth muscle layers; extra outer longitudinal layer is seen in lower part.
- Adventitia: Loose connective tissue layer with blood vessels and nerves.

22. Name the layers of urinary bladder.

Ans. Layers (*refer* **Figure 14.9**)
- Mucosa
  - Has transitional epithelium.
  - Lamina propria—made of connective tissue and supports the epithelium.
- Muscle layer (detrusor)—made of inner longitudinal, middle circular and outer longitudinal smooth muscle layers.
- Adventitia—loose connective tissue layer with blood vessels and nerves.
- Serosa—seen in areas where peritoneum covers bladder.

23. Urethral sphincters.

Ans. Internal and external **(Fig. 14.20)**
- Internal urethral sphincter:
  - Consists of circular smooth muscle fibers
  - Situated around internal urethral orifice
  - Involuntary
  - Function—closes internal urethral orifice during ejaculation.

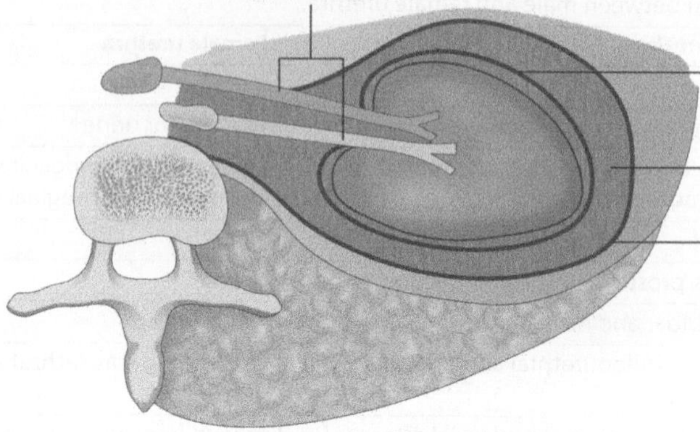

Fig. 14.19: Coverings of kidney (left).

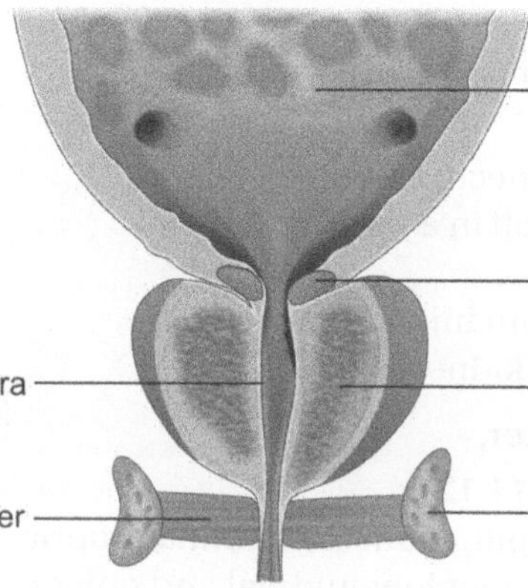

Fig. 14.20: Urethral sphincters.

- External urethral sphincter:
  - Seen below internal sphincter
  - Located around membranous urethra
  - Made of circular skeletal muscle
  - Under voluntary control.

24. What is the total length of male urethra and what are its parts?

Ans.
- Parts—prostatic, membranous and spongy urethra **(Fig. 14.13)**.
- Length—20 cm.
- Prostatic:
  - Wide
  - In prostate
  - Has openings of ejaculatory duct, prostatic utricle and prostate glands.
- Membranous:
  - In urogenital diaphragm.
- Spongy:
  - Longest part
  - Has opening of bulbourethral glands.

25. Name the structures opening in male urethra.

Ans.
- Prostatic glands
- Ejaculatory ducts
- Bulbourethral glands
- Urethral glands

26. Female urethra.

Ans.
- Female urethra is short, measures 4 cm
- It begins at neck of the urinary bladder, passes through urogenital diaphragm.
- Its course is close to the anterior wall of vagina.
- It opens into the vestibule between the labia minora, above the vaginal opening.
- Since it is short, urinary tract infections are more common in females.

27. Stress incontinence.

Ans.
- Most common type of incontinence.
- Presents as leakage of urine from urinary bladder.
- Due to weakness of pelvic floor.
- Seen usually in multiparous women.
- Leakage occurs during activities that increase abdominal pressure like coughing, laughing, sneezing, exercising and lifting heavy objects.

28. Kidney biopsy.

Ans.
- A biopsy needle is used to obtain tissue from kidney in cases of suspected renal cancer.
- To avoid damage to pleura, needle is inserted in the lower part of kidney to get the tissue sample.

29. Name the openings in urinary bladder.

Ans.
- Two ureteric orifices
- One internal urethral opening.

30. What are the two main functions of urinary bladder?

Ans.
- Is a reservoir for urine
- Releases urine from the bladder once it is full.

31. List the differences between renal cortex and medulla.

Ans. *Refer* **Table 14.3.**

Table 14.3: Differences between renal cortex and medulla.

Renal cortex	**Renal medulla**
Outer	Inner
Made of cortical arches and columns	Made of renal pyramids
Granular	Striated
Contains renal corpuscles, convoluted tubules and medullary rays	Contains nephron loop, collecting tubules and ducts of Bellini
Light red	Darker reddish-brown

32. Name accessory organs of urinary system.

Ans.
- Ureters
- Urinary bladder
- Urethra

33. What is the order of fluid flow through nephron?

Ans.
- Glomerulus-blood gets filtered.
- PCT, loop of Henle, DCT— reabsorption occurs
- Collecting duct—secretion and reabsorption
- Finally, the filtrate becomes urine and enters ureter.

34. Bowman's capsule.

Ans.
- A cup-shaped structure made of double layer of epithelium.
- It surrounds the glomerulus.
- Two layers of capsule are: Inner visceral and outer parietal.
    1. Inner layer—contains podocytes which send foot-like processes around the capillary endothelial cells.
    2. Parietal layer—formed by flat cells of simple squamous epithelium.
- Capsular space—between two layers.

35. Glomerulus.

Ans.
- A capillary network shaped like a ball.
- Covered by Bowman's capsule.
- The capillaries start from afferent arteriole and end in efferent arteriole.
- Afferent arteriole usually larger than efferent arteriole.
- Mesangial cell are seen between capillaries of glomerulus.

36. What are the various types of nephrons?

Ans.
- Two types: Cortical and juxtamedullary.
- Cortical: 85%.
- Juxtamedullary: 15%.
- Function:
    - Cortical nephrons: Sodium absorption.
    - Juxtamedullary nephron: Water absorption.

37. Cystitis.

Ans.
- Inflammation of urinary bladder.
- Cause—bladder stone, infection and tumors.
- More common in females due to short urethra.
- Leads to pelvic pain, frequent urination and hematuria.

38. Pyelonephritis.

Ans.
- Inflammation of renal pelvis and kidney tissue.
- Causes—infection (bacterial, fungal or viral), calculi (stone) and tumors.

39. Nephrotic syndrome.

Ans.
- Glomerular disorder.
- Passage of protein in urine (proteinuria).
- Low albumin levels in blood (hypoalbuminemia).
- Collection of fluid in tissues (edema).

40. Glomerulonephritis.

Ans.
- Damage to membrane of glomerular capsule.
- Causes—immune disorder, heredity, etc.

41. Pyelography.

Ans.
- A radiological study of kidney and urinary tract using a contrast medium.
- It is used to examine calyces, renal pelvis and ureter.
- Types—intravenous and retrograde.
  1. Intravenous pyelography: Iodine containing contrast medium is injected in a vein and it is excreted by kidney. X-ray is taken after few minutes to visualize the calyces and ureter.
  2. Retrograde pyelography: A cystoscope is used to locate the ureter opening in urinary bladder. An iodine solution is injected into ureteric opening via catheter and X-ray is taken to see ureter and calyces.

15
CHAPTER

Reproductive System

LONG ESSAYS — 10 MARKS

1. Draw a neat labeled diagram of the parts of male reproductive system. Describe testes under—external features, coverings, internal structure, blood supply and applied anatomy.

Ans. *Refer* **Figure 15.1**.

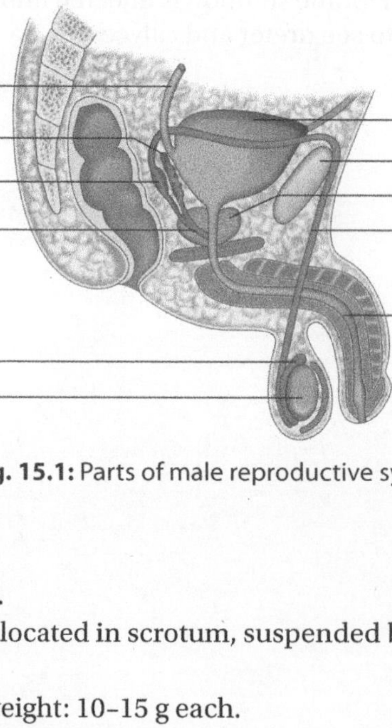

Fig. 15.1: Parts of male reproductive system.

Testis:

- Is the male gonad.
- It is paired organ, located in scrotum, suspended by spermatic cords.
- Shape: Oval.
- Size: 5 × 2.5 cm; weight: 10–15 g each.
- Function: Formation of sperms and synthesis of male hormones like testosterone.

External features (Fig. 15.2):

- Two ends—upper and lower.
- Two surfaces—medial and lateral.
- Two borders—anterior and posterior.
- Upper pole—related to head of epididymis.
- Epididymis (body) and vas deferens seen on the posterior aspect.

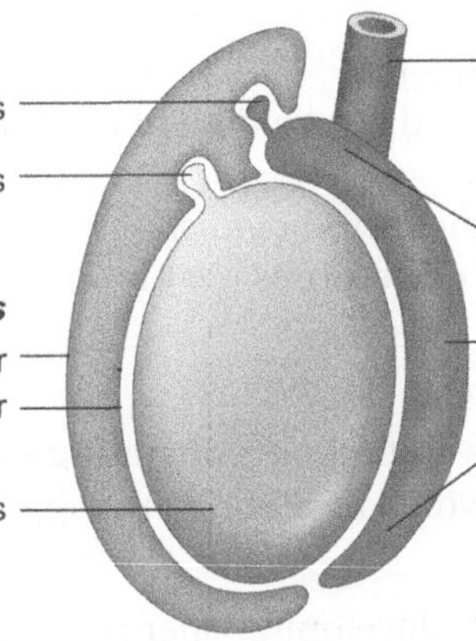

Fig. 15.2: Testis and epididymis with tunica vaginalis.

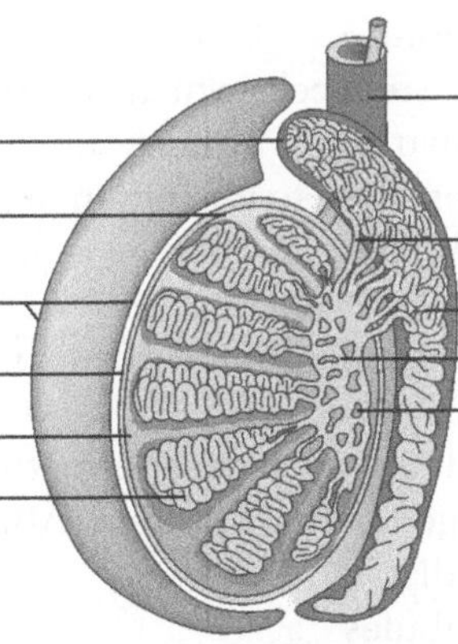

Fig. 15.3: Coverings and internal structure of testis.

Coverings—from outside to inside (Fig. 15.3):

- Layers of scrotum—skin, dartos muscle, external spermatic fascia, cremasteric fascia, internal spermatic fascia.
- Tunica vaginalis—has outer parietal and inner visceral layers and in between is a potential space **(Fig. 15.2)**.
- Tunica albuginea—tough, fibrous layer. It forms a thick mediastinum testis on posterior aspect.
- Tunica vasculosa—is the innermost layer that contains blood vessels.

Sinus of epididymis: A small recess of tunica vaginalis between testis and epididymis on the posterolateral aspect.

Internal structure (Fig. 15.3):

- Below tunica albuginea, the fibrous septa divide the testis into lobules.
- In each testis, 200-300 lobules are seen.
- Each lobule contains highly coiled, one to three seminiferous tubules.
- **Rete testis**—a network formed by seminiferous tubules in the mediastinum testis.
- **Efferent ductules:**
  - Arise from rete testis

  - 12–20 in number
  - Form head of epididymis
- Efferent ductules join and form a **duct of epididymis**.
- **Duct of epididymis**:
  - Forms body and tail of epididymis.
  - Continues as **ductus deferens** near lower pole of testis.

Seminiferous tubules:
- Site of **spermatogenesis.**
- Lined by seminiferous epithelium containing sperm forming cells (spermatogonia and spermatocytes), which lie among the supporting sertoli cells.

Blood-testis barrier:
- Separates blood from developing sperms to prevent immune reaction against sperm antigens.
- Formed by tight junctions between Sertoli cells.

Cells in seminiferous tubule:
1. Spermatogonia are the stem cells which give rise to spermatocytes.
2. Spermatocytes are of two types: primary and secondary.
3. Mature sperms are seen close to the lumen of tubules.
4. Sertoli or sustentacular cells:
   - Large cells.
   - Extend from basement membrane to the lumen of tubule.
   - Functions:
     i. To support and to protect the spermatogonia cells.
     ii. To secrete antigen binding protein (ABP) and inhibin.
5. Interstitial cells of Leydig:
   - Located between tubules
   - Produce testosterone

Blood and nerve supply:

Arterial supply: Testicular artery—branch of abdominal aorta.

Venous drainage:
- By pampiniform plexus—network of 8–12 veins in the spermatic cord.
- These veins join and form a testicular vein.
- Right testicular vein—opens into inferior vena cava
- Left testicular vein—drains into left renal vein.

Lymphatic drainage—lumbar and preaortic lymph nodes.

Nerve supply—testicular nerve plexus.

Applied anatomy:
- Cryptorchidism—undescended testis.
- Hydrocele—accumulation of excess fluid in tunica vaginalis.
- Varicocele—enlargement of veins of pampiniform plexus.

2. Draw a neat labeled diagram of the female reproductive system. Describe the uterus under—position, parts, relations, blood supply and applied anatomy.

Ans. Uterus is a hollow, muscular organ of female reproductive system **(Fig. 15.4).**

Location: In the pelvic cavity between urinary bladder and rectum.

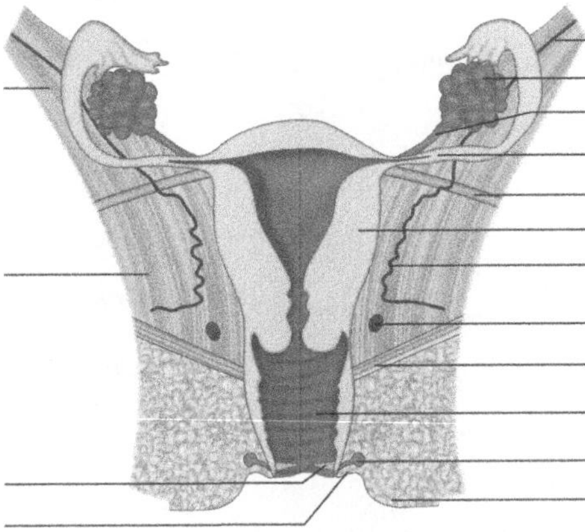

Fig. 15.4: Parts of female reproductive system.

Shape and size:

- Inverted pear-shaped.
- 7.5 × 5 × 2.5 cm (3 × 2 × 1 inches).
- Increases in size in pregnancy due to hypertrophy.
- Larger in multiparous than nulliparous.
- Smaller after menopause.

Position (Fig. 15.5):

- Anteflexion and anteversion.
- Anteflexion—the forward bend of uterus in relation to the cervix (125°).
- Anteversion—the forward bend of cervix to form a right angle (90°) with the axis of vagina.

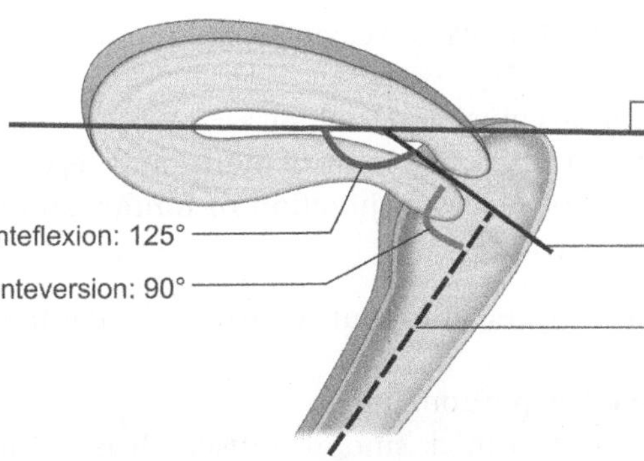

Fig. 15.5: Normal position of uterus.

Function: Site for implantation of a fertilized ovum and its further development till fetus is fully formed.

Parts: Fundus, body and cervix (**Fig. 15.6**).

- **Fundus**
  - Region above the attachment of uterine tubes.

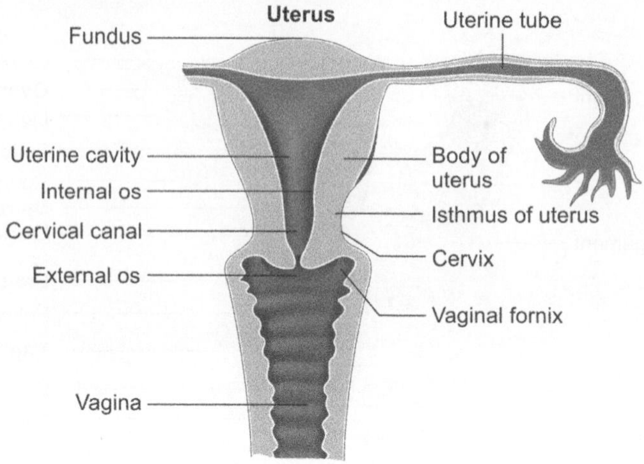

Fig. 15.6: Parts of uterus.

- Covered with peritoneum.
- Uterine cavity does not extend into fundus.

- **Body**
  - Large central portion.
  - Contains triangular uterine cavity.
  - Covered with peritoneum.
  - Two surfaces: Anterior and posterior.
  - Two lateral borders.
  - Broad ligament is attached to lateral margins.
- **Cervix**
  - Lower, cylindrical part.
  - Contains cervical canal.
  - Cervical canal opens into uterine cavity by an internal os and into vagina by an external os.
  - Parts of cervix: Supravaginal and vaginal.
- Isthmus—constricted part between body of uterus and cervix.
- Cornua—lateral angles of uterus at junction of fundus and body. Uterine tubes open here into uterine cavity.

Layers—Uterus has **three** layers. From outside to inside: Perimetrium, myometrium and endometrium.

1. Perimetrium—formed by peritoneum.
2. Myometrium—made up of thick smooth muscle. It is arranged in three layers: inner longitudinal, middle oblique and outer longitudinal.
3. Endometrium—mucous membrane lined with simple columnar epithelium. Uterine glands and spiral arteries are seen in endometrium. Forms decidua in pregnancy.

Relations (Fig. 15.7):

- *Anterior surface:*
  - Vesicouterine pouch and urinary bladder.

- Peritoneum covers anterior aspect of body of uterus up to isthmus and reflects to bladder anteriorly. Supravaginal part of cervix is not covered with peritoneum.
- *Posterior surface:* Rectouterine pouch (pouch of Douglas), sigmoid colon and small intestine. Peritoneum covers supravaginal part of cervix.
- *Lateral*: Broad ligament and uterine vessels.

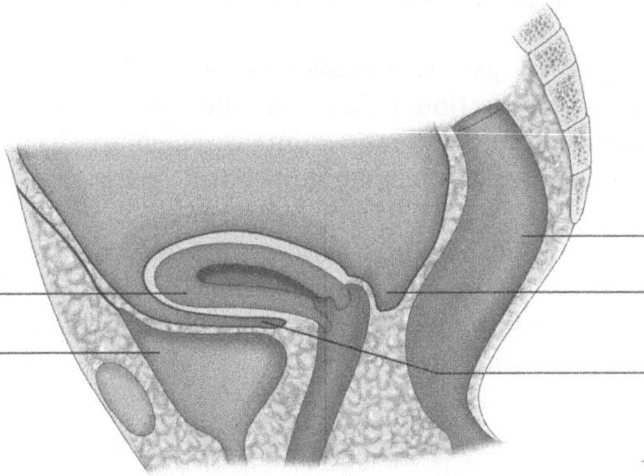

Fig. 15.7: Peritoneal relations of uterus.

Blood supply (Fig. 15.4):

- Arteries—uterine and ovarian arteries.
- Veins—uterine and ovarian venous plexus.
- Lymphatics—
  - Fundus: Superficial inguinal lymph nodes
  - Body of uterus and cervix: Preaortic and lateral aortic lymph nodes.

Applied anatomy:

1. Hysterectomy:
   - The surgical removal of uterus.
   - Uterus is removed through abdominal wall or vagina.
   - It is done in cases with carcinoma of uterus and cervix.
2. Prolapse of uterus:
   - Supports of uterus become weak after multiple childbirths.
   - In subjects with weak uterine support, any increase in intra-abdominal pressure, leads to prolapse of uterus (uterus is pushed through the vagina).
3. Endometriosis:
   - The presence of endometrial tissue outside the uterine cavity.
   - This tissue can be seen on the ovary, or on the peritoneum between uterus and rectum.
   - It goes through cyclical changes like the endometrium in uterus.
   - The patient can complain of infertility or pain during menstruation.

SHORT ESSAYS 5 MARKS

3. Spermatogenesis.

Ans. *Refer* **Figure 15.8.**

Spermatogenesis is the process of formation of mature sperms from spermatogonia.

- Starts at puberty.
- Takes place in seminiferous tubules of testis. Tubules are lined by spermatogonia, spermatocytes and spermatids. After formation sperms are released into the lumen of tubules.
- Each cycle of spermatogenesis requires 64 days.
- Requires high concentration of testosterone and low temperature. Luteinizing hormone (LH) from pituitary gland stimulates Leydig cells to secrete testosterone.
- During spermatogenesis, spermatogonia and spermatocytes are supported by Sertoli cells.

Spermatogonia—multiply by mitosis and produce **primary spermatocytes**.

- Primary spermatocyte—gives rise to secondary spermatocytes by meiosis.
- Each secondary spermatocyte—divides to form two spermatids.
- Spermatid forms a mature sperm by a process called as spermiogenesis.

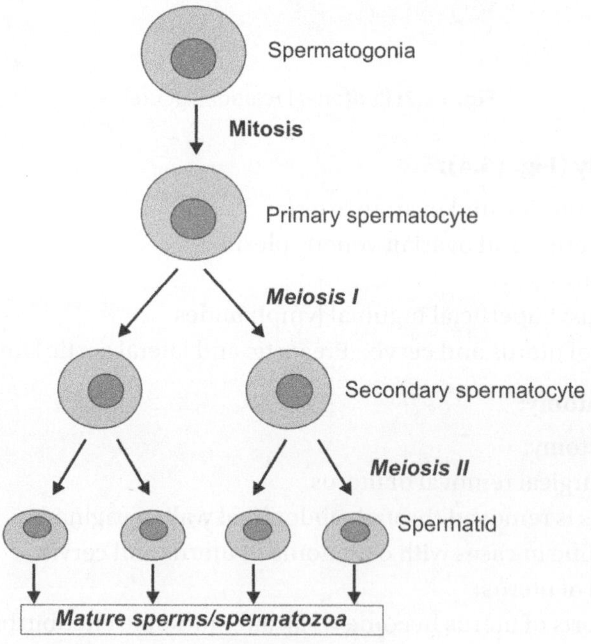

Fig. 15.8: Spermatogenesis.

4. Vas (ductus) deferens.

Ans. Vas deferens is a thick, cord-like tube and most important content of the spermatic cord.

- Easily palpable in spermatic cord through the skin.
- Length: 45 cm.
- Function—transports sperms to urethra for ejaculation.

Origin, course and termination of Vas deferens (Fig. 15.9):

Origin:
- At lower pole of testis
- From tail of epididymis

Termination:
- Behind urinary bladder
- Joins duct of seminal vesicle

Course:
- Upward after origin
- Located behind testis and medial to epididymis
- Passes through spermatic cord, inguinal canal and pelvic cavity
- Reaches posterior aspect of urinary bladder
- Ampulla of vas—dilatation of vas before termination.

Structure of vas deferens:
- Small lumen
- Thick smooth muscle in the wall
- Contraction of muscle helps in transport of sperms.

Applied anatomy:

Vasectomy
- Method of family planning.
- Vas deferens of both sides is ligated so that sperms cannot reach urethra during ejaculation.
- This procedure does not affect the sperm production in testis.

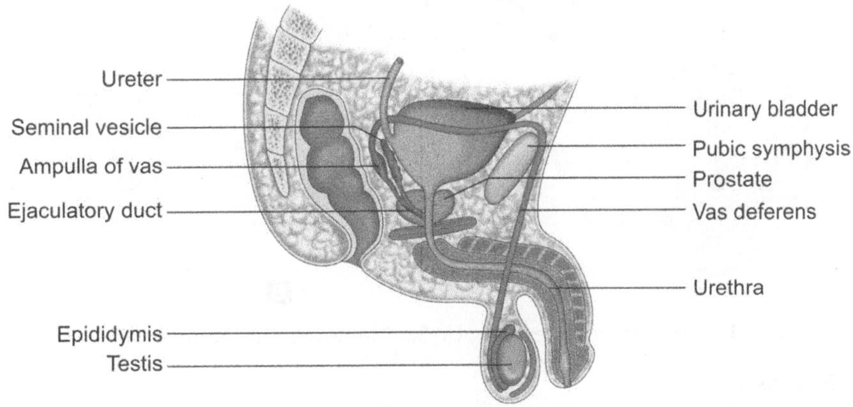

Fig. 15.9: Vas deferens.

5. Prostate gland.

Ans. Prostate gland is the single, largest accessory male reproductive gland **(Fig. 15.10)**
- Location—below urinary bladder, around the prostatic urethra
- Size—3 × 4 × 2 cm
- Capsules—inner true capsule and outer false capsule.

Parts (Fig. 15.10):

A. **Base**: Located above and related to the neck of urinary bladder.
B. **Apex**: Located below and related to urogenital diaphragm.
C. **Surfaces**:
   i. Anterior surface is related to pubic symphysis.
   ii. Posterior surface is related to rectum.
   iii. Inferolateral surfaces related to levator ani muscle.
D. **Lobes: Five lobes (Figs. 15.11A and B):**
   i. Anterior
   ii. Posterior
   iii. Two lateral
   iv. Median

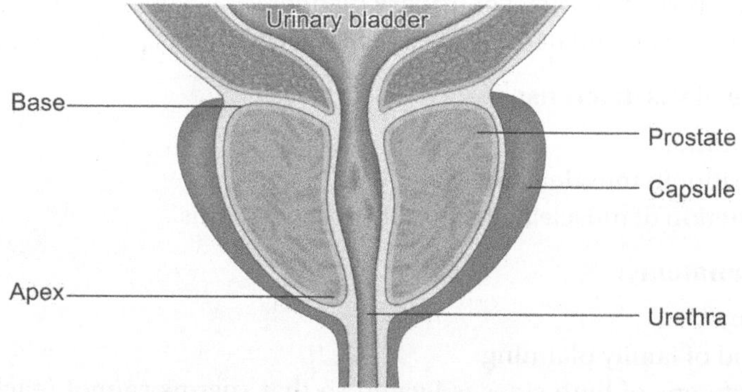

Fig. 15.10: Prostate—location and parts.

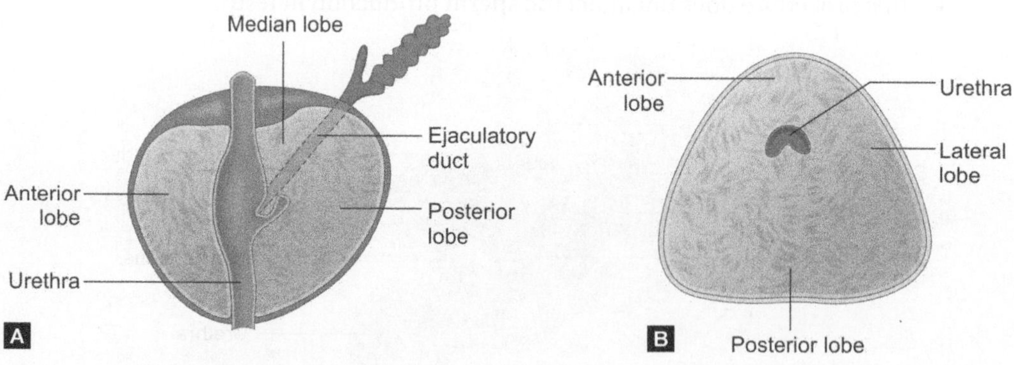

Figs. 15.11A and B: Prostate lobes. (A) Sagittal section; (B) Transverse section.

- **Microstructure:**
   i. Consists of fibrous, muscular and glandular tissue.
   ii. Prostatic glands open into prostatic urethra.
- **Structures passing through prostate (Fig. 15.12)**
   i. Prostatic urethra
   ii. Two ejaculatory ducts
   iii. Prostatic utricle.
   iv. Ejaculatory ducts and utricle—open in prostatic urethra.

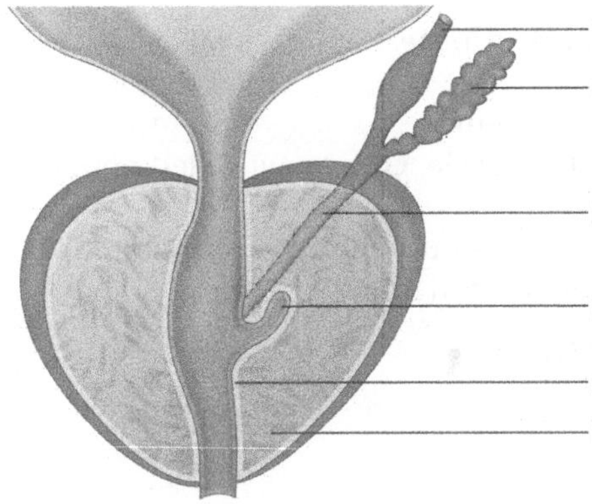

Fig. 15.12: Structures passing through prostate.

Blood supply:

Arterial: Inferior vesical, middle rectal and internal pudendal.

Venous:

i. Prostate venous plexus- between two capsules
ii. Drains into internal iliac veins
iii. Communicates with vesical plexus and vertebral Batson's plexus.

Functions:

i. Produces milky, slightly acidic fluid
ii. Produces enzyme—prostatic specific antigen (PSA).

Prostate secretions:

i. Make 25% of semen volume.
ii. Rich in acid phosphatase.
iii. Important for sperm motility and survival.

Applied anatomy:

- Benign prostatic hypertrophy (BPH): Involves inner zone of the gland.
  i. Enlargement of median lobe in old age.
  ii. Obstructs the outflow of urine from bladder.
  iii. Patient complains of difficulty in passing urine—prostate enlargement is the most common cause of this complaint in the elderly.
- Prostate cancer—involves outer zone of the gland. It can spread via venous blood and result in metastasis to vertebral column.

6. Scrotum.

Ans. Testes are located outside abdominal cavity in a sac called scrotum. The word scrotum is derived from Latin and means a purse-like covering or skin for testes.

- **Location**—continues below from inguinal region of abdominal wall, and seen below and behind penis.
- **Contents**—testes, epididymis and lower part of spermatic cord.
- **Function**—to protect the testis.

This is essential since the sperm formation needs low temperature (2–3°C below the body core temperature). In warm temperature, dartos muscle relaxes to move testes away from body. In cold climate, dartos contracts to move testes closer to body to maintain temperature.

Features:

a. Skin—thin, dark in color and loose. Raphe—a raised, narrow band on outer aspect in the midline.
b. The subcutaneous fat is absent.
c. Dartos muscle—smooth muscle. Gives a wrinkled appearance to scrotum when contracts.
d. Scrotal septum—each testis is present in a sac separated in the middle by a scrotal septum. The skin will not extend into the septum.

Layers of scrotum (Fig. 15.13):

1. Skin
2. Dartos
3. External spermatic fascia
4. Cremasteric fascia
5. Internal spermatic fascia
6. Parietal layer of tunica vaginalis

Nerve supply—from lumbar and sacral plexus of nerves.

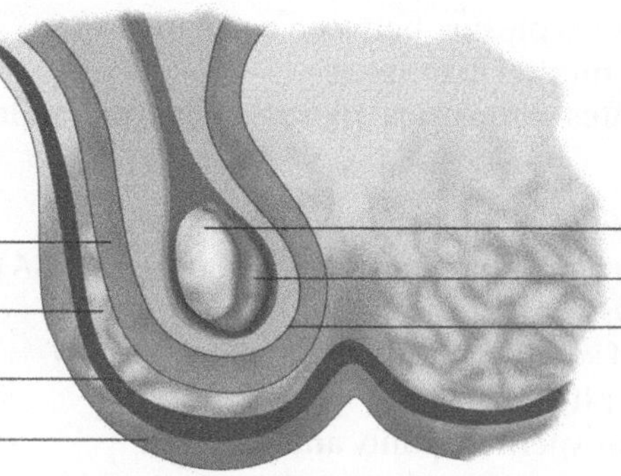

Fig. 15.13: Layers of scrotum.

7. Spermatic cord.

Ans.
- It is a cord-like structure of the male reproductive tract containing the vas deferens, and associated blood vessels and nerves.
- Extent—from upper end of testis to the deep inguinal ring of inguinal canal.
- Length: 7.5 cm.
- Coverings of spermatic cord (inside to outside):
  i. Internal spermatic fascia.
  ii. Cremasteric fascia.
  iii. External spermatic fascia.
- **List of contents (structures passing through spermatic cord) (Fig. 15.14)**
  1. Ductus (vas) deferens
  2. Three arteries (testicular artery, artery to ductus deferens and cremasteric artery)
  3. Nerves (genital branch of genitofemoral nerve and testicular plexus)
  4. Veins (pampiniform plexus)
  5. Lymphatics
  6. Remnant of processus vaginalis
  7. Loose connective tissue

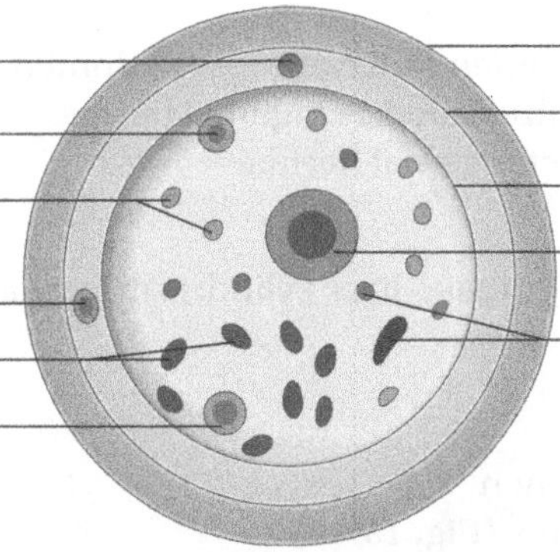

Fig. 15.14: Coverings and contents of spermatic cord.

8. Inguinal canal.

Ans. Inguinal canal is an oblique canal in anterior abdominal wall, above the medial part of inguinal ligament.

- Extent of inguinal canal—deep inguinal ring to the superficial inguinal ring **(Fig. 15.15)**
- Length: 4 cm.
  A. Superficial inguinal ring—opening in external oblique aponeurosis.
  B. Deep inguinal ring—opening in fascia transversalis (fascia lining inside of transversus abdominis muscle of abdominal wall).

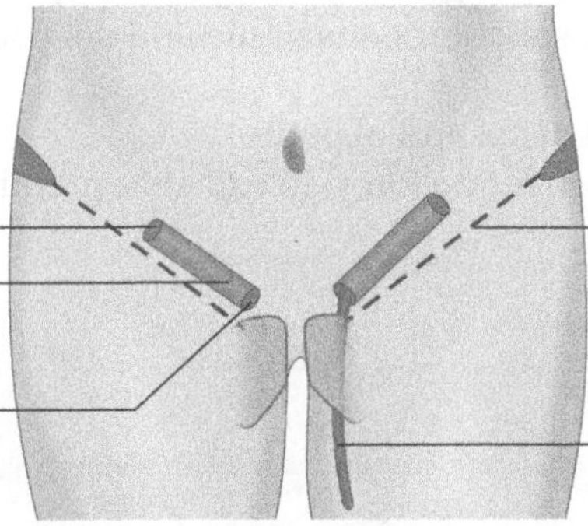

Fig. 15.15: Inguinal canal.

Boundaries:

- Floor—inguinal ligament.
- Roof—by fibers of internal oblique and transversus abdominis.
- Anterior wall—external oblique aponeurosis.
- Posterior wall—fascia transversalis.

Contents (structures passing through the canal):

- Males: Spermatic cord and ilioinguinal nerve.
- Females: Round ligament of uterus and ilioinguinal nerve.

Importance:

- Before birth, testis descends through the inguinal canal to reach scrotum.
- This makes canal well developed in males as compared to females.

Inguinal hernia:

- Weakness in anterior abdomen wall can cause abdomen contents to bulge through inguinal canal into scrotum; called as inguinal hernia.
- Types—direct and indirect inguinal hernia.

9. Structure of penis.

Ans. Penis is a male copulatory organ. It is cylindrical in shape and contains urethra **(Fig. 15.16)**.

Function:

- Copulatory organ
- Passage for ejaculated semen
- Parts—root, body and glans **(Fig. 15.16)**
- Ligaments—fundiform and suspensory
- Root—is attached to perineal membrane and consists of a bulb and two crura.

A. Bulb:

- Expanded posterior part of corpus spongiosum
- Attached to the deep muscles of perineum
- Covered by bulbospongiosus muscle.

B. Crus:

- Posterior narrow part of corpus cavernosum
- Attached to ischiopubic ramus
- Covered by ischiocavernosus muscle.

C. Body:

- Dorsal—two masses called as corpora cavernosa
- Ventral—a corpus spongiosum and contains spongy urethra
- Coverings—skin, subcutaneous tissue and deep fascia (Buck's fascia).

D. Glans penis:

- Slightly enlarged distal end of penis
- Covered by a loose fitting foreskin called as prepuce.

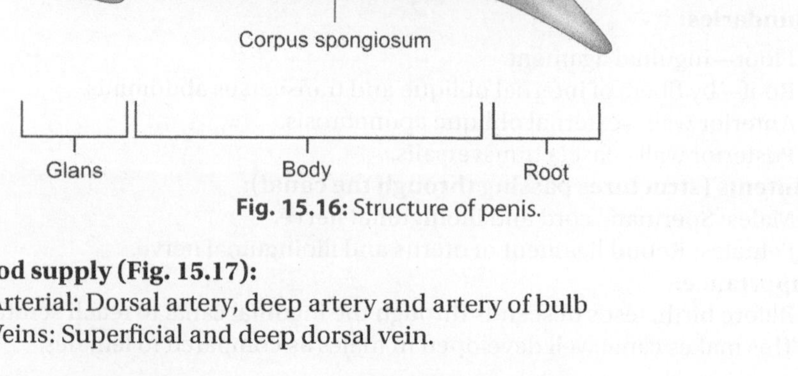

Fig. 15.16: Structure of penis.

Blood supply (Fig. 15.17):

- Arterial: Dorsal artery, deep artery and artery of bulb
- Veins: Superficial and deep dorsal vein.

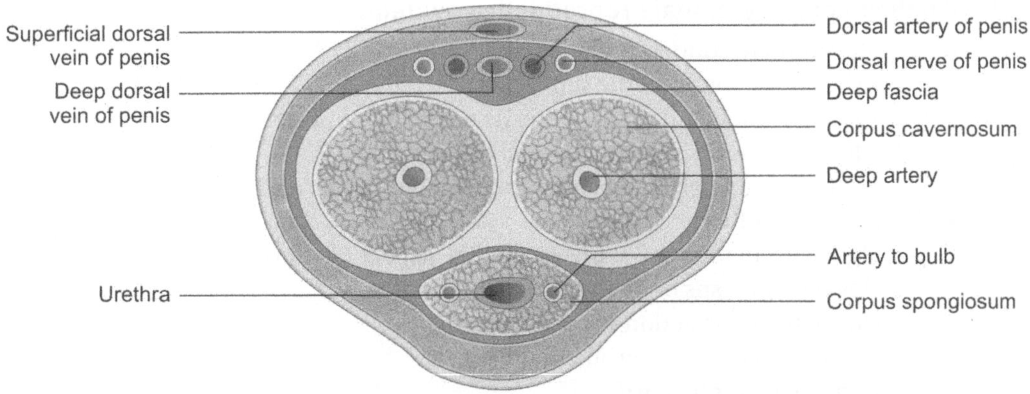

Fig. 15.17: Cross section of penis.

Nerve supply:
- Dorsal nerve of penis
- Nervi erigentes (pelvic splanchnic nerves)
- Superior hypogastric plexus.

10. Structure of a spermatozoon.

Ans. *Refer* **Figure 15.18:**
- Male gamete.
- Length—60 μm.
- Function—to reach, penetrate and fertilize the secondary oocyte.
- Parts:
  - Head:
    - Contains genetic material.
    - Covered with an acrosomal cap.
    - The enzymes (hyaluronidase and protease) in acrosome help sperm to digest and penetrate through outer covering of the oocyte.
  - Neck—contains centrioles.
  - The middle piece or body—contains mitochondria to provide energy for sperm movement.
  - Tail:
    - Similar in structure to flagella.
    - Contains microtubules for movement.

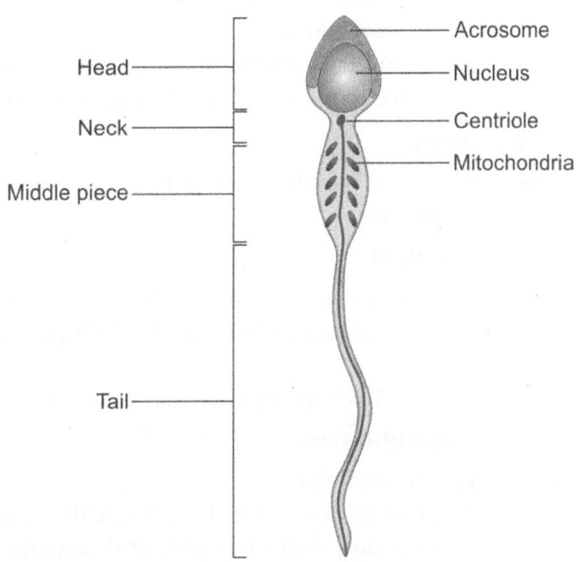

Fig. 15.18: Structure of spermatozoon.

11. Applied anatomy of male reproductive system.

Ans.
- **Cryptorchidism** (undescended testis)
  1. Testis is not found in the scrotal sac.
  2. Can be present anywhere along its normal path of descent.
  3. Most commonly seen in inguinal canal.
     - ¤ Increased risk of testicular cancer if it remains undescended.
- **Cremasteric reflex:**
  - Light stimulation of skin on medial aspect of upper part of thigh causes elevation of testis on the same side.
  - Due to the contraction of cremaster muscle.
  - This reflex is very active in children.
- **Torsion of spermatic cord:**
  - Twisting of spermatic cord contents.
  - Surgical emergency due to obstruction of blood supply of testis.
  - If not corrected on time, then necrosis of testis may occur.
- **Hydrocele:**
  - Accumulation of excess fluid in the tunica vaginalis between parietal and visceral layers.
  - Presents as the enlargement of scrotal sac.
  - The patient may complain of discomfort.
  - Can be surgically corrected.
- **Varicocele:**
  - Dilation of pampiniform plexus of testicular veins.
  - Feels like a bag of worms on palpation.
  - The enlargement of veins is visible when patient stands and usually disappears after patient lies down due to emptying of veins.
  - Mostly occurs on the left side.
- **Circumcision:**
  - Surgical procedure to remove prepuce partially or completely.
  - It can be done for cultural, religious or medical reasons.

12. Ovary.

Ans. Ovary is a female gonad and is involved in production of female gametes (ova) and hormones.

Location:

1. It is placed in pelvic cavity, related to ovarian fossa lateral to the uterus.
2. In pregnancy, it rises in abdomen with the uterus. It returns to pelvis after pregnancy.
3. Attached to the posterior surface of broad ligament by mesovarium.

Shape and size:

1. Almond-shaped.
2. Length—3 cm, width—1.5 cm, thickness—1 cm.
3. In young, surface is pink and smooth. After repeated ovulation, surface becomes grayish, irregular and scarred.

Gross structure (Fig. 15.19):

- Two surfaces—lateral and medial
- Two margins—anterior and posterior. Mesovarium—attached to the anterior margin of ovary.
- Upper end—related to the uterine tube.
- Lower end—gives attachment to the ligament of ovary. Ligament of ovary—connects ovary to the side of uterus.

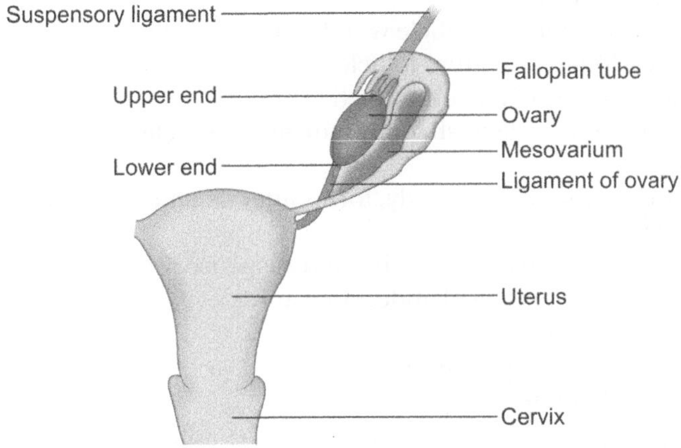

Fig. 15.19: External features and ligaments of ovary.

- As the ovulation starts after puberty, the surface of ovary becomes rough due to the discharge of oocyte.
- Blood vessels and nerves enter through hilum.
- Ovary is covered on the surface by a germinal epithelium (simple cuboidal epithelium).

Internal structure (Fig. 15.20):

- Tunica albuginea—present below the germinal epithelium and forms the capsule. Below the tunica, ovary is divided into outer cortex and inner medulla.

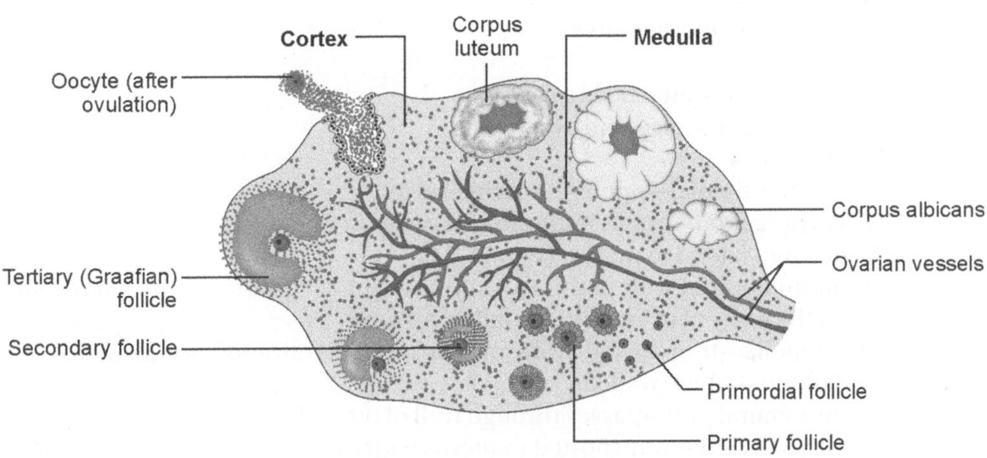

Fig. 15.20: Internal structure of ovary.

- **Cortex**—consists of ovarian follicles, stromal cells and connective tissue.
  Ovarian follicles—follicles in different stages of development are seen in the cortex.
  Types of follicles—primordial, primary, secondary and tertiary.
  1. Primordial follicle—consists of primary oocyte with a layer of flat follicular cells around it.
  2. Primary follicle—has primary oocyte with multiple layers of follicular or granulosa cells.
  3. Secondary follicle—follicle with fluid-filled cavity.
  4. Tertiary follicle—mature follicle.
- **Medulla**—consists of loose connective tissue.
  Corpus luteum—yellowish body, forms after release of oocyte from Graafian follicle.
  Corpus albicans—fibrous body, forms after degeneration of corpus luteum.

Blood vessels:
1. Ovarian vessels—reach ovary through suspensory ligament.
2. Ovarian artery—branch of abdominal aorta.
3. Ovarian venous drainage:
   Right vein → inferior vena cava.
   Left vein → left renal vein.

Applied anatomy:
- Ovarian tumors—teratoma can arise from pleuripotent cells in ovary. These tumors contain structures like cartilage or hair which are derived from multiple germ layers.
- Ovariectomy—surgical removal of ovary.

13. Uterine (fallopian) tube.

Ans. Fallopian tubes are paired structures, attached to the sides of uterus **(Fig. 15.21)**.
- Location—in upper free margin of the broad ligament
- Length—10 cm.

Mesosalpinx—encloses uterine tube. It extends between the tube and ligament of ovary.

Gross anatomy of uterine tube:
- Two ends:
  1. Medial end—attached to uterus.
  2. Lateral end—related to ovary
- Two openings:
  1. Uterine/medial—opens in uterine cavity.
  2. Pelvic/lateral—opens in peritoneal cavity.
- **Parts**: From lateral to medial **(Fig. 15.21)**
  1. Infundibulum with fimbriae—funnel shaped. Fimbriae at the lateral end help in the entry of ovum into the fallopian tube.
  2. Ampulla—thin-walled, wide and tortuous. Fertilization occurs here.
  3. Isthmus—thick-walled.
  4. Intramural part—passes through wall of uterus.

  Fertilized ovum is transported to uterus with the help of cilia in the lining of tube and, muscle contraction of tubal wall.

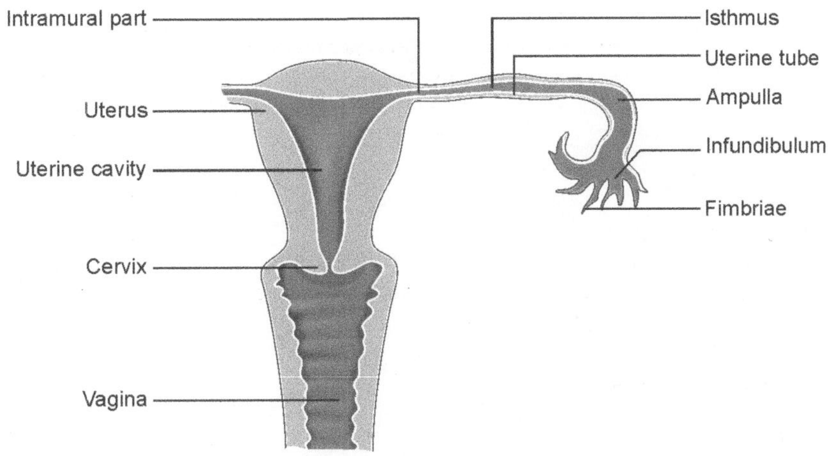

Fig. 15.21: Parts of uterine tube.

- **Microstructure**—three layers—inner mucous layer (with ciliated columnar epithelium), middle muscular layer and outer serous layer.
- Blood supply—arteries: branches from ovarian and uterine arteries. Veins: drain into ovarian and uterine veins.
- **Applied anatomy:**
  1. Tubectomy—a method of birth control. A clip or ring is placed on the uterine tube to close it. It can be done by laparoscopy method under local anesthesia.
  2. Hysterosalpingography—radiographic procedure to check the patency of uterine tubes.
  3. Ectopic pregnancy—the fertilized ovum is implanted outside the uterine cavity. Uterine tube is the most common site for ectopic pregnancy. Further development of embryo can cause rupture of the tube and heavy bleeding in first trimester of pregnancy.

14. Mammary gland.

Ans. Mammary gland is an accessory reproductive organ. It is well developed in females. Its function is to synthesize, and secrete milk.

Location—in subcutaneous tissue of anterior chest wall. The outer part of gland extending towards the axilla is called as the **axillary tail of Spence**.

- **Extent**—transversely from lateral sternal margin to midaxillary line. Vertically from 2nd to 6th ribs.
- **Shape**—hemispherical or conical.
- **Surfaces**:
  i. Superficial—covered with skin.
  ii. Deep—gland lies over fascia covering pectoralis major, serratus anterior and external oblique aponeurosis. The space between gland and underlying fascia is called as retromammary space.
- **Structure (Fig. 15.22)**
  - Modified sweat gland
  - Consists of glandular, fibrous and fatty tissue
  - Most prominent part is called as **nipple**.

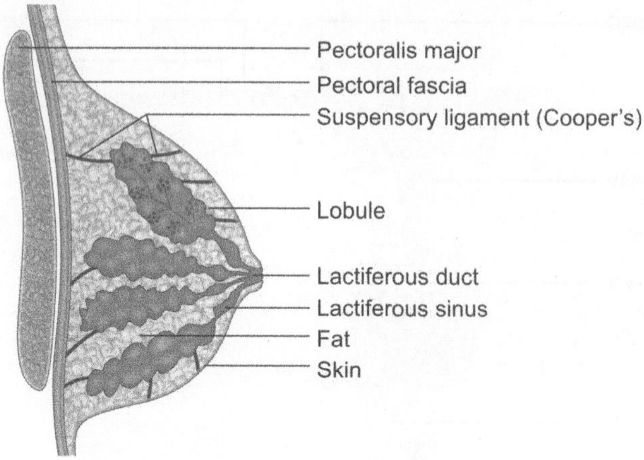

Fig. 15.22: Structure of a mammary gland.

- **Areola** is a circular pigmented area around the nipple. It has modified sebaceous glands.
- **Suspensory ligaments of Cooper** attach skin to the underlying fascia.

- **Parenchyma (functional/glandular part)**
  - Consists of 15–20 **lobules.**
  - Lobules consist of **alveoli** which secrete milk during lactation.
  - Each lobule is drained by a **lactiferous** duct which opens on the tip of nipple.
  - **Lactiferous** sinus is the dilated part of duct near nipple.
  - During pregnancy and lactation, the glandular part increases for the milk production.
- **Blood supply**
  - Arteries—lateral thoracic, internal thoracic, intercostal (3rd, 4th, 5th).
  - Veins—drain into internal thoracic, axillary and intercostal veins.
- **Lymphatic drainage:**
  - It is mostly by axillary lymph nodes.
  - Other lymph nodes draining the mammary gland are parasternal, infraclavicular and inferior phrenic.

Applied anatomy:

- Carcinoma breast—malignant tumor of breast. It presents as a painless and hard mass. It arises from the duct epithelium. It commonly spreads by lymphatic route and axillary lymph nodes are usually enlarged. If ligaments of Cooper are involved, the breast gets fixed to pectoral fascia and its skin becomes dimpled. The breast skin looks like an orange peel (peau d' orange) if lymphatics are blocked.
- Mastectomy—surgical removal of mammary gland.

15. Supports of uterus.

Ans.
- Function—to keep the uterus in its normal position in pelvic cavity.
- Types of supports—ligaments, muscles, viscera and pelvic fascia (**Figure 15.23, Table 15.1 and Flowchart 15.1**).
- The main support is given by the true ligaments and muscles.

Table 15.1: Supports of uterus.

True ligaments (Fig. 15.23)	False ligaments	Muscles	Viscera
Round ligaments: • Attach on the side of uterus, below and in front of uterine tube • Course between two layers of broad ligament, through inguinal canal and then attach to labia majora	*Broad ligaments:* • Double fold of peritoneum • Attach on the lateral margins of uterus and extends to the pelvic wall • Contents: Uterine tube, round ligament, ligament of ovary, uterine vessels, ovarian vessels, lymphatics, nerves, epoophoron and paroophoron	*Pelvic diaphragm:* Levator ani muscle	Urinary bladder
Uterosacral ligaments: From uterus to sacrum	Vesicouterine fold between bladder and uterus	• Perineal body—gives attachment to the perineal muscles and levator ani • Maintains the pelvic floor • Perineal body damage during childbirth can cause prolapse of uterus	Anorectal junction
Lateral cervical ligaments (Mackenrodt or Cardinal): From cervix to the pelvic wall	Rectouterine fold between rectum and uterus		Posterior wall of vagina
Pubocervical: Between cervix and pubis bone			

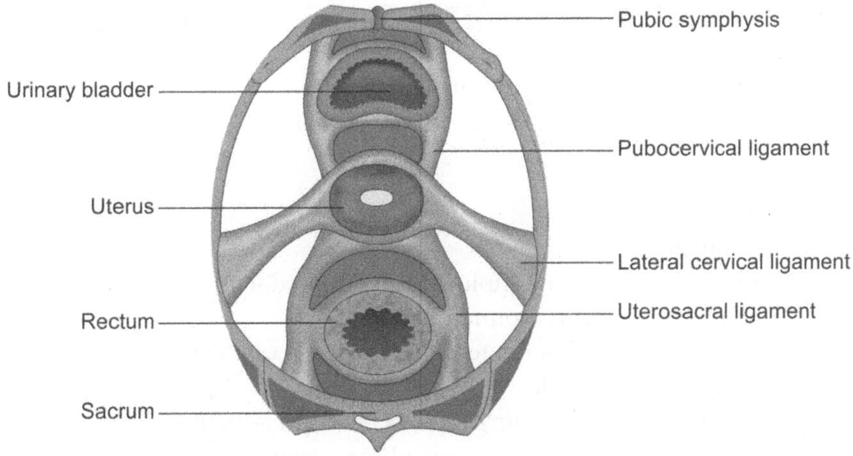

Fig. 15.23: Supports of uterus.

16. Name the types of ovarian follicles.

Ans. *Refer* **Figure 15.24.**

- Primordial follicle:
  - Primary oocyte with single layer of flat follicular cells
  - Follicular cells surround the oocyte.

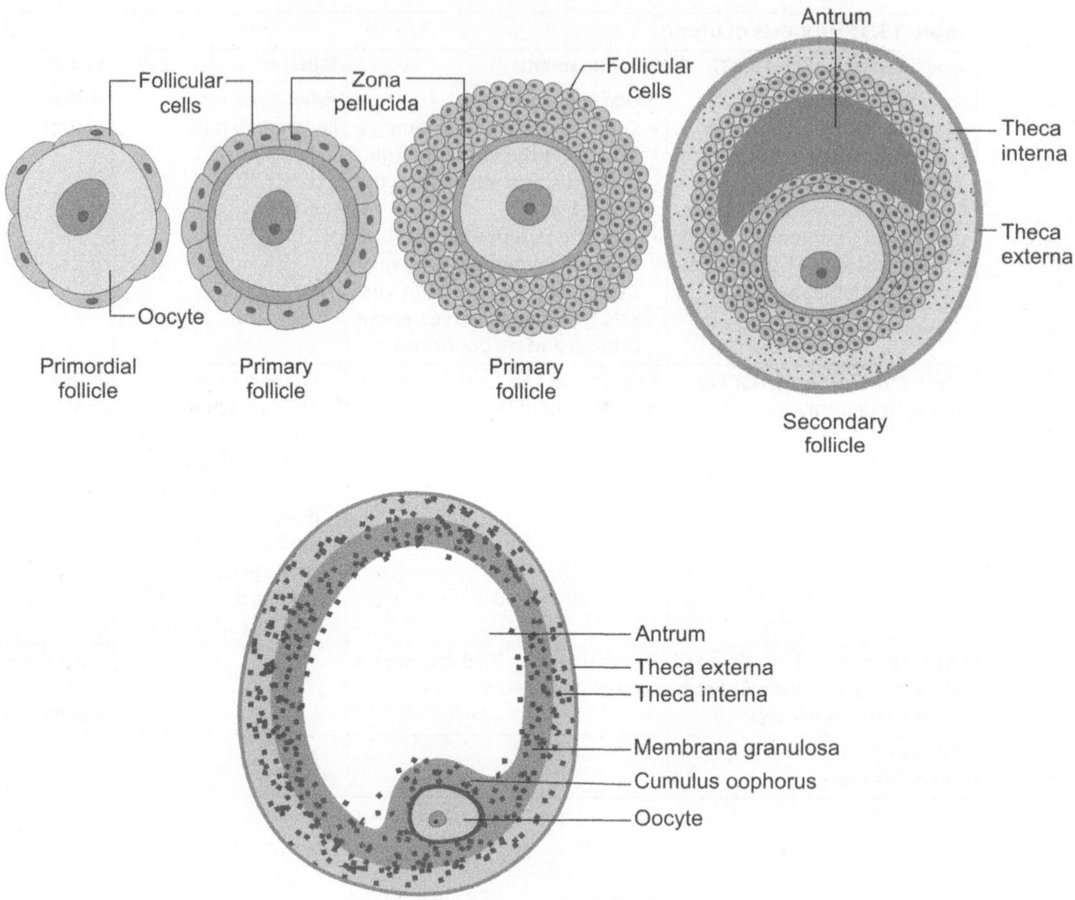

Fig. 15.24: Types of ovarian follicles.

- Primary follicle:
  - Primary oocyte with multiple layers of cuboidal follicular cells
  - Zona pellucida forms around oocyte
  - Theca interna and externa form outside follicular cells.
- Secondary or antral follicle:
  - Fluid-filled cavity (antrum) appears between follicular cells.
  - Follicular cells divided into—membrana granulosa and cumulus oophorus
  - Membrane granulosa—lines the antral cavity
  - Cumulus oophorus—around oocyte.
- Tertiary or Graafian follicle:
  - Large, mature follicle with secondary oocyte and large antral cavity
  - Size—10 mm
  - Releases oocyte during ovulation.

17. Menstrual cycle.

Ans.
- Endometrium of uterus undergoes changes during menstrual cycle **(Fig. 15.25).**
- Duration—28 days.
- Menstrual cycles start at puberty and stop after menopause.
- Three stages in menstrual cycle are—follicular, secretory and menstrual.
  1. Menstrual or flow phase:
     - If ovum is not fertilized, the upper layer of endometrium breaks down and is released with blood into vagina.
     - Functional layer is shed and basal zone is not affected.
     - This phase starts 14 days after ovulation and lasts for 4–5 days.
     - First day of this phase marks the start of menstrual cycle.

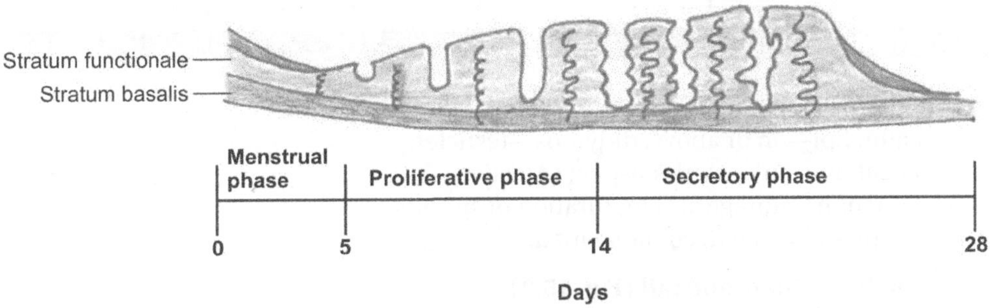

Fig. 15.25: Menstrual cycle.

  2. Follicular or proliferative phase:
     - From the end of menstrual phase till secretory phase (9 days).
     - After menstrual phase, stratum basalis regenerates to form stratum functionalis.
     - Endometrium grows under influence of estrogen from ovarian follicles.
  3. Secretory or luteal phase:
     - Starts after ovulation and lasts for 13 days.
     - Endometrium grows further in thickness under influence of progesterone.
     - Large uterine glands and spiral arteries are seen in endometrium.

18. Ovarian cycle.

Ans. The ovarian cycle refers to the series of changes in the ovary during which the ovarian follicle matures, and the ovum is shed.
- Corresponds with menstrual cycle.
- Starts at puberty.
- In each cycle, ovarian follicles grow due to hormones and an oocyte is released from ovary at the time of ovultion on 14th day **(Fig. 15.26)**
- At the start of an ovarian cycle, follicle stimulating hormone (FSH) stimulates few primary follicles to grow.
- A **zona pellucida** separates oocyte from the surrounding granulosa cells.
- Primary follicles accumulate fluid and form secondary follicles. One of these follicles becomes a mature or Graafian follicle and rest of follicles become atretic. The mature follicle ruptures during ovulation to release oocyte. Ruptured follicle forms a corpus luteum and secretes progesterone.

Primary follicle → secondary follicle → tertiary/Graafian follicle

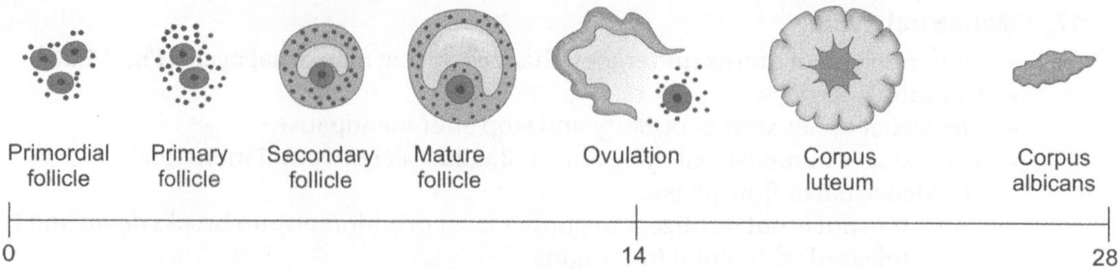

Fig. 15.26: Ovarian cycle.

SHORT ANSWERS — 2 MARKS

19. Epididymis.

Ans.
- Latin: Epi—on or above, didymos—testicles.
- Location—on posterior aspect of testis.
- Function—storage and maturation of sperms.
- Shape—elongated, coma-shaped.

Parts: Head, body and tail (Fig. 15.2).
- Head: Upper part at superior pole of testis. Made of lobules formed by 12–14 efferent ductules.
- Body and tail: Made of highly coiled, single duct of epididymis.
- The duct of epididymis—continues as ductus (vas) deferens.
- Sinus of epididymis—separates epididymis from testis on lateral side.
- Appendix of epididymis—embryological remnant.

20. Seminal vesicle.

Ans.
- Paired structure
- Elongated, pyramidal in shape
- Length—5 cm
- Function:
  - Produces thick, alkaline secretions rich in fructose and prostaglandin
  - Secretions form bulk of the semen
- Location:
  - Posterior aspect of urinary bladder
  - Lateral to ampulla of vas deferens
- Termination:
  - At the base of prostate
  - Joins the ductus deferens to form an ejaculatory duct

21. Name the coverings of testis.

Ans. Three layers from outside to inside: tunica vaginalis, tunica albuginea and tunica vasculosa.
- **Tunica vaginalis (Fig. 15.2)**
  - Serous membrane
  - Outer parietal and inner visceral layer

- **Tunica albuginea:**
  - Thick, white fibrous layer
  - Divides testis into lobules
- **Tunica vasculosa:** Contains blood vessels.

22. Ejaculatory ducts.

Ans.
- Paired ducts
- Length—2.5 cm
- Formation—union of vas deferens and duct of seminal vesicle **(Fig. 15.12).**
- Forms near neck of urinary bladder or base of prostate.
- Course:
  - Passes downwards and forwards through the prostate gland
  - Open into the prostatic urethra.

23. Name common disorders of prostate.

Ans.
- Benign prostatic hypertrophy (BPH):
  - Noncancerous enlargement of prostate in old men.
  - Pressure on urethra causes difficulty in emptying bladder and leads to urinary retention.
  - Treatment—surgical removal of prostate called as prostatectomy.
- Prostate cancer: Associated with high levels of prostate specific antigen (PSA).

24. Name the accessory organs of male reproductive system.

Ans.
- Accessory ducts:
  - Epididymis
  - Vas deferens
  - Ejaculatory ducts
- Accessory glands:
  - Seminal vesicles
  - Prostate
  - Bulbourethral glands
- Supporting structures:
  - Scrotum
  - Penis
  - Pair of spermatic cords

25. Name the genital ducts of male reproductive system.

Ans.
i. Epididymis—contains duct of epididymis.
ii. Vas deferens—continuation of epididymis.
iii. Ejaculatory ducts—open into prostatic urethra.

26. Name the contents of spermatic cord.

Ans. The contents of spermatic cord are **(Fig. 15.14):**
- Vas deferens
- Pampiniform plexus of veins
- Arteries—testicular artery, artery to vas deferens and cremasteric artery
- Lymphatics
- Nerves—testicular plexus and genital branch of genitofemoral nerve
- Loose connective tissue
- Remnant of processus vaginalis.

27. Name the cylindrical masses of erectile tissue in penis.

Ans. Three erectile tissue masses **(Fig. 15.17)**
- A corpus spongiosum
- Two corpora cavernosa.

Corpus spongiosum
- On ventral aspect of body of penis
- Contains spongy urethra

Corpora cavernosa
- Dorsal to corpus spongiosum
- Consists of spaces lined by endothelium

28. List of ducts in sequence, sperm passes through from formation to ejaculation.

Ans. List of ducts in sequence for passage of sperms:
- Rete testis
- Efferent ductules
- Epididymis
- Vas deferens
- Ejaculatory duct
- Urethra

29. Bulbourethral glands/Cowper glands.

Ans.
- Paired glands
- Pea-sized
- Compound tubuloalveolar glands
- Location—below prostate gland in urogenital diaphragm, on the side of membranous urethra.
- Duct—passes through perineal membrane and opens into spongy (penile) urethra.
- Functions:
  - Alkaline secretions of the gland neutralize the acids from urine.
  - Mucus secretions lubricate penis.

30. Name the organs/parts of male reproductive system.

Ans.
- Male gonad—testes.
- Ducts:
  - Epididymis
  - Vas deferens
  - Ejaculatory ducts
- Urethra
- Accessory glands:
  - Seminal vesicles
  - Prostate
  - Bulbourethral glands
- Supporting structures:
  - Scrotum
  - Penis
  - Spermatic cord

31. Functions of various parts of male reproductive system.

Ans.
- Gonads—testes.
  - Produce gametes (sperms).
- Genital ducts—epididymis, vas deferens and ejaculatory duct.
  - Transport sperm
- The urethra serves as common passage for urine and semen.
- Accessory glands—seminal vesicle, prostate and bulbourethral gland. These glands produce secretions for nourishment, transport and maturity of sperms.

32. Name the glands contributing secretions to semen.

Ans.
- Quantity—2-3 mL
- Sperm count—200-300 million
- Secreted from:
  - Prostate—slightly acidic, rich in acid phosphatase.
  - Seminal vesicle—alkaline secretion with fructose and prostaglandin.
  - Bulbourethral gland—alkaline secretions
  - Testis and epididymis—secretions with sperms.

33. What is the relationship between prostate and urethra?

Ans.
- Urethra—prostatic part passes through prostate gland.
- Prostate enlargement will compress upon the urethra and will cause urinary retention.

34. What are the functions of dartos and cremaster muscles?

Ans.
- Dartos:
  - Slight elevation of testis
  - Wrinkling of scrotal skin
- Cremaster—pulls testis upwards towards perineum and elevates it.

Both muscles act when stimulated by cold temperature and sexual arousal.

35. Spermiogenesis.

Ans. It is a process of development of mature sperm from a spermatid.
- Last phase of spermatogenesis
- No cell division
- Spermatids go through morphological changes
- Stages:
  - Acrosome formation
  - Nucleus condensation
  - Formation of neck, middle piece and tail
  - Reduction of cytoplasm

36. Descent of testis.

Ans.
- Passage of testis from lumbar region to scrotum.
- Starts in fetal life and testis reaches scrotum at birth.
- Significance—sperm development in testis requires a lower temperature than body core temperature. Testis in abdomen is prone to cancer.
- Factors for descent:
  - Increase pressure in abdomen pushes testis down
  - Hormones from anterior pituitary
  - Growth of parietal peritoneum

  - Gubernaculum testis—connects testis to scrotum and pulls testis down by contraction
- Cryptorchidism—undescended testis.

37. Name the organs of female reproductive system.

Ans. The organs are internal and external.

a. Internal organs—ovaries, uterine tubes, uterus, cervix and vagina.
b. External organs—mons pubis, pudendal cleft, labia majora and minora, bulb of vestibule, clitoris, Bartholin's glands.

38. Name the supports of uterus.

Ans. *Refer* **Flowchart 15.1.**

Flowchart 15.1: Supports of uterus.

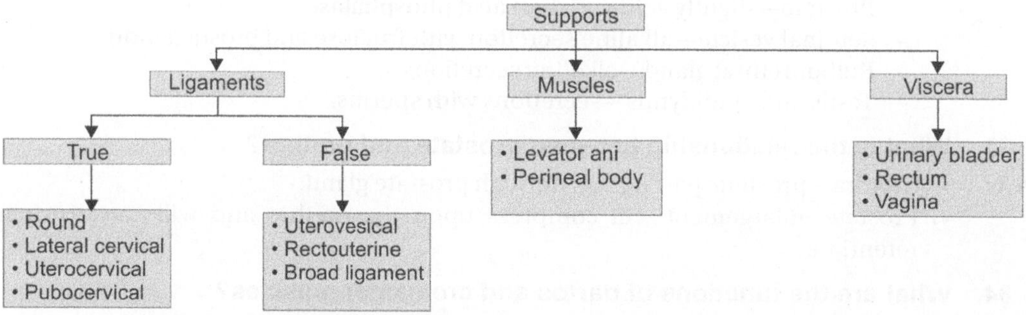

39. Name the essential and accessory organs of female reproductive system.

Ans.
- Essential organs—ovaries.
- Accessory organs:
  - Ducts—uterine tubes, uterus and vagina.
  - External genitalia—vulva that includes mons pubis, labia majora, labia minora, clitoris, bulbs of vestibule, greater and lesser vestibular glands.
  - Additional sex glands—mammary glands.
- Internal genitalia—ovaries, uterine tubes, uterus and vagina.

40. Name the layers of uterus.

Ans. From inside to outside: Endometrium, myometrium and perimetrium.
- Endometrium:
  - Inner mucosa layer
  - Lines the uterine cavity
  - Consists of simple columnar epithelium and lamina propria
  - Uterine glands and spiral arteries are within the lamina propria
  - Undergoes changes during menstrual cycle and is shed at the beginning of each menstrual cycle
  - Site of implantation for developing embryo
- Myometrium: Middle, thick layer consisting of smooth muscles. The smooth muscles undergo hypertrophy and hyperplasia during pregnancy.
- Perimetrium:
  - Outer layer
  - Formed by peritoneum

41. Layers of endometrium.

Ans.
- Consists of simple columnar epithelium and lamina propria.
- It is divided into a superficial stratum functionalis and a deep stratum basalis zone **(Fig. 15.25)**.
- Functional layer consists of two layers:
  1. Stratum compactum—near the lumen
  2. Stratum spongiosum
- Stratum functionalis undergoes cyclic changes during menstrual cycle.

42. Tubectomy.

Ans.
- A method of sterilization for family planning.
- Uterine tubes are cut and ligated at both ends.
- Can be done laparoscopically.
- Prevents sperms from reaching the ovum and fertilizing it.

43. Blastocyst.

Ans.
- After fertilization, zygote divides by mitotic division to form a mass of cells called as morula.
- A cavity, blastocele, filled with fluid appears between cells of morula and embryo is now called as a blastocyst.
- Blastocyst reaches the uterine cavity.
- After the zona pellucida surrounding the blastocyst disappears, it implants in endometrium.

44. Ovulation.

Ans.
- The release of oocyte from Graafian follicle into the peritoneal cavity is called ovulation **(Fig. 15.26)**.
- Related to increase in levels of luteinizing hormone (LH) surge
- Before ovulation, primary oocyte divides by meiosis to form a secondary oocyte
- At the time of ovulation, a secondary oocyte is released by rupture of Graafian or mature follicle:
  1. Oocyte is captured by fimbriae of the uterine tube and is transported into the tube.
  2. If oocyte is not fertilized, corpus luteum degenerates after 14 days to form corpus albicans.

45. Corpus luteum.

Ans. Formation (Fig. 15.26):
- After ovulation, wall of ovarian follicle folds and a blood clot forms inside it.
- Granulosa lutein cells are formed by enlargement of granulosa cells and accumulation of yellowish carotenoid pigment.
- LH stimulates formation of corpus luteum.
- If no fertilization occurs, it degenerates after 12–14 days and forms corpus albicans.
- If pregnancy occurs, corpus luteum is active for 6 months.
- Function—secretes progesterone, estrogen and relaxin.

46. Name the blood vessels supplying uterus and ovary.

Ans. Arteries: Uterine and ovarian artery **(Fig. 15.4)**
- Uterine artery:
  - A branch of internal iliac artery
  - Tortuous

- Runs in broad ligament
- Along lateral margin of uterus
- Related to ureter near cervix
- Branches—ureteric, vaginal, cervical, to uterine tube and to uterus
- Ovarian artery:
  - Branch of abdominal aorta
  - Enters broad ligament through suspensory ligament of ovary
  - Anastomoses with uterine artery
  - Supplies—ovary, uterine tube and uterus

Veins:
- Uterine veins
- Ovarian veins

47. What is the normal position of uterus?

Ans. Normal position—anteflexion and anteversion (*refer* **Fig. 15.5**).
- Anteflexion:
  - The forward bend of uterus in relation to the cervix.
  - Angle—120°
- Anteversion:
  - The forward bend of cervix with the axis of vagina
  - Angle—90°

48. Name the parts of uterus.

Ans. Fundus, body and cervix **(Fig. 15.6)**
- Fundus:
  - Upper part
  - Above uterine tubes
- Body:
  - From fundus to isthmus.
  - Contains uterine cavity
- Isthmus—narrow part between body and cervix.
- Cervix:
  - Lower part
  - Contains cervical canal
  - Divisions: supravaginal and vaginal
  - Cervical canal opens into uterine cavity by internal os and into vagina by external os.

49. Name the adnexa of female reproductive system and their function.

Ans. Adnexa: Fallopian tube and ovary.
- Ovary:
  - Female gonad
  - Releases secondary oocyte
  - Produces hormones.
- Fallopian tube:
  - Receives the oocyte from ovary
  - The site of fertilization
  - Transports fertilized ovum to uterus

50. Classify and name the ligaments which hold uterus in position.

Ans. Ligaments—true and false.

- True ligaments:
  - Round ligament
  - Lateral cervical
  - Uterocervical
  - Pubocervical
- False ligaments:
  - Uterovesical fold
  - Rectouterine fold
  - Broad ligament

51. Name the parts of broad ligament.

Ans.

- Mesometrium:
  - Extends from ovary and its ligament to the base of broad ligament
  - Contents—uterine vessels
- Mesovarium:
  - Attached from anterior border of ovary to posterior layer of broad ligament
  - Contents—ovarian vessels and nerves.
- Mesosalpinx:
  - Upper part.
  - Between uterine tube and ligament of ovary.
  - Contents—uterine tubc, anastomosis of uterine and ovarian arteries, epoophoron and paroophoron.
- Suspensory ligament of ovary:
  - Attached from ovary to pelvic wall
  - Contents—ovarian vessels and nerves

52. Name the ligaments attached to ovary.

Ans. Three ligaments (*refer* **Fig. 15.19**)

- Ligament of ovary: Between uterus margin to ovary.
- Suspensory ligament of ovary:
  - Between ovary and pelvic wall
  - Ovarian vessels and nerves pass through it
- Mesovarium:
  - Attaches ovary to broad ligament
  - Ovarian vessels and nerves pass through it and enter hilum of ovary.

53. Functions of various parts of female reproductive system.

Ans.

- Ovary:
  - Releases secondary oocyte
  - Produces hormones like estrogen and progesterone.
- Uterine tubes:
  - Site for fertilization
  - Transport fertilized ovum to uterus.
- Uterus: Implantation of fertilized ovum and its development.
- Vagina:
  - Receives penis in sexual intercourse
  - Forms lower part of birth canal during childbirth.

- Transports blood and endometrial tissue from uterus to outside during menstruation
- Mammary glands: Synthesize and secrete milk for the newborn.

54. Oogenesis.

Ans. Formation of oocyte from oogonia by cell division **(Fig. 15.27).**

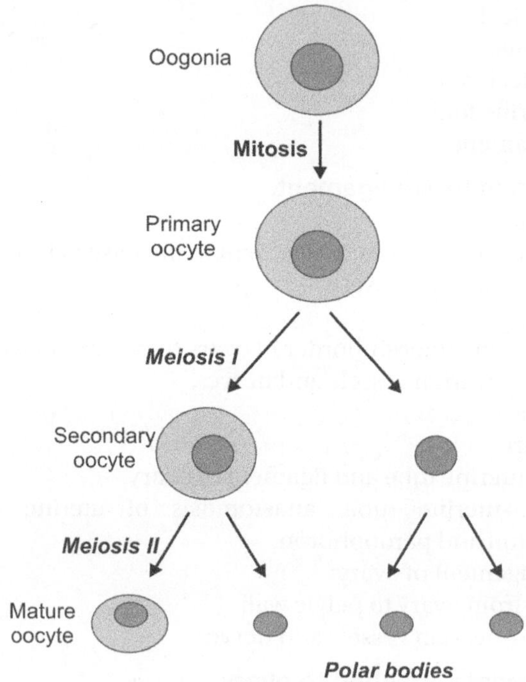

Fig. 15.27: Oogenesis.

55. Name the parts of uterine tube.

Ans. Uterine tube has four parts **(Fig. 15.21):**

1. From lateral to medial—infundibulum, ampulla, isthmus and intramural part. Total length of uterine tube is 10 cm.
2. Infundibulum—1 cm long, has fimbriae.
3. Ampulla—5 cm, longest and widest part. Site for fertilization.
4. Isthmus—3 cm, thick walled.
5. Intramural—1 cm, inside wall of uterus.

56. Perineal body.

Ans.
- Center point of perineum
- Pyramidal shape, 1.25 cm
- Fibromuscular body
- Location: Between vagina and anal openings
- Muscles attached to perineal body: Levator ani, superficial and deep transverse perinei, external anal sphincter and bulbospongiosus.

Function: Supports and maintains pelvic floor. If torn during child birth, it causes prolapse of uterus.

57. Greater vestibular glands/Bartholin's glands.

Ans. *Refer* **Figure 15.4.**

- Homologous to bulbourethral glands in the male
- Paired, bean-shaped
- Location—on each side of vaginal opening
- Duct opens in space between hymen and labium minus
- Infected gland leads to Bartholin abscess

58. Vagina.

Ans

- Tubular and fibromuscular canal **(Fig. 15.4).**
- Length—10 cm.
- Location—between urinary bladder and rectum
- Extent—cervix to vaginal opening.
- Course—upwards and backwards from vaginal opening.
- Fornices (singular: fornix)
  - Upper part of vagina around cervix.
  - Four in number and are named as anterior, posterior and two lateral.
- Layers: Inner mucosa, middle muscle layer and outer adventitia.
- Functions:
  - Receives penis in sexual intercourse
  - Forms lower part of birth canal during childbirth.
  - Transports blood and endometrial tissue from uterus to outside during menstruation
- Hymen:
  - Fold of mucosa
  - Partially closes vaginal opening
  - Imperforate hymen—in this anomaly hymen completely covers vaginal opening.

59. Pap smear.

Ans.

- Tissue from cervix is obtained and is studied under microscope by preparing a pap smear.
- This helps to screen for cervical cancer.
- Procedure: A spatula is placed in the external os. The spatula is rotated and tissue obtained is placed on a glass slide.

16
CHAPTER

Endocrine System

LONG ESSAYS — 10 MARKS

1. Name the endocrine glands in the body. Describe thyroid gland under the following: Location, gross features, relations, blood supply and applied anatomy.

Ans. Endocrine glands in the body are: Pituitary, thyroid, parathyroid, adrenal, pancreas and pineal glands.

Thyroid gland

It is the largest endocrine gland in the body.

Location (Fig. 16.1):

- In front and sides of lower part of neck.
- At level of vertebrae C5, C6, C7 and T1.

Gross features:

- Brownish-red in color.
- Size and shape: 25 g, H-shaped.
- Increases in size during pregnancy and menstruation.

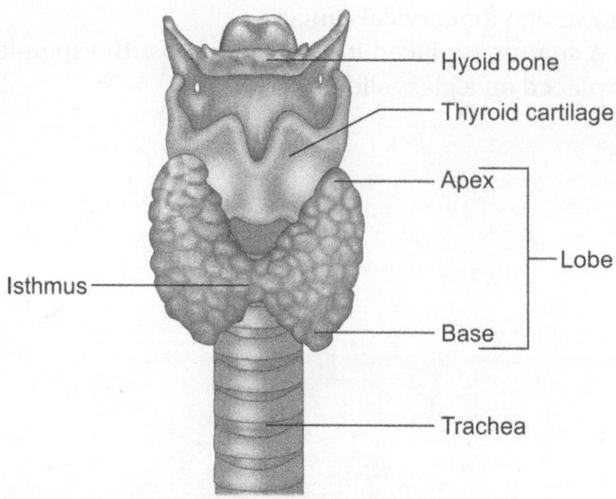

Fig. 16.1: Parts of thyroid gland.

- Capsules: Outer false and inner true.
  - False capsule—formed by pretracheal layer of deep cervical fascia.
  - True capsule—fibrous tissue.
- Suspensory ligament of Berry:
  - Thickening of false capsule.
  - Connects thyroid gland to larynx, so it moves during swallowing.

Parts (Fig. 16.1):

- Two lateral lobes and one isthmus.
- **Isthmus:**
  - Connects lobes.
  - Borders: Upper and lower.
  - Surfaces:
    - Anterior—covered by skin, superficial and deep fascia.
    - Posterior—related to 2nd, 3rd, 4th tracheal rings.
- Pyramidal lobe—extends from upper border of isthmus towards hyoid bone.
- Levator glandulae thyroideae—fibromuscular band from hyoid bone to isthmus.
- **Lobes:**
  - Each lobe is conical.
  - Size—5 × 3 × 2 cm.
  - It has apex, base, three surfaces and two borders.
  - Apex—upwards, reaches till oblique line of thyroid cartilage.
  - Base—at level of 5th tracheal cartilage.
  - Surfaces: Anterolateral, medial and posterolateral.
  - Borders: Anterior and posterior.
- **Relations (Fig. 16.2):**
  - Lobes:
    - Anterolateral surface: Sternohyoid, sternothyroid muscles.
    - Posterolateral surface: Carotid sheath.
    - Medial surface: 2 tubes (trachea, esophagus), 2 cartilages (thyroid, cricoid), 2 muscles (cricothyroid, inferior constrictor) and 2 nerves (external and recurrent laryngeal).

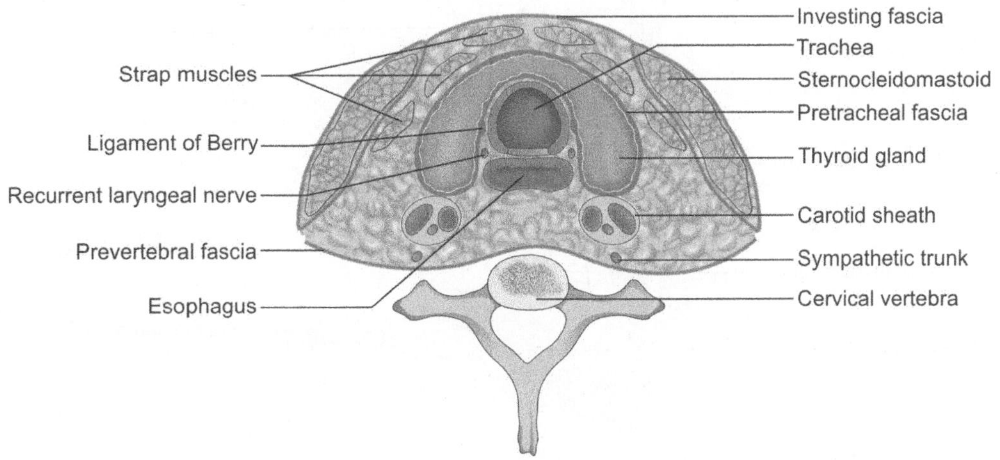

Fig. 16.2: Cross-section passing through neck showing relations of thyroid gland.

- ¤ Anterior border: Superior thyroid artery.
- ¤ Posterior border: Anastomosis between superior and inferior thyroid arteries, and parathyroid glands.

- **Internal structure (histology):**
  - Below the capsule, gland is divided into lobules.
  - Follicles are present inside each lobule.
  - Thyroid follicle- filled with colloid.
  - The hormones are produced and stored in thyroid follicles as colloid.
  - **Cells:** Follicular and parafollicular cells.
  - **Follicular cells** are present around the follicles, and parafollicular cells (C cells) are seen between follicles.
  - Follicular cells produce thyroxine and triiodothyronine hormones.
  - **C cells produce calcitonin.**

Blood supply (Fig. 16.3):

- Highly vascular.
- Arteries:
  - Superior and inferior thyroid arteries.
  - Superior thyroid—branch of external carotid artery.
  - Inferior thyroid—branch of thyrocervical trunk (from subclavian).
  - Thyroidea ima—sometimes present. Branch of aorta.
  - Relation to nerves: Superior thyroid—to external laryngeal nerve; inferior thyroid—to recurrent laryngeal nerve.
- Veins:
  - Superior, middle and inferior thyroid veins form thyroid plexus.
  - Superior and middle veins drain into internal jugular vein.
  - Inferior thyroid—drains into brachiocephalic vein.
- Lymphatic drainage: Deep cervical lymph nodes.

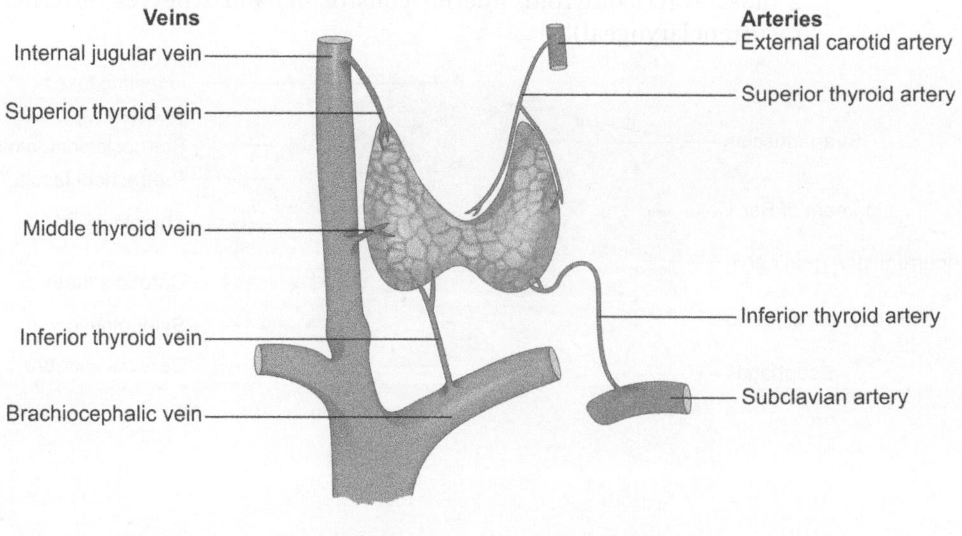

Fig. 16.3: Blood supply of thyroid gland.

Applied anatomy:

- Goiter—is the enlargement of thyroid gland. It can result due to iodine deficiency.
- Thyroidectomy:
  - Surgical removal of a part or whole of thyroid gland.
  - Posterior part of the gland is not removed to save parathyroid glands.

2. Name the endocrine glands in the body. Describe pituitary gland (hypophysis cerebri) in detail.

Ans. Endocrine glands in the body are: Pituitary, thyroid, parathyroid, adrenal, pancreas, and pineal glands. These glands pour their secretion directly into the blood circulation.

Pituitary gland (Fig. 16.4):

- Small, ovoid and reddish-gray gland.
- Attached to hypothalamus by a stalk called as **infundibulum**.
- Location: **Pituitary fossa** (Sella turcica) of sphenoid bone.
- Size: 12 × 8 mm. Weight: 0.5 g.
- Covered by a capsule.

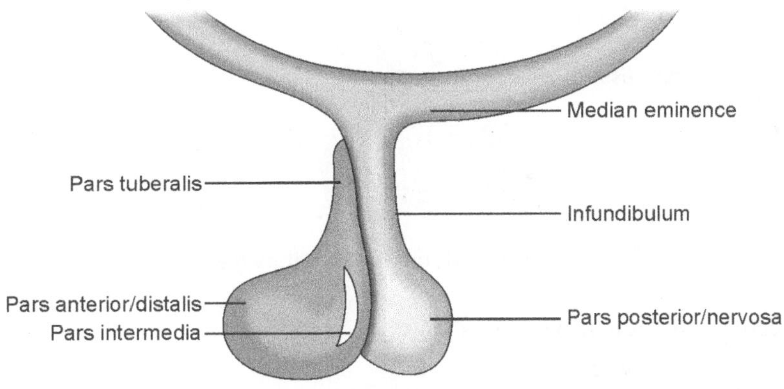

Fig. 16.4: Parts of pituitary gland.

Parts:

Anterior lobe (adenohypophysis) and posterior lobe (neurohypophysis).

Relations:

- Below—sphenoid air sinus.
- Above—dura mater (diaphragm sellae), optic chiasm and floor of third ventricle.
- Sides—cavernous sinus.

Blood supply:

Superior and inferior hypophyseal arteries **(Fig. 16.5)**.

Anterior lobe/adenohypophysis:

- It consists of glandular tissue and forms 75% of total weight of the gland.
- Develops in embryo from the **Rathke's pouch** which is an upward growth from the pharynx wall.

- Has 3 parts: Pars anterior, pars tuberalis and pars intermedia **(Fig. 16.4)**.
- Contains secretory cells and large number of capillaries.
- *Cells of adenohypophysis and their secretions*:
  - Types of cells—chromophobes and chromophils.
    - Chromophobes are pale cells without granules. Chromophils have granules that contain hormones.
    - Chromophils—mostly acidophils and few basophils.
      - Acidophils—secrete growth hormone and prolactin.
      - Basophils—secrete thyroid stimulating hormone, follicle stimulating hormone, luteinizing hormone, adrenocorticotrophic hormone and melanocyte stimulating hormone.
- Hypothalamus controls its secretions by releasing and inhibitory hormones through hypophyseal portal system **(Fig. 16.5)**.

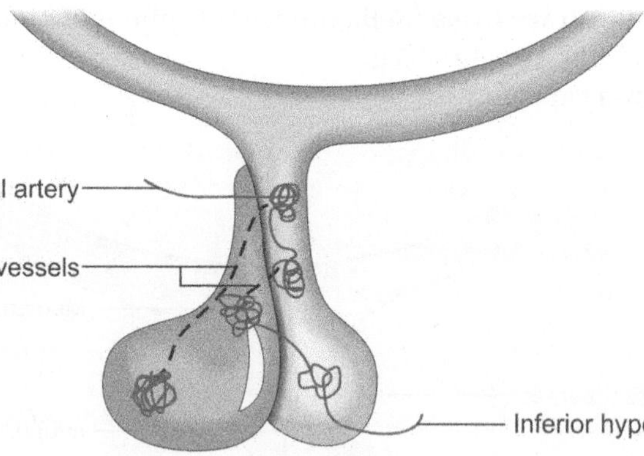

Fig. 16.5: Blood supply of pituitary gland.

Posterior lobe/neurohypophysis:

- Consists of nerve tissue.
- It only stores and releases hormones synthesized by cells in hypothalamus, namely—paraventricular and supraoptic neurons.
- Connected to hypothalamus by nerve fibers **(hypothalamo-hypophyseal tract)**.
- Develops in embryo as downward growth from the brain.
  Parts: **Pars nervosa, infundibular stem and median eminence (Fig. 16.4)**.
- Cells seen in neurohypophysis are called as pituicytes. These cells are a type of neuroglial cells.
  Hormones—oxytocin, vasopressin [antidiuretic hormone (ADH)].
- Hormones are produced in the *supraoptic and paraventricular nuclei of hypothalamus*.
- The axons of hypothalamo-hypophyseal tract carry the hormones with carrier protein to the pars nervosa.
- At nerve endings, hormones are stored in the vesicles called as **Herring bodies**.

Applied aspects:

- Hypophysectomy: Removal of pituitary gland by surgery or radiation. The hormone supplements are given to patient to compensate for the loss of pituitary hormones.

- Gigantism: Increased growth of bones due to excess release of growth hormone, before skeleton growth is complete.
- Acromegaly: Due to excess release of growth hormone, after skeletal growth is complete.
- Dwarfism: Poor skeleton growth due to decreased release of growth hormone from pituitary gland.
- Pituitary tumors: Arise from anterior pituitary. Increase in pituitary size causes raised intracranial pressure, compression of optic chiasma and hypothalamus.

SHORT ESSAYS 5 MARKS

3. Adrenal (suprarenal) gland.

Ans.
- Flat, golden-yellow colored gland.
- **Location**: Paired glands, above each kidney.
- **Weight**: 5 g.
- **Shape**: Right—pyramidal; Left—semilunar.
- Covered by a capsule.

a. Hilum:

i. A slit on anterior surface.
ii. Single suprarenal vein comes out of it.

b. Blood supply (Fig. 16.6):

i. Highly vascular.
ii. Three types of arteries: Superior, middle and inferior suprarenal arteries.
iii. Venous drainage:
  1. Right suprarenal vein → inferior vena cava.
  2. Left suprarenal vein → left renal vein.

c. Parts (Fig. 16.7):

i. Outer **cortex** and inner **medulla**.
ii. Both parts are different in structure, function and development.

d. Functions:

i. Adrenal cortex produces mineralocorticoids, glucocorticoid and androgens.
ii. Adrenal medulla produces epinephrine and norepinephrine.

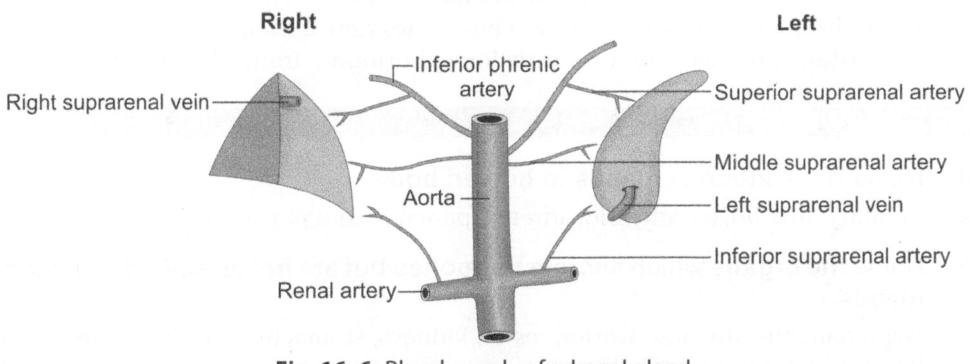

Fig. 16. 6: Blood supply of adrenal gland.

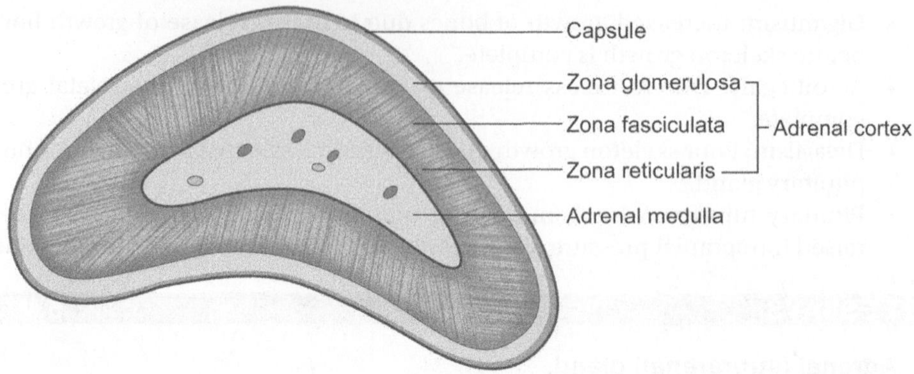

Fig. 16.7: Section of adrenal gland showing its parts.

Adrenal cortex:

a. Essential for life.
b. Forms outer, larger part of gland.
c. Three zones/layers—zona glomerulosa, zona fasciculata and zona reticularis.
   - Zona glomerulosa:
     - ¤ Outer layer, seen below capsule.
     - ¤ Contains round clusters of cells.
     - ¤ Secretes mineralocorticoids: Aldosterone.
   - Zona fasciculata:
     - ¤ Cells are placed in straight columns.
     - ¤ Secretes glucocorticoids: Cortisol.
   - Zona reticularis:
     - ¤ Inner layer.
     - ¤ Cells are arranged in branching and anastomosing network
     - ¤ Secretes androgens.

Adrenal medulla:

a. Inner part of gland.
b. Secretory cells are called as chromaffin cells (postganglionic sympathetic neurons).
c. Nerve supply—preganglionic sympathetic fibers synapse with chromaffin cells.

Applied anatomy:

a. Pheochromocytoma: Tumor of adrenal medulla.
b. Addison's disease—deficiency of hormones from adrenal cortex.
c. Cushing's disease—excess formation of hormones from adrenal cortex.

SHORT ANSWERS 2 MARKS

4. Name the endocrine glands in human body.

Ans. Pituitary, thyroid, parathyroid, adrenal, pancreas and pineal glands.

5. Name the organs which secrete hormones but are not classified as endocrine glands.

Ans. Hypothalamus, thymus, ovaries, testes, kidneys, stomach, liver, small intestine, skin, heart, adipose tissue and placenta.

6. What is the location of pituitary gland and its relation to the hypothalamus?.

Ans. • Location: Pituitary gland is attached to lower part of hypothalamus by pituitary stalk (infundibulum).
- Relations:
  - Anterior lobe:
    - The hormone secretion from anterior pituitary is controlled by releasing and inhibitory hormones of hypothalamus.
    - In this way, hypothalamus is 'master' of anterior pituitary.
    - Hypophyseal portal system **(Fig. 16.5)** connects anterior lobe to hypothalamus.
  - Posterior lobe:
    - Connected to hypothalamus by a hypothalamo-hypophyseal tract.
    - Hormones produced in hypothalamus are stored and released by posterior lobe.

7. Parathyroid gland.

Ans. *Refer* **Figure 16.8.**
- Small, oval glands.
- Located on posterior aspect of thyroid lobe.
- Total four in number— two superior and two inferior.
- Cells:
  - Contains chief and oxyntic cells.
  - Chief cells secrete parathormone which increases blood calcium levels.
- Blood supply:
  - Inferior thyroid artery.
  - Parathyroid vein drains into thyroid plexus.

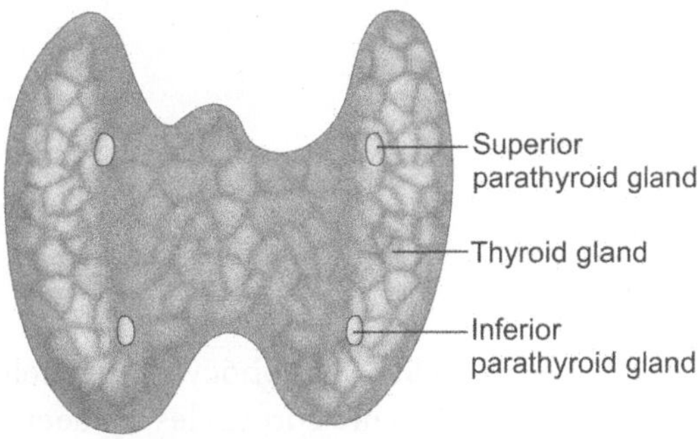

Fig. 16.8: Parathyroid glands (shown in posterior view of thyroid gland).

8. Pineal gland.

Ans. • Meaning: pinecone shaped.
- A small gland.
- Location: In midline and in the roof of third ventricle.
- The secretary cells are called as pinealocytes.
- The hormone secreted by pineal gland—melatonin.
- More amount of melatonin is secreted at night and it helps in maintaining body's biological clock.

9. Thymus.

Ans. • An important organ of immune system.
- It is a large organ in children.
- Size decreases at puberty.
- In adults—mostly adipose and areolar connective tissue.
- Location: In mediastinum, just above the heart **(Fig. 16.9)**.
- **Structure**:
  - The whole gland is covered by a capsule.
  - Fibrous tissue from capsule divides the gland into cortex and medulla.

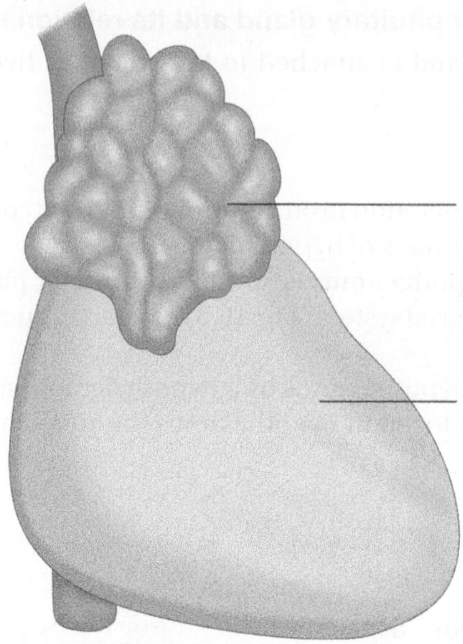

Fig. 16.9: Thymus (in a child).

- Cells: T lymphocytes, epithelioreticular cells.
- Hassall's corpuscles are seen in medulla.

- **Function:** T cell maturation takes place in the lobules of thymus.
- **Hormones**: Thymosin, thymic humoral factor, thymic factor and thymopoietin.

10. Pancreatic islets or islets of Langerhans.

Ans.
- Endocrine part of pancreas.
- Oval shaped collection of cells.
- Rich in capillaries.
- Number: 1-2 million.
- More in number in tail of pancreas.
- Cells:
  - Alpha (A) cells—glucagon.
  - Beta (B) cells—insulin.
  - Delta (D) cells—somatostatin.
  - F cells—pancreatic polypeptide.

11. Hypothalamo-hypophyseal tract.

Ans. *Refer* **Figure 16.10.**
- Formed by axons of cells in hypothalamus (supraoptic and paraventricular nuclei).
- These axons reach posterior pituitary near capillaries and pituicytes.
- Neurons in hypothalamus produce oxytocin and antidiuretic hormone (ADH).
- These hormones are packed in vesicles and are transported by this tract to posterior pituitary. Here, hormones are stored at axon terminals till release.

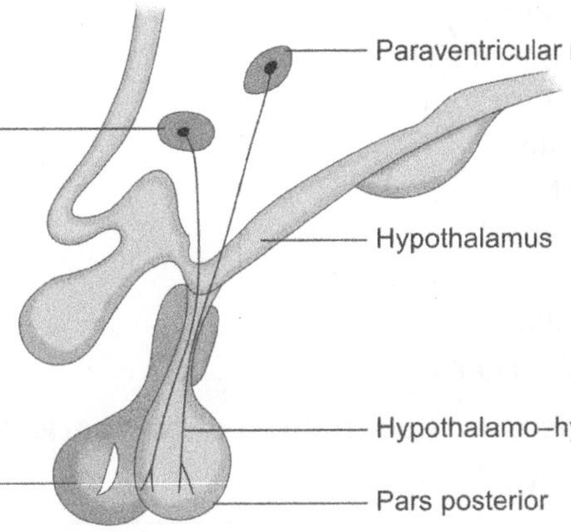

Fig. 16.10: Hypothalamo-hypophyseal tract.

12. Hypophyseal portal system.

Ans.
- Superior hypophyseal artery forms capillary plexus in infundibulum **(Fig. 16.5)**.
- Portal vessels arise from this plexus.
- These portal vessels then form another capillary plexus in anterior pituitary and supply it.
- Through portal vessels hormones from hypothalamus reach pituitary gland and control its secretion.

13. What is the location and shape of thyroid gland?

Ans.
- Location: In lower part of neck, on the front and sides of trachea.
- Shape: Butterfly or H-shaped. Two lateral lobes and one isthmus.

14. Name the parts of thyroid gland.

Ans.
- Two lateral lobes—conical.
- Isthmus—middle part which connects two lobes.
- Pyramidal lobe—sometimes seen. It is attached to isthmus and extends upwards towards hyoid bone.

15. Name the parts of pituitary gland.

Ans. *Refer* **Figure 16.4.**
- Two parts: Adenohypophysis and neurohypophysis.
- Adenohypophysis:
  - Glandular part
  - Consists of pars distalis, pars tuberalis and pars intermedia.
- Neurohypophysis:
  - Neural part.
  - Consists of pars nervosa, infundibular stem and median eminence.

16. Name the zones/layers of adrenal cortex.

Ans. *Refer* **Figure 16.7.**

Three parts/layers in adrenal cortex from outside to inside: Zona glomerulosa, zona fasciculata and zona reticularis.

1. Zona glomerulosa:
   - Just below the capsule
   - Secretes aldosterone
2. Zona fasciculata:
   - Widest part
   - Secretes cortisol
3. Zona reticularis:
   - Near medulla
   - Secretes androgens

17. List the differences in the structure of two parts of pituitary gland.

Ans. *Refer* **Table 16.1.**

Table 16.1: Differences between adeno- and neurohypophysis.

Features	Adenohypophysis	Neurohypophysis
Type of tissue	Glandular tissue	Neural tissue
Structure	Groups of secretory cells with capillaries	Nerve fibers and neuroglia with capillaries
Cells	Chromophils and chromophobes	Pituicytes
Blood supply	Hypophyseal portal system	Hypophyseal arteries
Function	Produces and secretes hormones	Stores and releases hormones
Connection to hypothalamus	Control through portal system	Nerve fibers from nuclei in hypothalamus
Parts	Pars anterior, pars tuberalis and pars intermedia	Pars nervosa, infundibular stem and median eminence
Development	Rathke's pouch (from roof of oral cavity)	Down growth from brain

18. List the differences in the structure of adrenal cortex and medulla.

Ans. *Refer* **Table 16.2.**

Table 16.2: Differences between adrenal cortex and medulla.

Features	Adrenal cortex	Adrenal medulla
Region	Outer	Inner
Parts	Three zones	None
Hormones	Aldosterone, cortisol and androgens	Epinephrine and norepinephrine
Contents	Endocrine tissue with sinusoids	Chromaffin cells with sinusoids
Function	Essential for life	Not essential for life

19. Name the hormones secreted by the tissues and organs other than endocrine glands.

Ans. *Refer* **Table 16.3**.

Table 16.3: List of hormones and their source.

Tissue	Hormone
Skin	Cholecalciferol
Ovary	Estrogen, progesterone, inhibin
Testis	Testosterone, inhibin
Placenta	Human chorionic gonadotropin, estrogen, progesterone, human chorionic somatomammotropin
Thymus	Thymosin, thymic humoral factor, thymic factor, thymopoietin
Gut mucosa	Gastrin, secretin, cholecystokinin
Heart	Atrial natriuretic peptide
Adipose tissue	Leptin
Kidney	Renin, erythropoietin, calcitriol

20. Name the endocrine glands in body and mention their location.

Ans.
- Thyroid gland:
  - Located in front and sides of lower neck.
  - At level of C5 to T1 vertebrae.
- Pituitary gland:
  - Located in pituitary fossa on the body of sphenoid bone.
  - Attached to base of brain by a stalk.
- Adrenal glands: Seen on the upper pole of each kidney.
- Parathyroid glands:
  - Related to posterior border of the thyroid lobe.
  - Close to anastomoses of superior and inferior thyroid arteries.
  - Superior parathyroid gland— near upper part of lobe.
  - Inferior parathyroid gland—close to lower pole of lobe.
- Pineal gland: In the roof of 3rd ventricle in midline.

SECTION 2

PHYSIOLOGY

Section Outline

17
CHAPTER

General Physiology

SHORT ESSAYS 5 MARKS

1. Define homeostasis.

Ans.
- It is defined as mechanisms that maintains the constancy of the internal environment of the body.
- Walter Canon coined the term homeostasis
- Homeostasis achieved through feedback mechanisms, negative and positive feedback mechanism.

Negative feedback mechanism

- Most of the regulatory mechanism of body is achieved through negative feedback mechanism
- Normally a stimulus produce a response, when the initial stimulus reverse the response it is said to be achieved through negative feedback mechanism
- Examples:
  - Temperature regulation
  - Regulation of blood glucose

Positive feedback regulation

- Only few situations in the body occur through this mechanism
- Initial stimulus accentuate the response
- Examples:
  - Parturition reflex
  - LH surge
  - Activation of coagulation cascade

2. Write short note on facilitated diffusion.

Ans.
- It is also known as carrier mediated transport.
- Transport of substance occur through the carrier protein
- It is a downhill transport and does not require ATP.

Example: Transport of glucose in RBC in skeletal muscle.

Features of facilitated diffusion (Fig. 17.1)

- Faster rate of transport
- Specificity (the binding site recognize a specific substance permit D-glucose but not L glucose)

- Saturation kinetics (if all carrier protein is occupied by the substance, saturation point is achieved, further transport does not occur).
- Competitive inhibition (chemically similar substance can compete for the same binding site D-galactose and D-glucose).

Factors affecting facilitated diffusion

- Availability of carrier protein
- In some tissues it is hormone mediated process (insulin-dependent glucose uptake in the skeletal muscle)

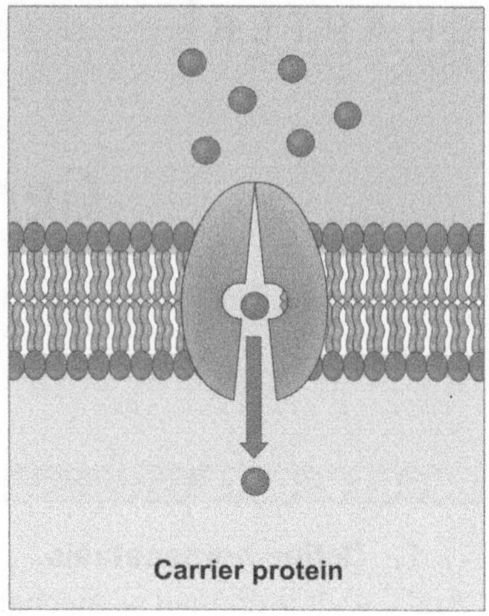

Fig. 17.1: Facilitated diffusion.

3. What is RMP and mention the causes for it?

Ans.
- The membrane potential recorded at rest is resting membrane potential (RMP).
- It is the difference in electrical potential between inside and outside the cell membrane under resting condition with inside negative to outside.
- It is –70 mV for neuron and varies in other tissue.
- RMP caused by difference in the permeability of membrane to various ions.

Causes for RMP being negative

- Potassium efflux from the cell due to high permeability of the membrane to K ion, therefore negativity is created inside the cell (main cause for RMP)
- The permeability of membrane to sodium is less than potassium, therefore K efflux is not balanced by Na influx.
- Exit of anion from the cell is low due to impermeability of the membrane to anion
- Sodium potassium pump is electrogenic pump that causes exit of 3 Na for 2 K.

4. Write a short note on sodium potassium pump.

Ans. **Structure of a Na, K ATPase/Na K pump (Fig. 17.2).**

- Sodium potassium pump is present in all the cells of the body.
- It has 2 subunit α and β subunit which spans the cell membrane.
- The intracellular portion of the α subunit has a Na^+-binding site (1), a phosphorylation site (4), and an ATP-binding site (5). The extracellular portion has a K^+-binding site (2) and an ouabain-binding site (3)
- It is an electrogenic pump in that pumps three positive charges ($3Na^+$) out of the cell for each two ($2K^+$) that it moves in, and therefore the coupling ratio of 3:2
- Na^+, K^+ ATPase catalyzes the hydrolysis of ATP to adenosine diphosphate (ADP) and uses the energy to expel three Na^+ from the cell and take two K^+ into the cell for each molecule of ATP hydrolyzed.

Functions

- Maintain cell volume
- Maintain high K and low Na ion concentration inside the cell
- Contribute to resting membrane potential.

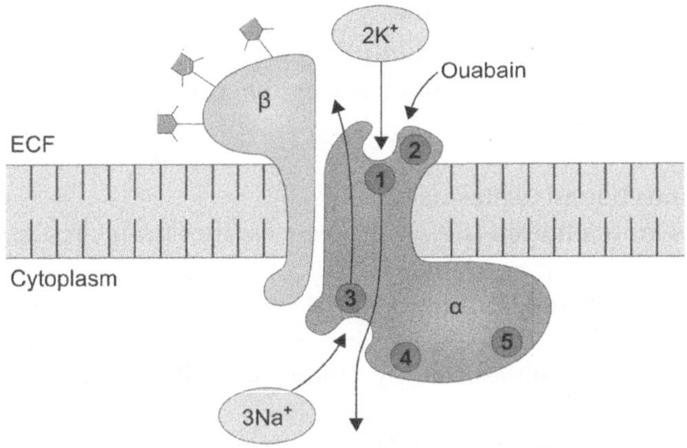

Fig. 17.2: Sodium potassium pump.

5. Give the distribution of total body water in different fluid compartments.

Ans. Distribution of total body water in a normal adult

Body fluid compartments	Volume (L)
Total body water (TBW)	42
Intracellular fluid (ICF)	28
Extracellular fluid (ECF)	14
ECF compartment comprises	
• Plasma	3.5
• Interstitial fluid and transcellular fluid	10.5

6. Describe the principle of measurement of body fluid compartment.

Ans. Volume of fluid compartment is measured by 'Indicator Dilution Principle' which is based on following relationship:

$$V = A/C$$

'A' is Amount of substance injected intravenously, 'V' is volume in which substance is distributed, 'C' is final concentration attained.

Principle of Measurement

Volumes of the fluid compartment are measured by determining the volume of distribution of a indicator substance. A known amount of a indicator is added to a compartment. The indicator concentration in that compartment is measured after allowing sufficient time for uniform distribution throughout the compartment. The compartment volume is calculated as: Amount of indicator injected—amount removed/final concentration of the indicator.

Characteristics of an indicator

- Should be nontoxic
- Should be easy to measure
- Should remain in compartment being measure
- Must mix throughout the compartment being measured
- Should remain unchanged by body during mixing period
- Should not change the fluid distribution in compartment being measured.

7. Describe the measurement of plasma volume.

Ans. Plasma volume is measured by two dilution methods:

First method—the indicator used should neither leaves the vascular system nor penetrate red cells.

Examples:

1. Evans blue dye that remains bound to plasma proteins
2. Radioiodinated human serum albumin (RISA): It slowly escapes from circulation into interstitial fluid
3. Radioiodinated gamma globulin and fibrinogen: These substances do not leak out of the blood

Volume of fluid compartment is measured by 'Indicator Dilution Principle'. Accordingly

Volume = Amount injected - amount removed/final concentration of substance.

Second method — radioisotopes of phosphorus, iron and chromium are used that penetrate and bind to red cells. Therefore red cells volume can be measured by injecting tagged red cells intravenously. After thorough mixing the fraction of RBC tagged is measured.

Plasma volume measured by using formula:

$$\text{Plasma volume} = 100 - \text{PCV}/100 \times \text{Blood volume}$$

Packed cell volume is practically red cell volume.

SHORT ANSWERS 3 MARKS

8. Write short notes on intercellular communication.

Ans. Cells communicate with one another via chemical messengers.

4 types of intercellular communication are **(Fig. 17.3)**:

1. **Synaptic communication**, in which neurotransmitters are released from nerve cells and act across a narrow synaptic cleft on a postsynaptic cell.
2. **Endocrine communication**, in which hormones reach target tissues via the circulating blood.
3. **Paracrine communication**, in which the products of cells diffuse in the ECF to affect neighboring cells that may be some distance away the cells that secrete chemical messengers.
4. **Autocrine communication:** The chemical messengers released by the cell act on the same cell.

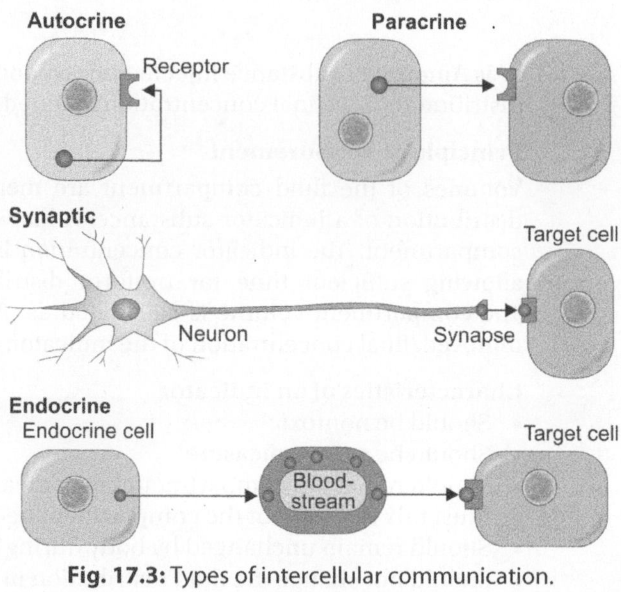

Fig. 17.3: Types of intercellular communication.

9. Define passive transport and name the passive transport process.

Ans. It is defined as transport of substance down the concentration gradient without utilization of energy.

Passive transport process

- Simple diffusion
- Facilitated diffusion
- Osmosis
- Filtration
- Bulk flow and solvent drag

10. Write short note on active transport.

Ans.
- It is defined as transport of substance against electrochemical gradient with utilization of energy **(Fig. 17.4)**:
- Example: Sodium potassium pump
- It is of two types:
  1. Primary active transport—uses chemical energy like ATP to transport solutes against concentration gradient.
  2. Secondary active transport—here transport of ions brings about electrochemical gradient across a membrane, which helps in transport of molecules.

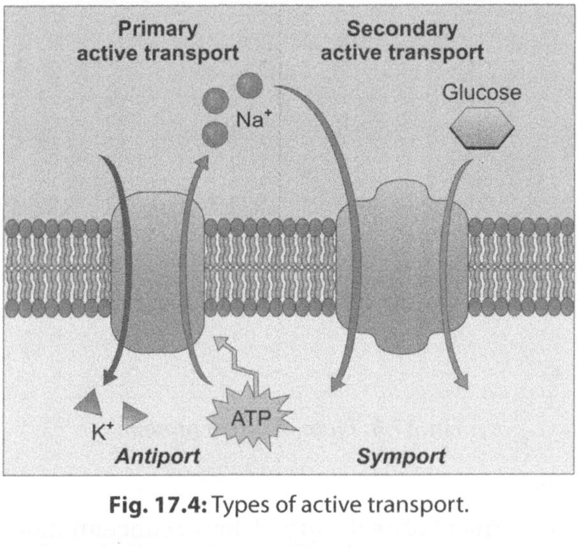

Fig. 17.4: Types of active transport.

11. What is secondary active transport?

Ans.
- In this mechanism, the active transport of sodium is coupled to the transport of other substances.
- Reabsorption of glucose in the intestinal enterocyte or renal tubule is an example for secondary active transport.
- The sodium potassium pump create an electrochemical gradient for sodium (higher outside than inside) this facilitate sodium movement into the cell through a carrier protein which is a symport, hence along with sodium it transport glucose and energy is utilized indirectly in this process, since its function depends on the primary active transport it is known as secondary active transport **(Fig. 17.5)**.

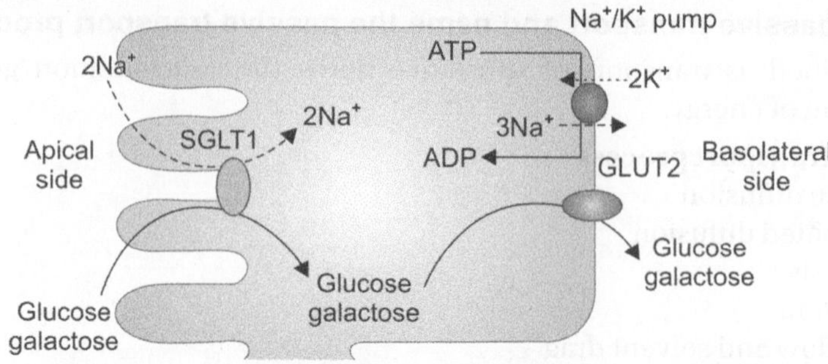

Fig. 17.5: Mechanism of secondary active transport.

12. What are types of carrier protein?

Ans. The types of carrier protein is given in **Figure 17.6**.

Uniport: It transport only one substance at a time

Cotransport or symport: Transport of two or more substance in the same direction

Counter transport or antiport: Transport of two substances in opposite direction

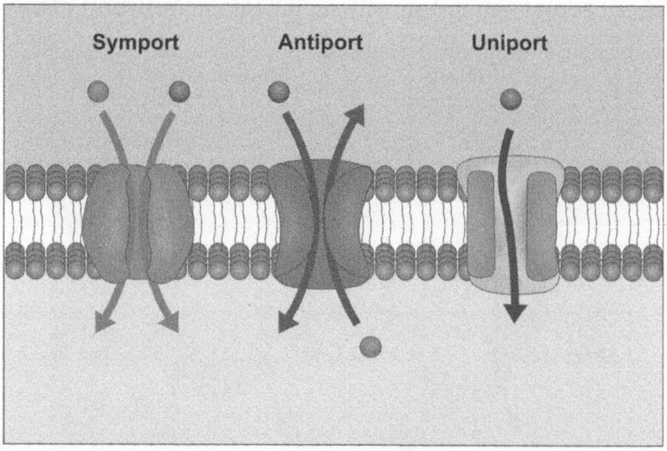

Fig. 17.6: Types of carrier protein.

13. Define osmosis.

Ans. It is the passive movement of a solvent with lower concentration of solutes to a solution of higher solute concentration through a semipermeable membrane **(Fig. 17.7)**.

The osmotic properties are defined by:

- **Osmolarity:** mOsm (milliosmoles)/L = concentration of particles per liter of solution.
- **Osmolality:** mOsm/kg = concentration of particles per kg of solvent.

14. Write a note on vesicular transport.

Ans. It is of two types **(Figs. 17.8 and 17.9)**:

1. Endocytosis
2. Exocytosis

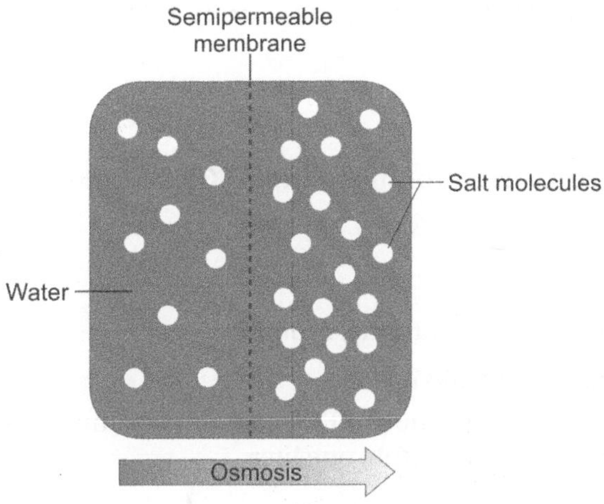

Fig. 17.7: Osmosis.

Endocytosis (Fig. 17.8)

- It is the process of transferring macromolecule into the cell.
- Internalization occur through engulfing the substance inside the cell
- It is of two type:
  1. Phagocytosis (cell eating)
  2. Pinocytosis (cell drinking)

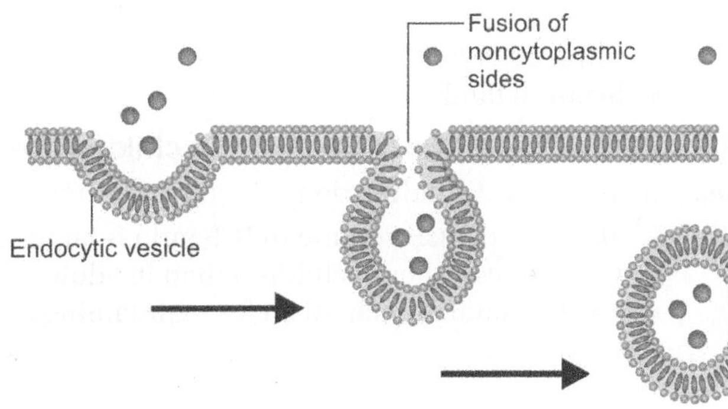

Fig. 17.8: Endocytosis.

Exocytosis (Fig. 17.9)

Seen in secretory cells where the secretory vesicle fuse with the cell membrane, then the region of fusion break and release the content of the granule outside the cell, which utilize ATP and calcium. Exocytosis occur via 2 pathways—(1) nonconstitutive and (2) constitutive pathway.

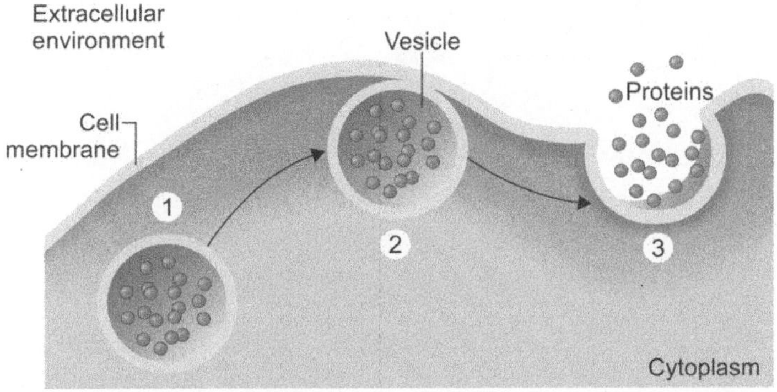

Fig. 17.9: Exocytosis.

15. Mention the indicators used for measuring total body water.

Ans.
- Deuterium oxide
- Tritium oxide
- Aminopyrine

16. List the indicators used for measuring ECF volume.

Ans.
- Inulin
- Mannitol
- Sucrose
- Radioactive isotopes of chloride, bromide

17. What is transcellular fluid?

Ans. Transcellular fluid is the portion of ECF contained within the epithelial-lined spaces. It is a part of ECF and it constitute one liter.
- Peritoneal fluid
- Pericardial fluid
- Pleural fluid
- CSF
- Intraocular fluid
- Synovial fluid

18. Why dehydration is common in children compared to adult?

Ans. In infants and children dehydration is common following small loss of fluid because:
- The ratio of ECF volume to ICF ratio is larger than the adult. But the absolute ECF volume is smaller in children than in adult
- The regulatory mechanism for maintaining ECF volume are not well developed.

18
CHAPTER

Blood and Immunity

BLOOD

LONG ESSAYS — 10 MARKS

1. Explain in detail the various stages of erythropoiesis. Add a note on the factors which regulate erythropoiesis.

Ans. Red blood cells (RBCs) are biconcave shaped cells which are 7.5 μm and with thickness in the center being 1μm and 2.2 μm in the periphery. The shape is maintained by the structural proteins like spectrin, ankyrin, actin. Its advantages are the RBCs can squeeze through the capillaries without getting deformed assuming a parachute like shape, increases the surface area. Energy is derived from the glycolytic pathway (80%) and pentose phosphate shunt pathway (20%). It is essential for the maintenance of the volume of RBC.

Erythropoiesis is the formation of red cells. There are four cell stages of erythropoiesis: Stem cells, progenitor cells, precursor cells and mature cells. Pluripotent stem cells give rise to committed stem cells. Mesoblastic stage, hepatic stage and medullary stage are discussed below.

Mesoblastic stage: During fetal development erythropoiesis takes place in the mesoderm of yolk sac. Hence erythropoiesis is intravascular during this stage.

Hepatic stage: From 5th week of intrauterine life erythropoiesis takes place in the liver and spleen.

Medullary stage: During third month of intrauterine gestation the bone marrow becomes the sole region for production of RBCs.

Erythropoiesis during adolescence occurs in all the bones. Later erythropoiesis ceases in the limb bones. After 20 years flat bones produce RBCs. The marrow in the long bones are replaced by yellow marrow.

Stages in RBC development:

Colony forming unit-spleen (CFU-S): The cell is supposed to be a pluripotent stem Cell with 15–22 μm diameter. They have a large nucleus and a thin rim of cytoplasm. They are capable of renewing themselves. They are also referred to as uncommitted stem cells.

Burst-forming unit-erythroid (BFU): This is referred to as burst forming unit. This gives rise to CFU (erythrocytic). This is a premature cell. This cell is not very sensitive to erythropoietin.

Colony forming unit-erythroid (CFU-E): This stage is colony forming unit erythrocytic and is very sensitive to erythropoietin. Proerythroblast, polychromatophil erythroblast, orthochromatic erythroblast formation **occurs in the bone marrow for 4–5 days. Reticulocyte and erythrocyte formation occurs in blood for 1–2 days (Fig. 18.1).**

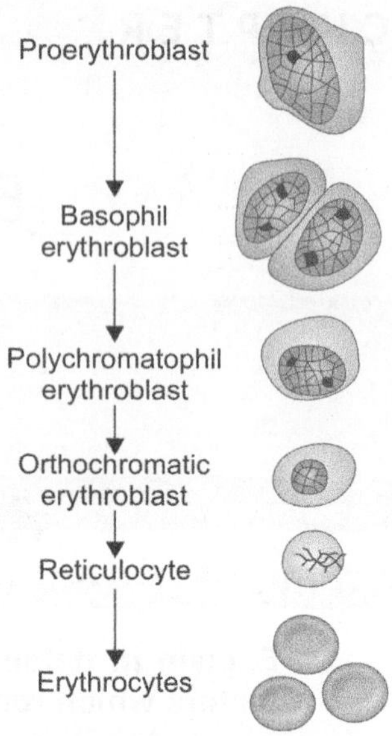

Fig. 18.1: Colony forming unit-erythroid.

- **Proerythroblast:** No hemoglobin, nucleus large and contain nucleoli.
- **Basophil erythroblast:** Early normoblast, nucleoli disappear, show mitosis, cytoplasm deep blue and there is increase in RNA and hemoglobin (Hb) starts appearing.
- **Polychromatophil erythroblast**: Late normoblast where nucleus appears smaller, coarse chromatin. There is hemoglobin increase. RNA takes up basophil stain.
- **Orthochromatic erythroblast:** Normoblast where nucleus appears smaller. This is followed by nuclear lysis and nuclear extrusion.
- **Reticulocyte:** Reticulum is seen, remnant of ER and GA. They synthesize Hb. Few mitochondria are seen. 1% of red cells. In another two days mature red blood cells are formed.

Factors regulating erythropoiesis:

1. General factors
   - Erythropoietin
   - Thyroxine
   - Hemopoietic growth factors
   - Vitamins
2. Dietary factors
   - Proteins
   - Minerals
3. Hormonal factors
   - Androgens
   - Estrogen
   - Growth factor
   - Thyroid-stimulating hormone (TSH)
4. Other factors
   - Intrinsic factor
   - Hypoxia
   - Chemical factor
   - Environmental (hypoxia)
   - Drugs

A. Tissue oxygenation:

Most important regulator of erythropoiesis: Any condition which decrease tissue oxygenation and **increases erythropoiesis**

- **Anemia:** Immediately increases RBCs production
- **Bone marrow destruction**: Causes hyperplasia of the remaining cells and increase production of RBCs
- **High altitudes:**
  - Partial pressure of **oxygen in air is less**
  - Decrease in oxygen transport to tissues
  - **Causes hypoxia**
- **Cardiac failure:**
  - Inefficient pumping by heart
  - Decreased blood flow to peripheral vessels
  - **Causes tissue hypoxia**
- **Lung diseases:** Failure of oxygen absorption in lungs, as a result blood carries less oxygen causing tissue hypoxia.

Erythropoietin

- Glycoprotein
- Molecular weight—34,000
- **Sites of production:**
  - Kidneys
  - Liver
  - Brain, uterus

Stimulants of erythropoietin production:

Renal mechanism: Anemic blood to kidney leads to less oxygen supplied. This in turn causes renal tubular cells to consume high O_2. This stimulates production of erythropoietin.

Role of erythropoietin in erythropoiesis

- Formed in response to hypoxia within minutes
- RBC production in 5 days
- Erythropoietin stimulates proerythroblasts formation
- Causes cells to pass through various stages of erythropoiesis rapidly.

B. Vitamins

- **Vitamin B_{12} and folic acid:**
  - Essential for formation of thymidine triphosphate
  - Essential building block of DNA
  - Diminished DNA causes failure of nuclear maturation and inadequate erythropoiesis.
- **Vitamin C:** Potentiates the effect of folic acid and assists in iron absorption and reducing ferric to ferrous form
- **Pyridoxine:**
  - Coenzyme for condensation of glycine and succinyl-CoA
  - Riboflavin and pantothenic acid help in heme formation and cell growth and division.
- **Minerals:**
  - Ceruloplasmin is necessary for iron transfer from storage sites like bone marrow, liver and spleen
  - Cobalt forms a part of vitamin $B_{12.}$
- **Proteins:** Formation of globin
- **Hormones:** Growth hormone, thyroxine, cortisol and testosterone stimulate production of erythropoietin.

SHORT ESSAYS 5 MARKS

2. Write a brief note on synthesis of hemoglobin (Hb).

Ans.
- Synthesis begins in proerythroblast
- Around 65% of Hb synthesis occurs during erythroblast stage and 35% occurs during reticulocyte stage
- It has two parts namely—heme and globin
- Heme is produced in mitochondria and globin in polyribosomes **(Figs. 18.2 to 18.4)**

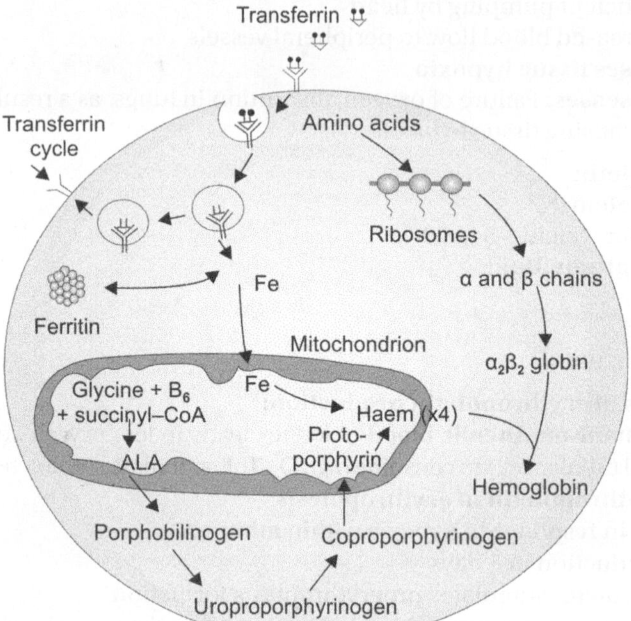

Fig. 18.2: Synthesis of hemoglobin.

- Various types of globin combines with haem to form different types of hemoglobin
- Eight functional globin chains, arranged in two clusters:
  1. β- cluster (b, g, d and e globin genes) on the short arm of chromosome 11
  2. α- cluster (a and z globin genes) on the short arm of chromosome 16

Globin synthesis, starts at 3rd week of gestation.

- Embryonic:
  - Hemoglobin Gower I
  - Hemoglobin Portland
  - Hemoglobin Gower II
- Fetal: HbF ($\alpha_2\gamma_2$), HbA ($\alpha_2\beta_2$)

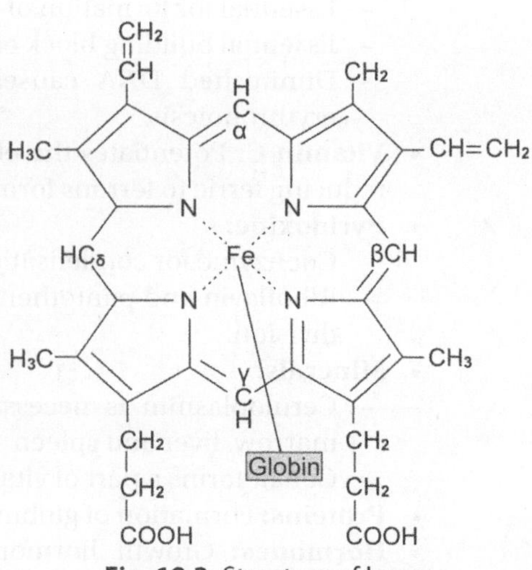

Fig. 18.3: Structure of heme.

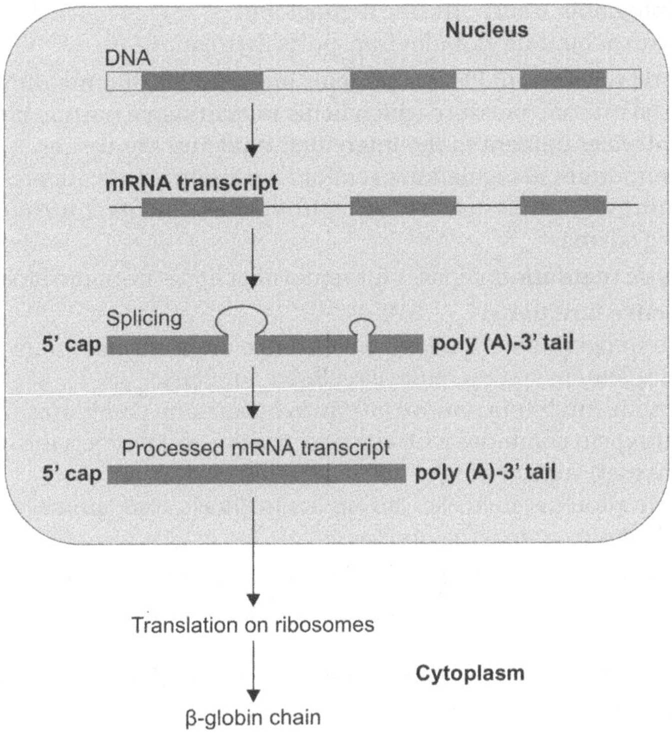

Fig. 18.4: Synthesis of globin.

- Adult: HbA, HbA_2, HbF
- Adult hemoglobin

	HbA	HbA_2	HbF
Structure	$\alpha_2\beta_2$	$\alpha_2\delta_2$	$\alpha_2\gamma_2$
Normal %	96–98%	1.5–3.2%	0.5–0.8%

3. What are the types and functions of plasma proteins?

Ans. Plasma proteins constitute:

- 7.6 g/100 mL plasma
- Large size and globular shape
- Prevents them from leaving vessels
- Three classes of proteins: Albumins, globulins and fibrinogen.
- The normal serum protein level is 63–83 g/L.

The following are the functions of plasma proteins:

1. **Transport functions:**
   - Transferrin transports iron.
   - Ceruloplasmin transports copper.
   - Albumin transports fatty acids, bilirubin calcium, many drugs, etc.
   - Transcortin transports cortisol and corticosterone
   - Retinol binding protein transports retinol.
   - Lipoproteins transport lipids.

- Haptoglobin transports free hemoglobin.
- Thyroxin binding globulin transports thyroxin.

2. **Osmotic regulation:** Plasma proteins are colloidal and nondiffusable and exert a colloidal osmotic pressure which helps to maintain a normal blood volume and a normal water content in the interstitial fluid and the tissues. Albumin content is most important in regulation of colloidal osmotic or oncoticpressure. Decrease in albumin level results in loss of water from blood and its entry into interstitial fluids causing edema.
3. **Catalytic regulation:** Lipases for removal of lipids from the blood.
4. **Protective functions:**
   - Immunoglobulins combine with foreign antigens and remove them.
   - Complement system removes cellular antigens.
   - Enzyme inhibitors remove enzymes by forming complexes with them, e.g., α_1-antitrypsin combines with elastase, trypsin and protects the hydrolytic damage of tissues, such as lungs.
   - Some proteins increase during acute phase and protect the body, e.g., α_1-antitrypsin, α_2-macroglobulins.
5. **Blood clotting:** Many factors are involved in clotting mechanism and prevent loss of excessive amount of blood, e.g., clotting factors IX, VIII, thrombin, fibrinogen, etc.
6. **Anticoagulant activity (thrombolysis):** Plasmin breaks down thrombin and dissolves the clot.
7. **Buffering capacity:** Proteins in plasma help to maintain acid-base balance.

4. Write in brief about blood coagulation.

Ans.
- It consists of an enzymatic cascade (amplification)
- Several serine proteases are involved.
  - Produced by liver (most)
  - Require vitamin K (several)
- Requires Ca^{2+}
- Localized to site of injury
- Reversible (via production of plasmin)
- Intrinsic pathway
- Hemostasis involves four main steps:
  1. Vascular spasm
  2. Platelets reaction
  3. Formation of platelet plug
  4. Blood coagulation
- The ultimate step in clot formation is the conversion of fibrinogen → fibrin **(Fig. 18.5)**.

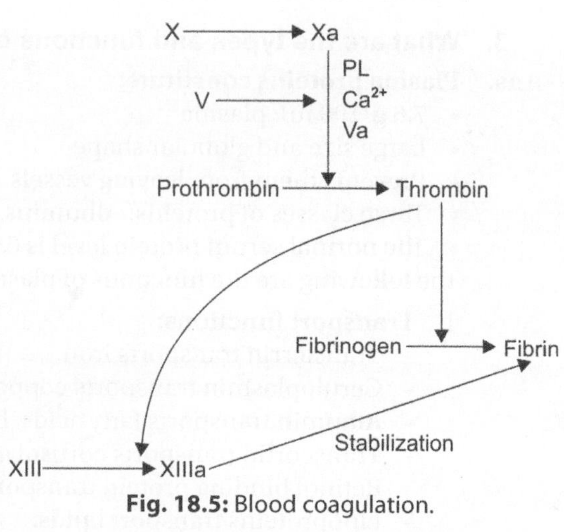

Fig. 18.5: Blood coagulation.

Intrinsic pathway:
- The initial reaction is the conversion of inactive factor X to active factor Xa.

- Factor X is activated in vitro by exposing blood to foreign surface (glass test tube).
- Activation in vivo occurs when blood is exposed to collagen fibers underlying the endothelium in the blood vessels.

Extrinsic pathway:
- Requires contact with tissue factors external to blood.
- This occurs when there is trauma to the vascular wall and surrounding tissues.
- The extrinsic system is triggered by the release of tissue factor (thromboplastin from damaged tissue) that activates factor VII.
- The tissue thromboplastin and factor VII activate factor X.

Figure 18.6 shows the clothing mechanism.

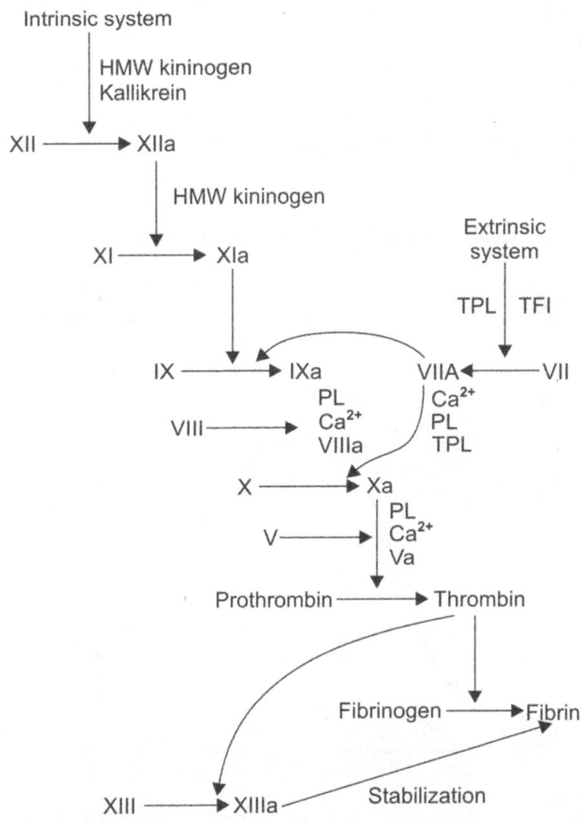

Fig. 18.6: The clotting mechanism. a, is active form of clotting factor. (TPL: tissue thromboplastin: TFI: tissue factor pathway inhibitor)

SHORT ANSWERS — 3 MARKS

5. Write the functions of hemoglobin.

Ans.
- The main function of red blood cell is transfer of O_2 from lungs to the tissue
- Transfer of CO_2 from tissue to lungs
- To accomplish this function red cells have hemoglobin
- Each red cell has 640 million molecules of Hb.

6. Write a brief note on oxyhemoglobin dissociation curve.

Ans.
- O_2 carrying capacity of Hb at different PO_2
- Sigmoid shape:
  - Binding of one molecule facilitates the second molecule binding
  - P 50 (partial pressure of O_2 at which Hb is half saturated with O_2) 26.6 mm Hg
- The normal position of curve depends on:
  - Concentration of 2,3-DPG
  - H^+ ion concentration (pH)
  - CO_2 in red blood cells
  - Structure of hemoglobin
- Right shift (easy oxygen delivery):
  - High 2,3-DPG
  - High H^+
  - High CO_2
  - HbS
- Left shift (give up oxygen less readily):
  - Low 2,3-DPG
  - HbF

Figure 18.7 shows oxyhemoglobin dissociation curve.

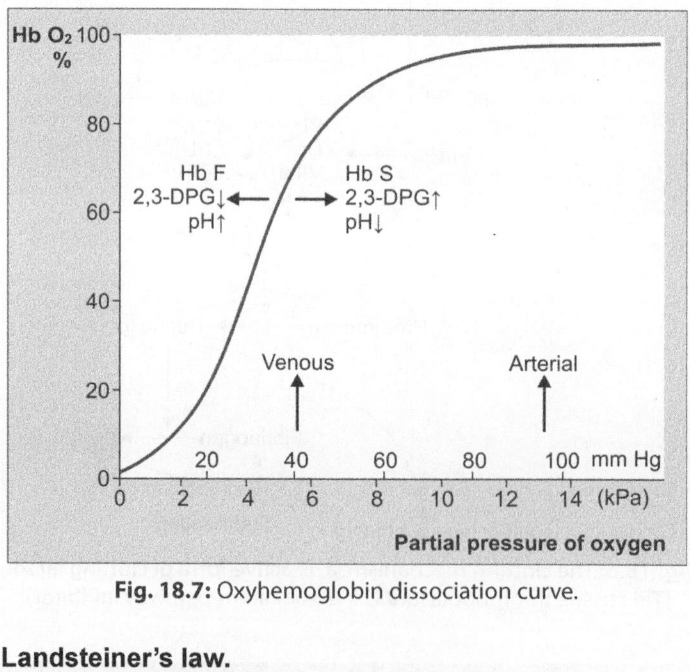

Fig. 18.7: Oxyhemoglobin dissociation curve.

7. Define Landsteiner's law.

Ans.
- If an agglutinogen is present on the RBC membrane the corresponding agglutinin is absent in the plasma.
- If an agglutinogen is absent on the RBC membrane the corresponding agglutinin is present in the plasma.
- Applicable to ABO blood group
- Not applicable to Rh system or other blood group system.

8. State the importance of abo blood group system.

Ans. The antibodies are "**naturally occurring**" antibodies, mostly **IgM class**. They are **capable** of agglutinating saline/low protein suspended red cell without enhancement and may activate complement cascade.

Antibodies are formed against most of the major group antigens and present in almost all individuals when the antigen is absent. In most other minor systems, natural antibodies to the antigens are found occasionally but as their antigenicity is low, the immune antibodies are also rare (except—Kell and Duffy). Mostly of them are IgM type. They react poorly at body temperature (except anti-A and anti-B), but agglutinate RBCs at 5–20°C and they usually do not cross placenta.

ABO group	Antigen present	Antigen missing	Antibody present
A	A	B	Anti-B
B	B	A	Anti-A
O	None	A and B	Anti-A and B

9. State the importance of universal donor and recipient.

Ans. **Universal donor**

- Group O
  - Carries no A or B antigens
  - Packed and processed units have little antibody

Universal recipient

- Group AB
  - Patient has no anti-A or anti-B present
  - Cannot lyse any transfused cells
  - Other antibodies may be present

10. Write briefly on erythroblastosis fetalis.

Ans. This immunologic disease occurs when an *Rh-negative mother* carries an *Rh-positive fetus*. The mother's immunological system is stimulated to produce antibodies to the Rh antigen on the fetal blood cell. These antibodies cross the placenta and destroy fetal red blood cells leading to fetal anemia. **Usually the fetus will not be affected if it is the first time** the mother has been exposed to the rhesus positive antigen. In the subsequent pregnancy, in-utero antigen-antibody reaction occurs on the RBCs surface leading to hemolysis and anemia. This leads to increased hepatic erythropoiesis and dysfunction. This causes portal and umbilical vein hypertension and ultimately heart failure. This causes hydrops fetalis and intrauterine death.

IMMUNITY

LONG ESSAYS — 10 MARKS

11. Explain the mechanism of cell-mediated immunity.

Ans.

- Cell-mediated immunity is mediated through T-lymphocytes.
- T-lymphocyte do not recognize the antigen directly.
- Signals to activate:

- The first signal is antigen recognition by antigen-presenting cells (APC) and binding of the processed antigen along with MHC protein in the T cell receptor, activate T cell
- The second signal is co-stimulation. (Some costimulators are cytokines)

Thus the process of cell-mediated immunity involves the following steps:

I. **Antigen recognition, processing and presentation by APC:**
- The cells that process and present antigen to the T cells are called antigen-presenting cells (APCs) which include macrophages, dendritic cells and B cells.
- Antigen processing involves conversion of an antigen into a form that can be recognized by lymphocytes.

Steps of antigen presentation and processing:
- **Ingestion of antigen by APC**
- Digestion of antigen and formation of vesicle containing the peptide fragment of antigen
- Formation of vesicle containing MHC
- Fusion of both vesicles
- Binding of peptide fragments with MHC-II molecules
- Insertion of antigen—MHC complex into the cell membrane of APC.

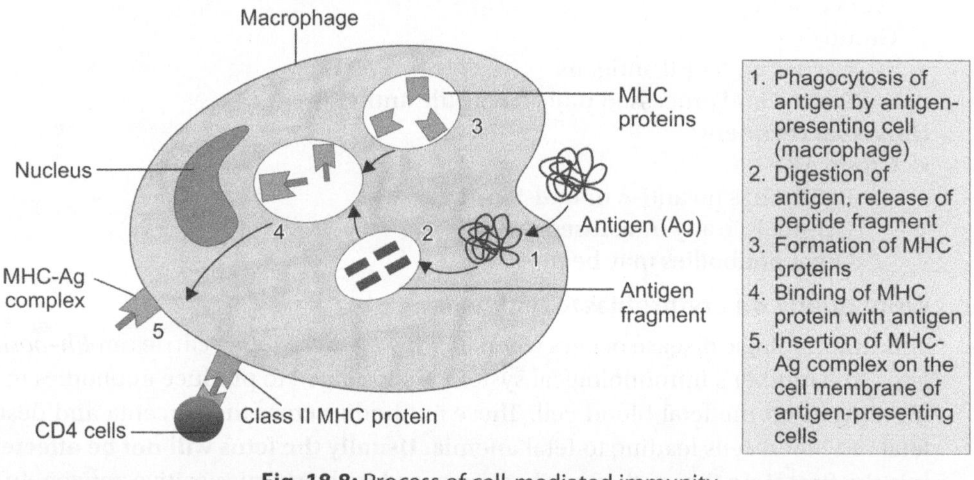

Fig. 18.8: Process of cell-mediated immunity.

II. **Antigen presentation to T- lymphocyte cells.**
- APC containing the MHC-II-Ag complex circulate in the blood. When it comes in contact with an immunocompetent
- T cell, the complex attaches to the T cell receptor, gets activated. That triggers cell mediated immunity.

III. **Activation and proliferation of T cells:** The T cells are produced in the bone marrow, do not contain any T cell receptors on their surface, once released into the blood, these T cells migrate to the *thymus for their maturation.* During the process of maturation the T cells acquire T cell receptors on their surface and ability to produce cytokines, however these cells are still not competent to fight with the antigen thus these cells are called *naïve cells.* When naïve cells are released in the blood they migrate to the lymphatics and come in contact with the antigen-presenting cells and get activated and proliferate to form the effector cells.

Proliferation and differentiation of T cells:

- The activated T cells with proper costimulation by helper T cells undergo proliferation and differentiated into two sets of T cells: cytotoxic T cells and memory T cells.
- This type of proliferation is called *clonal expansion* as a specific cell proliferate and expand to form a specific set of effector cells which will be active against a particular antigen.
  - ¤ Cytotoxic T cells or T_8 cells: These are the cells which contain CD8 proteins on their cell membrane. They are also known as killer cells. They kill the cells infected with viruses or other pathogens.
  - ¤ Memory T cells: Memory T cells are lymphocytes that become "experienced" by having encountered an antigen during a prior infection or a previous vaccination. Memory T cells are programed to recognize the subsequent exposure of same antigen and they mount faster and stronger immune response and kill the invading agent.

IV. **Removal of the pathogen:** The cytotoxic T cells kill the microbe by the following mechanisms:

- Cytolysis—killer cells synthesize and secrete perforins, and incorporate them into the membranes of the invader organisms. Perforins are water channels through which water enters the microbe and it swells and burst.
- Cytotoxic cells secrete lymphotoxin that kills the microbes.
- Cytotoxic T cells also kill their targets by programing them to undergo apoptosis.

Cell-mediated immunity is effective against:

1. Viral infections
2. Fungal infections
3. Tumor cells
4. Transplanted cells
5. Chronic bacterial infections like TB

12. Describe the mechanism of humoral immunity.

Ans.
- Humoral immunity is mediated by B cells, hence it is also called B cell-mediated Immunity
- B cells on specific antigenic stimulation, gets transformed to plasma cells and produces antibodies.

Steps of activation of humoral immunity:

1. **Presentation of antigen and activation of B lymphocyte**
   - B lymphocyte can identify antigen themselves, presentation of antigen by antigen presenting cells also induce humoral immunity.
   - **Activation of B cells:** When antigen binds directly to the receptors present on B cell surface, they get activated and B cells also gets activated when they come in contact with MHC -antigen complex on APC.
   - Activation of B cell is accentuated by the costimulation from type 2 helper cells by secreting IL-2 and IL-4
2. **Differentiation of B cells into plasma cells:** Activated B cells can differentiate into plasma cells that secrete antibodies.

   Proliferation of plasma cells and antibody production: Plasma cells undergo proliferation to form millions of plasma cells and secrete a large quantity of antibody.

Elimination of the invaders: Antibodies attack and destroys the antigen by following **mechanisms**

1. Neutralizing antigen: Antibodies neutralize the antigen.
2. Immobilization of microbes: Antibodies prevent the motility of bacteria thereby inhibit their spread to the surrounding tissue.
3. Activation of complement system: Antigen-antibody complex activate the complement system and kill the organisms.
4. Precipitation of antigen: Antibodies cause agglutination and precipitation of antigens.
5. Promotion of phagocytosis: Antibodies enhance phagocytosis by opsonizing the antigen.

Formation of memory B cells: After exposure to a given antigen, a small subset of activated B cells persist as memory B cells. These cells are readily converted to effector cells by a later encounter with the same antigen. This ability to produce a quicker response to a second exposure to an antigen is also called as secondary immune response, a prime feature of acquired immunity. This capacity persists for life-long.

SHORT ESSAYS — 5 MARKS

13. Define immunity. Describe the types of immunity.

Ans. **Immunity:** The process of defense of body against harmful elements that threaten our normal health is called immunity.

Types of immunity: There are two types of immunity:

1. **Innate or nonspecific immunity**—the innate immune responses are the first line of defense against invading pathogens. This is the inbuilt capacity of the body to fight against foreign harmful particles or organisms. Innate immunity present since birth and it do not require exposure to antigenic particles or organisms for their development. Innate immunity consists of:
   - Mechanical defenses—skin and epidermis, mucous membranes, hair, etc.
   - Chemical defenses—acidic pH of the skin, stomach
   - Defense by natural killer cells, granulocytes and mononuclear cells
2. **Acquired or specific immunity**—this form of immunity is formed by specific immune systems in the form of activated antibodies or lymphocytes that attack and destroy a specific set of antigens. Thus it is specific for each set of antigen and hence called specific immunity.

   This form of immunity is acquired during one's lifetime and develops on exposure to invading organisms or particles hence called the acquired immunity.

14. Write a short note on humoral immune response.

The humoral immune response of two types **(Fig. 18.9)**:

1. **Primary humoral immune response:**
   - Immune response when antigen enters into the body for the first time
   - The antibodies are formed slowly with a latent period of about 4 days to 4 weeks.
   - The concentration of antibodies rises gradually and attains smaller peak.
   - Though IgM and IgG antibodies contribute to the primary response, the response is mainly due to IgM.
   - Antibody titer in primary response returns back to normal within few days to week

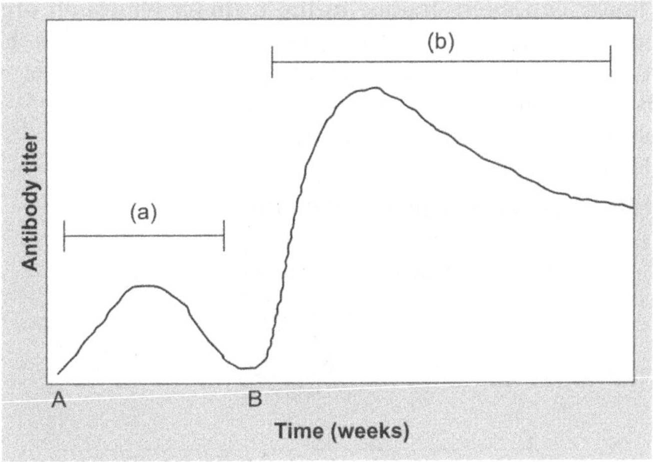

Primary response (a)
Secondary response (b)

Fig. 18.9: Types of humoral immunity response.

2. **Secondary humoral immune response**
   - The immune response produced by the same antigen entering the body for the second or subsequent time is called Secondary humoral immune response
   - It occurs quickly and intensely which is due to the immunological memory, i.e., due to persistence of memory B and T cells
   - Antibodies are formed rapidly. Therefore the concentration of antibody rises and reaches a greater peak.
   - Antibody titer falls very slowly and never returns to normal, rather remains elevated for a longer duration.
   - Antibodies in secondary humoral immune response are primarily of IgG type.

15. Write short note on major histocompatability complex (MHC) antigen.

Ans. Antigens are living organisms or substances that on entry into the body induce specific immune response. MHC antigens are self-antigens that help in identifying self from nonself protein. They are chemically glycoprotein. They are also called HLA antigens or human leukocyte associated antigens as they were first identified on the surface of leukocytes.

MHC antigens are of two types:

1. **MHC 1:** Found on all nucleated cell surface of all body cells except red cells
2. **MHC 2:** Found on surface of antigen presenting cells, thymus cells and activated T cells.

The function of the MHC antigen is to identify the foreign antigen and present them to T cells for induction of cell-mediated immunity. The MHC molecules is to bind peptide fragments derived from pathogens and display them on the cell surface for recognition by the appropriate T cells.

16. Describe the development of immunity.

Ans. Development of immunity is the development of lymphocytes.

Immunity develops in response to antigen, a specific antigen stimulates the development of a specific set of lymphocyte. The major sites of lymphocyte development are the primary lymphoid organs. In the primary lymphoid organs, lymphocytes differentiate from their precursors that originate from the bone marrow and proliferate and mature into functionally potent cells. T cells mature in thymus and B cells mature in the bone marrow. After maturation, they circulate in blood and migrate to secondary lymphoid organ, such as lymph nodes, spleen and gut associated lymph nodes.

Flowchart 18.1 shows development of immunity.

Flowchart 18.1: Development of immunity.

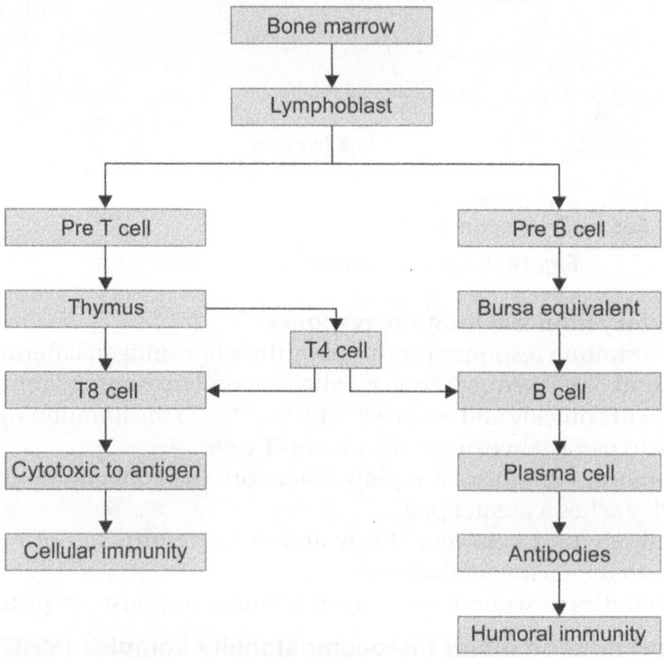

17. Write short note on immunoglobulins.

Ans. Immunoglobulins, also known as antibodies, they are glycoprotein molecules produced by plasma cells in response to an antigen invasion **(Fig. 18.10)**.

All immunoglobulins have a four chain structure as their basic unit. They are composed of two identical light chains (23kD) and two identical heavy chains (50–70kD), the heavy (H) and light chains and the two heavy chains are held together by interchain disulfide bonds. Depending on the type of H chain, antibodies are classified into five types: IgG, IgM, IgA, IgE and IgD. The general functions of immunoglobulin are:

- Activation of complement proteins
- Enhances phagocytosis
- Initiate immune response
- Secreted in body fluids and therefore provide local protection
- Plays a role in allergy by releasing histamine from mast cells.

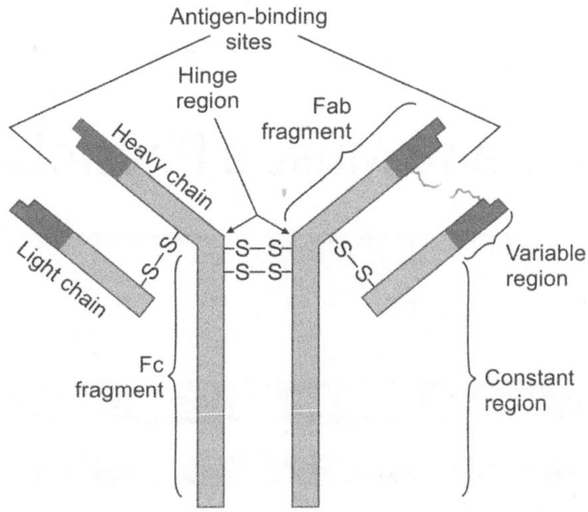

Fig. 18.10: Immunoglobulin structure.

SHORT ANSWER	3 MARKS

18. What are natural killer cells?

Ans. Natural killer cells (NK) are a third category of lymphocytes that are neither B nor T cells. NK cells form a part of the innate immunity and kill harmful antigens. It constitute 10–15% of the circulating lymphocytes. They lack surface receptors on their membrane like B and T lymphocytes. They do not involve major histocompatibility complex antigen for killing microorganism. They contain cytoplasmic granules (perforin and granzyme) it cause target cell to die by releasing the granules.

19
CHAPTER

Nerve and Muscle Physiology

SKELETAL MUSCLE

LONG ESSAYS — 10 MARKS

1. Explain in detail the molecular mechanisms involved in excitation-contraction coupling of skeletal muscle.

Ans. The action potential from sarcolemma spreads to the interior of the muscle through the T tubule system.

- This results in calcium release which in turn increases calcium in the sarcoplasmic reticulum (SR).
- Calcium diffuses to troponin C and causes muscle contraction.
- **Sliding filament theory**—AF Huxley proposed this theory in 1957.
- It is also known as cross-bridge theory. There are three types of troponin. *Troponin-I* attached to myosin binding site on actin. Other part of the site is covered by tropomyosin. *Troponin-T* is attached to tropomyosin. The tropomyosin-troponin complex act as a relaxing protein. When there is propagation of action potential calcium is released from sarcoplasmic reticulum raising its concentration and binding to *Troponin-C* causes a conformational change and results in shifting of *Troponin-I* from the actin allowing tropomyosin to move deeper into the actin groove—unmasking the myosin binding sites. This is referred to as *cross-bridge cycling*. During each cycle myosin attaches to thin filament causing displacement of thick filament over thin filament followed by detachment of myosin head in a repetitive fashion. These activities require ATP. All cross bridges do not undergo the same processes hence the contraction is smooth and sustained.
- Ca^{2+} ATPase pumps calcium from sarcoplasm to sarcoplasmic reticulum.

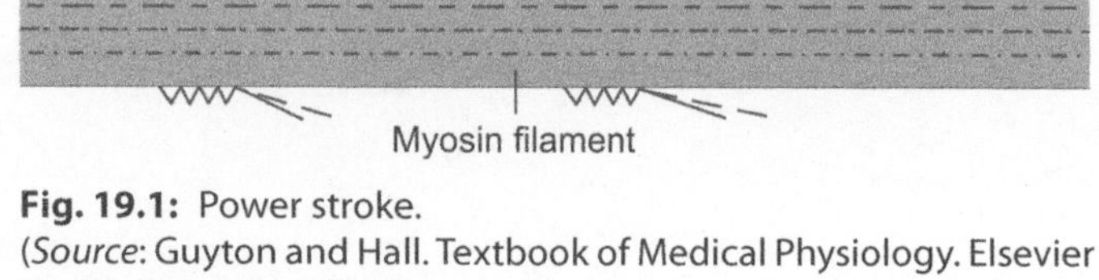

Fig. 19.1: Power stroke.
(*Source*: Guyton and Hall. Textbook of Medical Physiology. Elsevier Health Sciences, 2015)

- When an action potential does not arrive the level of calcium decreases and very few of them are available to bind with troponin. This leads to decreased cross-bridge formation. The contractile activity stops and relaxation ensues.

Rigor mortis: The detachment of the myosin head from the actin cannot take place until and unless a new ATP does not attach to the myosin head. This is important when death occurs, no more ATP is available and thus, *rigor mortis* occurs **(Fig. 19.1)**.

Steps in relaxation of skeletal muscle:

1. Signals at motor end plate stops which repolarizes the sarcoplasmic reticulum (SR) and T-tubules
2. Ca^{2+} ATPase closes. This leads to Ca pumped back into SR.
3. Decreased sarcoplasmic Ca^{2+} level
4. Detachment of Ca^{2+} from troponin
5. Cessation of actin myosin interaction
6. Muscle goes into a state of relaxation

2. Write a note on the sequence of events during neuromuscular events.

Ans. Transmission in a neuromuscular junction refers to the impulse transmission in three components **(Figs. 19.2 and 19.3)**:

1. **Presynaptic activities**: Arrival of a stimulus at this part of the terminal causes depolarization of the membrane and leading to opening of voltage gated calcium channels and calcium release.
   - Activation of molecular motors (microtubules and microfilaments) cause movement of neurotransmitter vesicles towards the presynaptic membranes.
   - The neurotransmitter gets released into the cleft by exocytosis.
   - There is interaction between the vesicular and synaptic membrane proteins—syntaxin and synaptobrevin.
2. **Synaptic cleft:** The acetylcholine diffuses across the synaptic cleft and binds to the receptor which gets acted upon by the acetylcholine esterase.

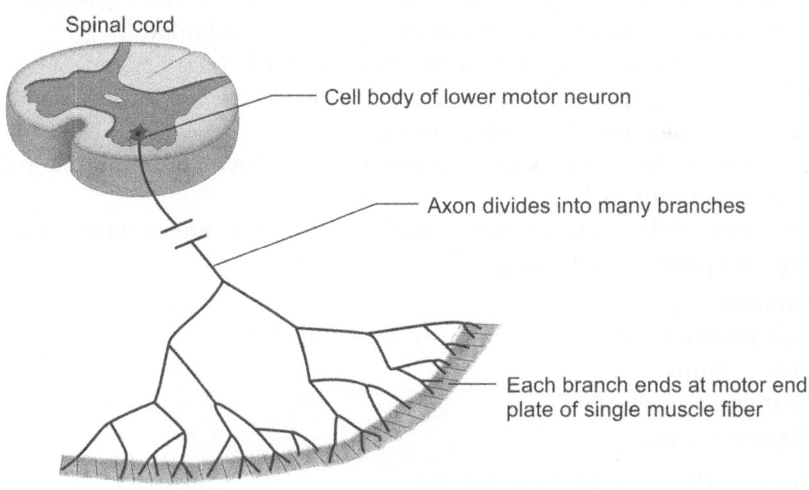

Fig. 19.2: Transmission of events in a neuromuscular junction.
(*Source*: Illustrated Physiology by Mackenna BR, R Callander, 6th edition)

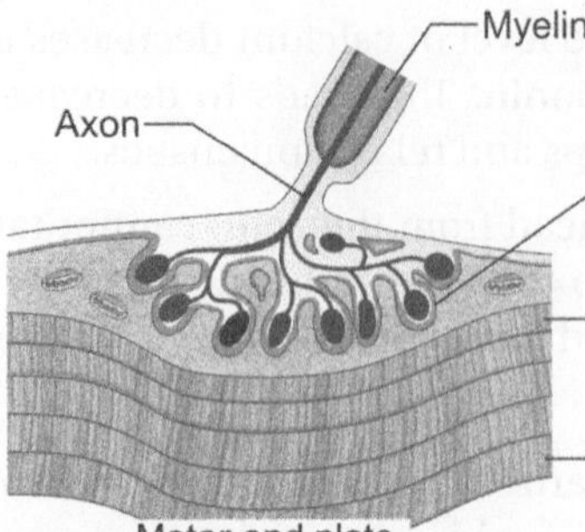

Fig. 19.3: Neuromuscular junction.
(*Source:* Illustrated Physiology by Mackenna BR, R Callander. Neuromuscular Junction, 6th edition)

3. **Postsynaptic events:** Acetylcholine after getting attached to its receptor causes influx of sodium ions. There is generation of end plate potential. This potential spreads across the sarcolemma and T-tubule and activating the motor endplate. Acetylcholine gets hydrolyzed and the end-plate potential (EPP) ceases and the membrane potential returns to normal. Acetate gets into the extracellular fluid (ECF) and choline is taken back for resynthesis of ACh. This processes takes place within a few milliseconds and the processes gets repeated several times.

Applied physiological aspects: Neuromuscular dysfunction

Myasthenia gravis:

- It is an autoimmune disorder, characterized by weakness and fatigability of skeletal muscles.
- It results from destruction of acetylcholine receptors due to production of circulating antibodies against the receptors.
- The postsynaptic folds are flattened. The acetylcholine receptor antibodies cause endocytosis of ACh receptors and damage the postsynaptic membrane. The antibodies compete with ACh to bind to ACh receptors, producing receptor blockade
- There is decremental response to repetitive nerve stimulation
- Women are more affected than men in ratio of 3:1
- Weakness increases during prolonged use of muscle and improves after rest
- Symptoms aggravate towards evening
- The extraocular muscles and eyelids are often involved, diplopia and ptosis are early symptoms
- Proximal limbs muscles are commonly affected and severe case respiratory muscles paralysis leads to death.

Treatment:

- Administration of acetylcholine esterase inhibitors
- Thymectomy
- Immunosuppresssion
- Plasmapheresis

Lambert-Eaton Myasthenic syndrome

- It is an autoimmune disorder
- Antibodies produced against voltage gated Ca^{++} channels

- The decreased Ca^{++} influx in the presynaptic axon terminal results in impaired ACh release from nerve endings
- There is incremental response to repetitive nerve stimulation as Ca^{++} level increases with each action potential.

SHORT ESSAYS — 5 MARKS

3. Name the types and characteristics of different types of muscles.

Ans. The different types of muscles are as follows **(Fig. 19.4)**:

Types

*Smooth muscle **(Fig. 19.5)**:*

- Located in the blood vessels, respiratory tract, iris of the eye, gastrointestinal tract
- The contractions are slow and uniform.
- Functions to alter the activity of various body parts to meet the needs of the body at that time.
- Is fatigue resistant
- Activation is involuntary.

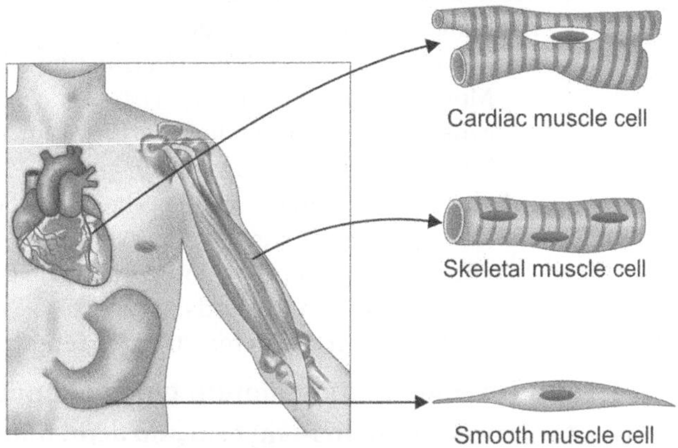

Fig. 19.4: Types of muscles.
(*Source*: Internet)

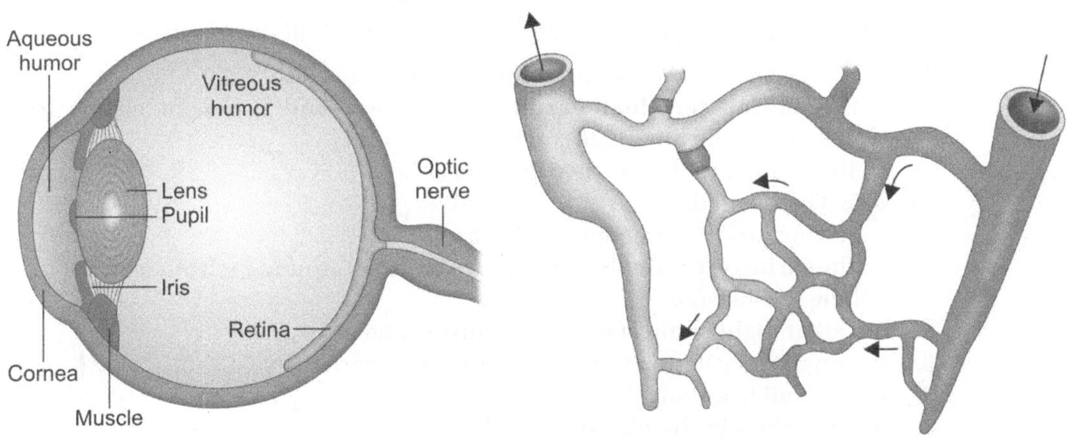

Fig. 19.5: Structure of the eye, blood vessels.
(*Source*: Internet)

Cardiac muscle:

- Has characteristics of both skeletal and smooth muscle
- Functions to provide the contractile activity of the heart
- Contractile activity can be gradated (like skeletal muscle)
- Is very fatigue resistant
- Activation of cardiac muscle is involuntary (like smooth muscle)

Skeletal muscle:
- They use chemical energy to generate force to produce movement (chemical energy is converted to mechanical energy)
- Movement is by muscle contraction
- The trigger for muscle contraction is a rise in cytosolic calcium concentration.

Each of the muscle is ultimately made up of:
- Skeletal/smooth muscle
- Muscle bundles/fascicles
- Large number of muscle fibers
- The connective tissue layer covering the:
  - Muscle is epimysium.
  - Muscle bundle/fascicle is perimysium
  - Muscle fiber is endomysium

  All the layers are made up of collagen and elastic fibers.

  In case of skeletal muscles:
  - The muscle fibers are long, cylindrical, multinucleated cells which attach to tendons at both the ends.
  - 10–100 μm in diameter, 20 cm in length.

4. Write a note on the different types of contractile proteins.

Ans. Contractile proteins—myosin and actin filaments

A. Myosin—is composed of:
- Two heavy (intertwined) chains
- Two regulatory light chains
- Two alkali light chains
- Myosin II has two globular heads, neck and a long tail

1. Myosin head (amino and carboxy terminal):
   - **Has amino terminal portion**—one heavy and two light chains (one regulatory and one alkali) forming a complex
   - The head portion has—two binding sites
     a. One for actin
     b. One for ATP (functions as ATPase)

     The **carboxy terminals** of the heavy chain coil around each other forming—a long rod-like tail
2. **The alkali light chain** stabilizes the myosin head
3. **The regulatory light chain** regulates its ATPase activity
4. **Myosin tail** lies along the long axis
5. **The two globular heads** extend to the sides
6. **Myosin hinge**—joins the head and tail.
   - The myosin molecule are placed in a definite directional arrangement.
   - The heads are directed away from the tails
   - Titin, myomesin and C-protein-maintain the bipolarity of the thick filaments.

B. Actin
- G-actin—globular protein
- Diameter—4–5 nm
- Molecular weight 42,000.

- G-actin molecules—joined from front to back
  - a double stranded alpha-helical filament
- F-actin (backbone of actin)

  Cytoskeletal protein—nebulin regulates the length of the F-actin molecule.
- Each actin monomer contains binding site for:
  - Myosin
  - Tropomyosin
  - Troponin-I
- Other actin monomers: The F-actin undergoes a half turn every seven G-actin monomers form a groove, where lies the long filamentous protein tropomyosin.
- Each thin filament contains 300–400 actin molecule and 40–60 tropomyosin molecules.

Tropomodulin:
- Located at the end of the thin filament towards the center of the sarcomere
- Maintenance of length.

5. Write a note on the different types of regulatory proteins.

Ans. Regulatory proteins (Fig. 19.6)

1. **Tropomyosin**
   - Rod-shaped molecule
   - Molecular weight—70,000
   - Length = seven active monomers

   Location
   - Molecules connected to one another serially
   - Along the entire length of the actin monomer
   - Covers the myosin binding site
   - Function is to prevent the binding of myosin with actin.

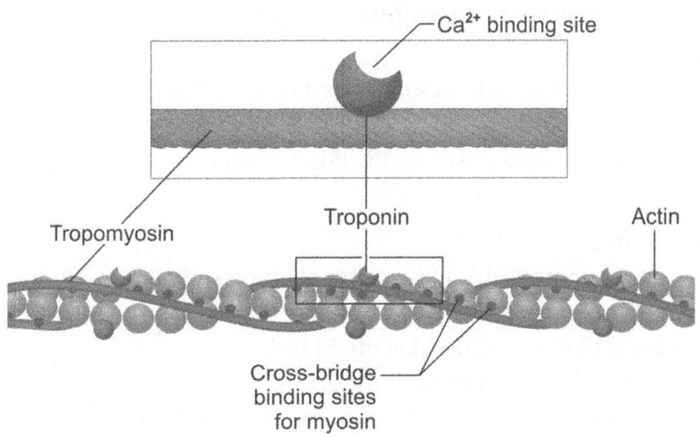

Fig. 19.6: Structure of tropomyosin and troponin.
(*Source:* Modified from Figure 11-13, in Vander, Sherman and Luciano. Human Physiology, 6th edition, McGraw-Hill, 1994, p. 313)

2. **Troponin**
   Composed of:
   Troponin T
   - Molecular weight—30,000
   - Binds troponin to tropomyosin

   Troponin I
   - Molecular weight—22,000
   - Inhibits the binding of actin to myosin.

   Troponin C
   - Molecular weight 18,000
   - Binds calcium

Attachment proteins

- Titin
  - Thin, elastic, filamentous protein—extends form the Z line to M line
  - Prevents over extension of the thick filaments.
  - Maintains central location of A band.
- Nebulin
  - Large filamentous protein
  - Helps in stabilizing the length of the actin during development
- Alpha actinin: Anchors the thin filaments to the Z line.
- Dystrophin
  - Rod-like protein
  - Anchors thin filaments to the membrane spanning protein beta-dystroglycan.
  - This in turn is connected to **laminin** (extracellular matrix protein) through alpha-dystroglycan
  - Helps in transferring the force from the contractile system to the extracellular regions
  - Genetic mutations—muscular degeneration, weakness and death—muscular dystrophies.

6. Describe sarcomere with a suitable diagram.

Ans. Sarcomere (Fig. 19.7)

- Each myofibril is made up of units—sarcomere. "Sarco" means muscle and "Mere" means part.
- It consists of the portion of myofibril between two successive Z lines. Its length is 2 µm.

Muscle structure

- The electron micrographic shows that each myofibril is made up of repeating dark and light bands
- In the middle of the dark band is the M line
- In the middle of the light band is the Z line
- The repeating unit from one Z line to the next is called the sarcomere
- The thin filament is 1 µm long and 7 nm in diameter (actin, troponin and tropomyosin—ratio 7:1:1)
- They project parallely from the Z line towards the center of the sarcomere.

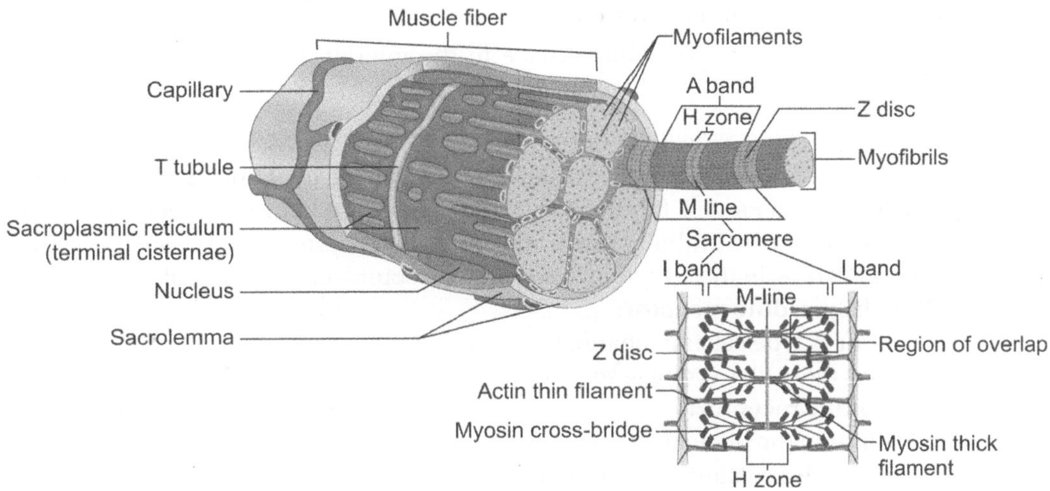

Fig. 19.7: Sarcomere.
(*Source:* Berne RM, Levy MN. Physiology; 4th edition. Mosby, 1998)

- The parallel array of thick filament in the center of the sarcomere produces A band
- Length—1.6 µm and 10 nm in diameter.
- I band —portion of the thin filament that lies between the ends of the A bands of the adjacent sarcomere.

During contraction the length of the sarcomere decreases.

- Length of I band changes. Length of A band remains unchanged.
- H zone—area of the A band where there is no overlap of thick and thin filaments.
- M line runs through the middle of the H band. It contains proteins that bind the parallel array of thick filaments.
- The protein titin binds the thick filament to Z line.
- A cross section of the overlap region shows—each thick filament is surrounded by a hexagonal array of thin filaments.
- The thin filament is surrounded by three thick filaments (triangular).

7. Describe the sarcotubular system.

Ans. Sarcotubular system (Fig. 19.8)

- In a muscle fiber the myofibrils are surrounded by sarcotubular system. It has T -tubules and sarcoplasmic reticulum.
- They are tubular extensions of sarcolemma 0.03 µm in diameter.
- It penetrates unto the center of the muscle fiber and surround the individual myofibrils at the junction of A and I band. ECF fills the lumen. Action potential travels to the interior of the fiber.
- The sarcoplasmic reticulum in the fiber is 0.04 µm in diameter.
- Runs parallel to the myofibril. And have elongated portion and dilated portion (terminal cisternae).
- The cisternae lie close to the T-tubules. T-tubules and the cisternae form a triad.

Functions of sarcotubular system

Transfers action potential from surface to the interior. Regulates calcium release. Calcium reuptake by SR enables muscle relaxation.

Role of sarcotubular system in muscle contraction

They are special receptors in the tubular system. Space of about 12–14 nm between terminal cisternae and T tubule. Areas of densities are known as 'feet'. Involve two proteins—one on the T tubule system and one on the terminal cistern. Dihydropyridine receptor (DHP)—in the T tubule. Ryanodine receptor—in the terminal cistern.

Dihydropyridine receptor:
- Is an 'L' type calcium channel
- Acts more like a voltage sensor

Ryanodine receptor:
- Binds to the plant alkaloid ryanodine
- Acts like a calcium release channel

Role of ST system during muscle contraction

Ca^{2+}ATPase pumps Ca^{2+} into longitudinal part of SR. Ca^{2+} is transferred and stored into the cisternae. Then action potential arrives and is transmitted into the T-tubules. Voltage gated calcium channels in the DHP receptors get activated followed by a conformational change in the ryanodine receptor causing release of Ca^{2+} into sarcoplasm. Ca^{2+} released binds with troponin C causing muscle contraction leading to autoactivation of Ca^{2+} ATPase which inturn pumps calcium into SR.

Ca^{2+} gets stored in the cisternal fluid bound to calsequestrin. This decrease in sarcoplasmic calcium concentration causes muscle to relax.

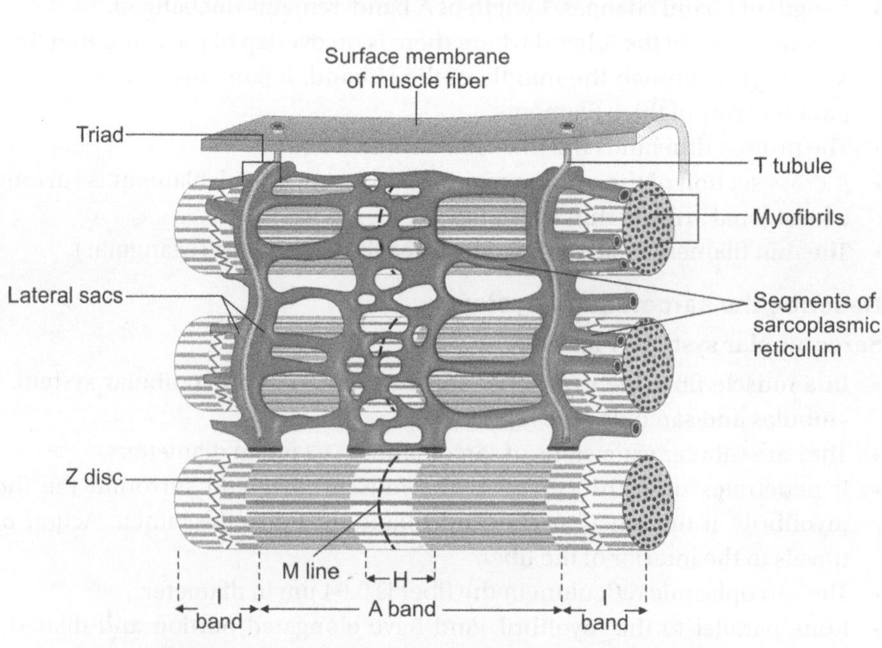

Fig. 19.8: Skeletal muscle with the sarcotubular system.
(*Source*: Modified from Fig. 10-8 in Sherwood, p. 222)

SHORT ANSWERS 3 MARKS

8. Functions of sarcolemma.

Ans. Sarcolemma transmits the wave of depolarization to the entire cell surface. Offers elastic resistance (resistance to stretch offered by all the connective tissue layers). Has no gap or tight junctions. Promotes electrical separation between fibers **(Fig. 19.9)**.

- Sarcoplasm is filled with myofibrils
- Extends along the axis of the cell
- Connected to the tendons at the ends
- Each is 1 μm in diameter
- Has two types of myofilaments
  1. Actin
  2. Myosin
- A severely damaged muscle may be replaced by hypertrophy of the existing fibers.
- Recently a transcription factor—myogenin is known to stimulate fibroblasts which then transforms into muscle cells.
- Existence of:
  - Dark bands: **A** band—anisotropic to polarized light
  - Light bands: **I** band—isotropic to polarized light
- Each myofibril is made up of units—sarcomere

9. Write a note on Duchenne's muscular dystrophy (DMD).

Ans. In this type of dystrophy there is defect in *dystrophin* gene. DMD results in muscular weakness, leading to cardiac and respiratory insufficiency.

- Dystrophin protein deficiency is seen in the skeletal muscle, eyes, brain and smooth muscle. The dystrophin glycoprotein complex provides a link between sub-sarcolemma cytoskeletal structures and the extracellular matrix.
- It stabilizes the sarcolemma and prevents contraction induced injury.
- Also serve as a scaffold for cell signaling cascades—promoting cell survival.

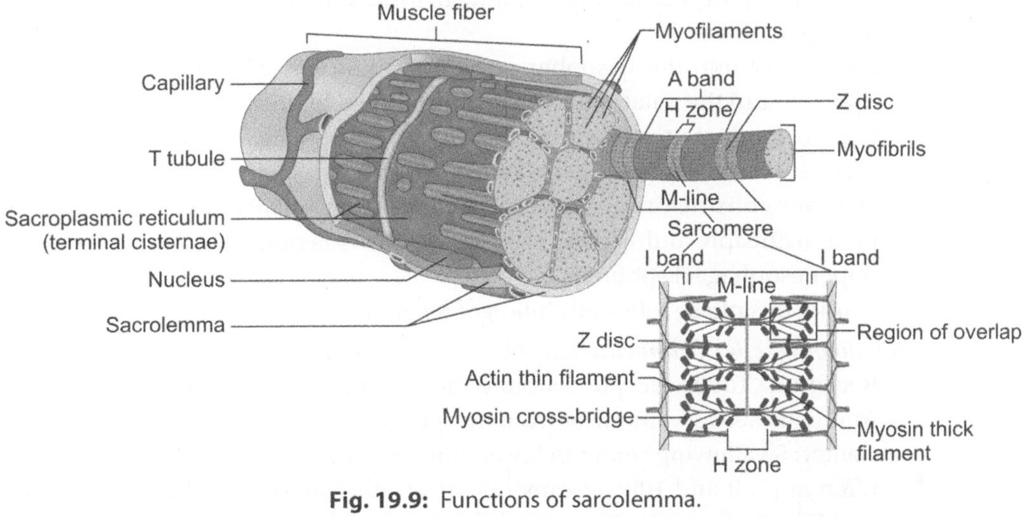

Fig. 19.9: Functions of sarcolemma.
(*Source*: Berne RM, Levy MN. Physiology, 4th edition. Mosby, 1998)

20

CHAPTER

Gastrointestinal System

LONG ESSAYS — 10 MARKS

1. Write short note on deglutition.

Ans.
- It is the process of swallowing.
- It is a sequence of events that propels food from the mouth to the stomach.
- A reflex phenomenon that is initiated voluntarily but terminates involuntarily.

It has three phases:

1. **Oral phase** (voluntary)
2. **Pharyngeal phase** (involuntary)
3. **Esophageal phase** (involuntary)

Oral Phase → Pharyngeal phase → esophageal phase

1. **Oral phase:**
   - Voluntary phase
   - Conversion of food material to bolus (with the help of salivary enzymes)
   - The tongue presses the hard palate and pushes the bolus into pharyngeal opening
   - Touch receptors stimulated resulting in initiation of swallowing reflex.
2. **Pharyngeal phase:**
   - Food entry into the nasopharynx is prevented by soft plate which is pulled upwards and the palatopharyngeal folds pulled in inwards direction.
   - Entry of food into trachea is prevented by closure of laryngeal opening by vocal cords and larynx moves against the epiglottis
   - Superior constrictor muscle of pharynx constrict which passes the food into pharynx deeply and then to esophagus, this is facilitated by the relaxation of upper esophageal sphincter.
   - During this phase reflex inhibition of respiration occurs.

   *Swallowing reflex (**Flowchart 20.1**):*
   - Receptors: Touch receptors around the opening of the pharynx
   - Afferents: Sensory impulses from the receptors
   - Center: Swallowing center in lower pons and medulla
   - Efferent (5, 9 and 10th): Cranial nerves to the pharynx and upper and lower esophagus.

Flowchart 20.1: Swallowing reflex.

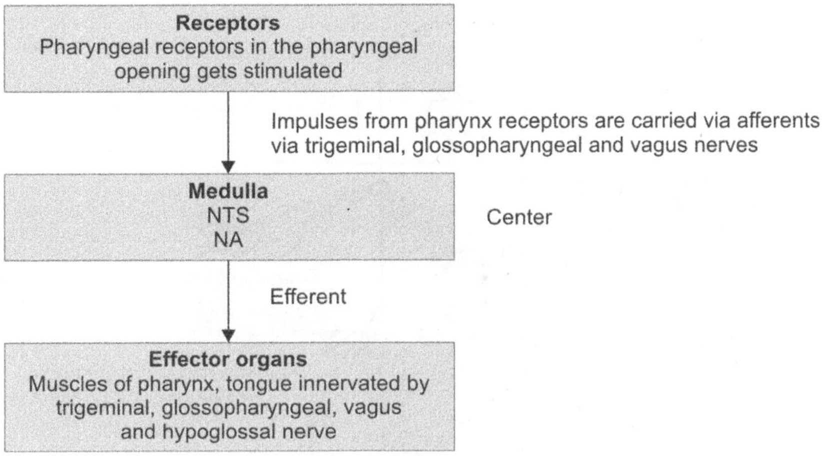

(NTS: nucleus tractus solitarius; NA: nucleus ambiguus)

3. **Esophageal phase:**
   - Once the food enters into the esophagus, the upper esophageal sphincter (UES) contracts which prevent regurgitation of food into the pharynx
   - Primary peristaltic wave initiated at 4 cm/s and takes 10 seconds for the food to pass through entire esophagus
   - Relaxation of the lower esophageal sphincter and entry of bolus into the stomach.

2. Write short notes on defecation.

Ans. When mass peristalsis of colon move the content to rectum, rectal distention causes reflex relaxation of the anal sphincter and initiate defecation reflex **(Fig. 20.1)**.

Defecation is a spinal reflex with voluntary component:

- *Stimulus*: Rectal distention
- *Receptor*: Stretch receptor located in the rectal wall
- *Afferent*: Pelvic nerve
- *Center*: S3 segment of the spinal cord
- *Efferent*: Parasympathetic fibers of pelvic nerve to rectum and internal anal sphincter
- Pudendal nerve to external anal sphincter
- *Response*: Expulsion of the feces
- *Higher center*: Cortex via corticospinal tract influence defecation.

Before defecation both the sphincters are in a state of tonic contraction therefore the anal canal remains closed. Once the defecation reflex signal reaches the spinal cord, contraction of rectum and relaxation of internal anal sphincter, external anal sphincter (EAS) opening depends on the situation (voluntary control).

Other effects include:

- Contraction of the abdominal muscle
- Relaxation of the puborectalis muscle opening of EAS
- Anorectal angle decreased.

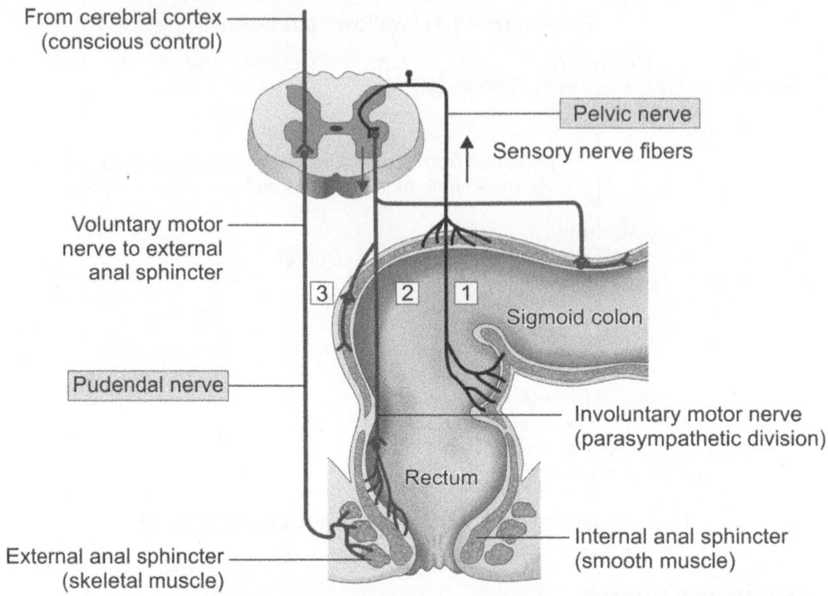

Fig. 20.1: Neural pathway in defecation reflex.

SHORT ESSAYS 5 MARKS

3. Discuss the composition and functions of saliva.

Ans. Daily output 1.5 L/day, pH; 7

Enzymes
- Ptyalin
- Lysozymes
- Kallikrein
- Lipase
- Mucin

Ions
- Na^+, K^+, Ca^{++}, Cl^-, HCO_3^-
- Organic constituents urea, uric-acid, creatinine, aminoacids

Functions
- Salivary amylase helps in digestion starch
- Keep the mouth moist
- Aids in speech
- Proline in saliva protects the enamel of teeth
- Mucin in saliva lubricates the food, it therefore helps in mastication and swallowing
- Lysozyme and lactoferrin has a protective role. It prevent oral infection
- Plays a role in temperature regulation in animals.

4. Enumerate the stomach functions.

Ans.
- Storage of food
- Gastric glands secrete gastric juice and hydrochloric acid.
- Grinding, mixing of chyme and regulated emptying of food.

- Parietal cell of gastric gland secrete intrinsic factor which is required for the absorption of vitamin B_{12}.
- Pepsinogen produced from chief cell, is converted into pepsin by HCL, which initiate protein digestion.
- Mucin produced from mucous gland protects the gastric epithelium.

5. Composition and function of gastric juice.

Ans.
- Volume: 1.5–2 L
- pH: Acidic.

Functions (Flowchart 20.2):

- HCl—kills microorganism, activate pepsinogen, convert ferric form iron into ferrous form (absorbable form)
- Pepsin: Activate pepsinogen to pepsin
- Lipase: Digestion of lipids
- Mucin-for protection
- Intrinsic factor helps in vitamin B_{12} absorption.

Flowchart 20.2: Composition of gastric juice.

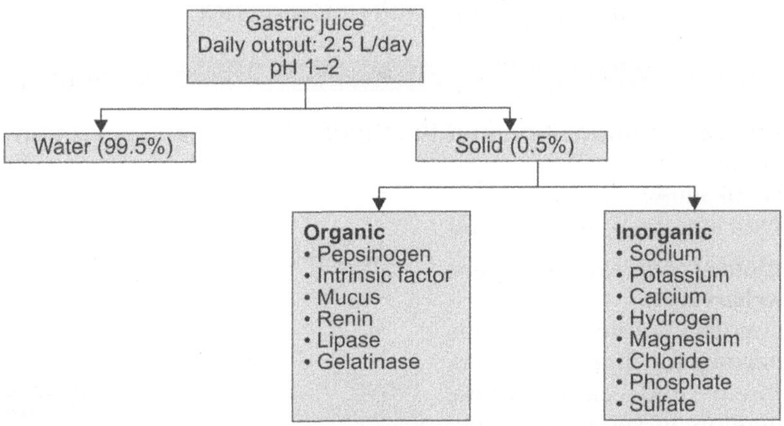

6. Describe the mechanism of hydrochloric acid secretion in the stomach.

Ans.
- Hydrochloric acid is *secreted from parietal cell* located in the stomach due to the presence of H^+/K^+ ATPase.
- Carbon dioxide derived from cellular metabolism, combines with water to form carbonic acid in the presence of carbonic anhydrase.
- Carbonic acid dissociate into H^+ and HCO_3
- HCO_3 is exchanged for Cl through HCO_3. Cl exchanger located on the basolateral membrane of the parietal cell.
- Hydrogen ion is pumped out of the cell through H^+/K^+ ATPase to the gastric lumen.
- For each hydrogen pumped out of the cell one bicarbonate is reabsorbed into the blood, as a result the pH of the blood increases as blood become alkaline, the urine also becomes alkaline. This is called as postprandial alkaline tide
- The potassium that enter in the cell through H^+–K^+ antiport is transported back to the gastric lumen which is reutilized **(Fig. 20.2)**.

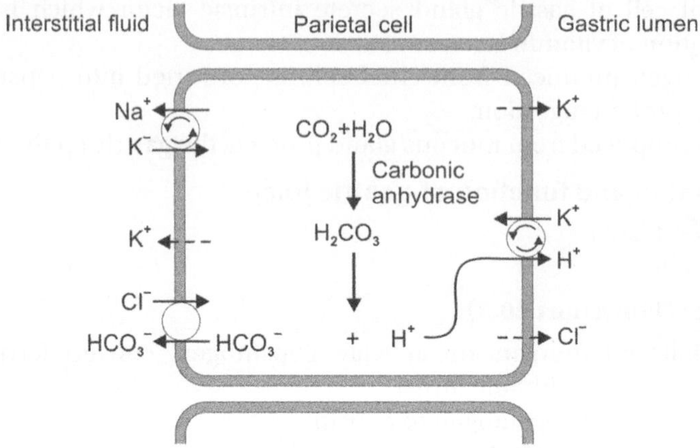

Fig. 20.2: Mechanism of HCl secretion.

- Chloride is extruded down its electrochemical gradient through a channel to the gastric lumen.
- In the lumen chloride combines with H^+ to form HCL.

SHORT ESSAYS — 5 MARKS

7. Describe the composition and functions of pancreatic secretion.

Ans.
- Volume: 1–2 L
- pH: Alkaline

It consist of water—98% and solid—2%.

Functions of pancreatic secretions (Flowchart 20.3)

- Pancreatic juice contains enzymes for digestion of fat, protein and carbohydrate. Therefore its secretion is necessary for digestion, absorption of nutrients.
- It contains bicarbonate and water that neutralizes the acidic content of the chyme

Flowchart 20.3: Composition of pancreatic secretion.

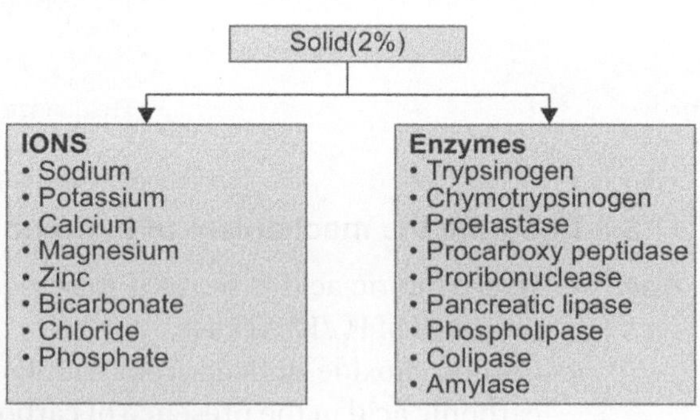

8. Describe the regulation of pancreatic secretion.

Ans. It is controlled by hormonal and neural mechanism.

Neural:
- Parasympathetic stimulation increases the pancreatic secretion
- Sympathetic stimulation decrease the pancreatic secretion

Hormonal:
- Cholecystokinin and secretin are the principal regulators of pancreatic secretion
- Secretin is produced by S cells of duodenum
- **Acidic chyme** in the duodenum activates S cells and increases the pancreatic secretion rich in bicarbonate and water

- **Products of digestion in the duodenum** activate I cells of small intestine to release CCK which increase the pancreatic secretion rich in enzymes.

9. Describe mechanism of pancreatic secretion.

Ans. The secretion of the pancreatic juice occurs by the entry of acidic chyme into the duodenum.

The columnar cells lining the pancreatic duct produce the aqueous component of the juice. CO_2 combines with water to form carbonic acid in presence of enzyme carbonic anhydrase. Carbonic acid dissociates into H^+ and HCO_3^- ions., via bicarbonate-chloride exchanger HCo_3 ions are actively transported from the cell to the lumen of the duct and chloride enters inside the cells. The hydrogen ions are exchanged for sodium ions through hydrogen sodium exchanger in the basolateral surface. The bicarbonate in the lumen neutralize the acid chyme.

Pancreatic enzymes are produced in the acinar cells released on appropriate stimuli **(Fig. 20.3)**.

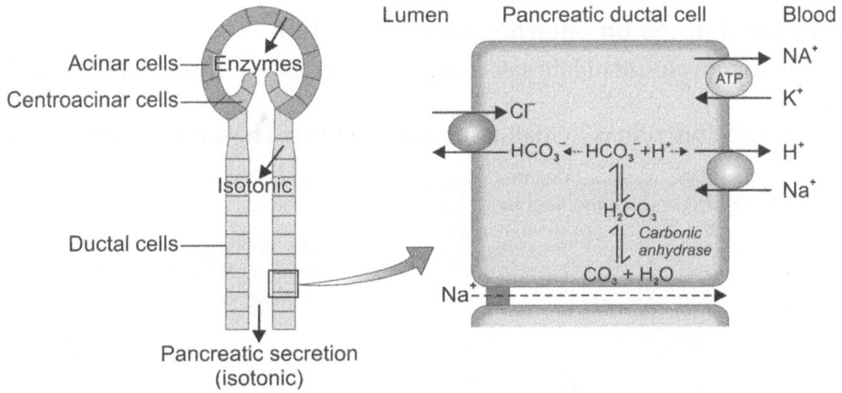

Fig. 20.3: Mechanism of pancreatic secretion.

10. Write short note on peptic ulcer.

Ans. Peptic ulcer is seen in the lining of stomach and/or duodenum. It is due to break in mucosal lining of stomach and duodenum.

Causes:

- *H. pylori* infection of the gastric mucosa
- Hypersecretion of acid due to stress, disease and tumor (gastrinomas)
- Prolonged intake of non-steroidal anti-inflammatory drug.

Features

- Patient present with abdominal pain, nausea, vomiting
- May present with peritonitis due to perforation of ulcer.

Treatment

Medical management is the first line therapy:

- H_2 receptor blocker—ranitidine, famotidine
- Proton pump inhibitors—omeprazole, pantoprazole
- Agents that strengthen the gastric lining—sucralfate
- Gastrin receptor blockers—proglumide
- Antibiotic to eradicate *H. pylori* infection
- Antacid—neutralizes acid in the stomach.

Surgical treatment is indicated in failure of medical management
Vagotomy (cutting the trunk of vagus nerve in abdomen just below the diaphragm)

11. Describe the regulation of gastric secretion.

Ans. Gastric secretion is controlled by neural and hormonal mechanism.

Phase	Stimulus	Mechanism	Gastric juice secretion (%)
Cephalic	Sight, smell, thought of food	Activate vagal nuclei in medulla through its vagally mediated response	30–50%
Gastric	Distention of stomach and products of digestion	Primarily local responses and response to gastrin	50–60%
Intestinal	Chyme in duodenum	Enterogastric reflex and also release of GI hormones, GIP and VIP	Less than cephalic and gastric phase

(GI: gastrointestinal; GIP: gastric inhibitory polypeptide; VIP: vasoactive intestinal polypeptide)

12. Write short notes on enterohepatic circulation.

Ans. It refers to movement of bile salt from liver to small intestine and recirculated back to liver.

The primary function is to maintain proper bile acid homeostasis **(Fig. 20.4)**.

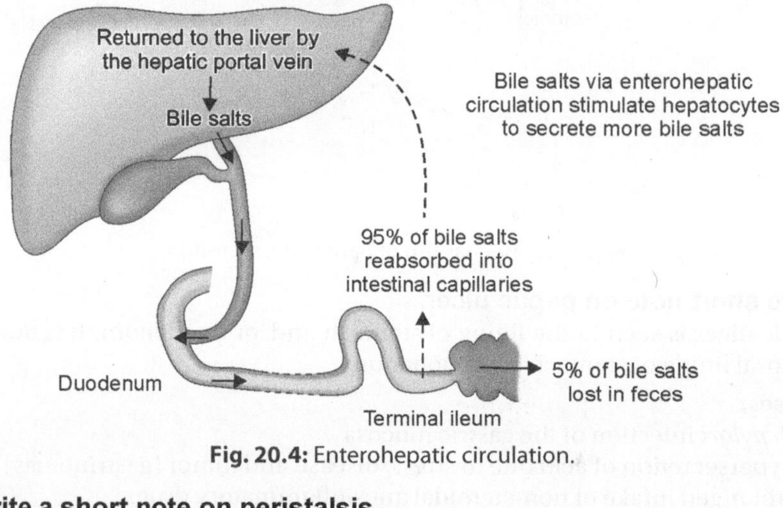

Fig. 20.4: Enterohepatic circulation.

13. Write a short note on peristalsis.

Ans.
- Peristalsis is a distinctive pattern of smooth muscle contractions that propels the chyme distally towards the colon **(Fig. 20.5)**.
- First described by Bayliss and Starling in 1899 as a type of motility in which there is contraction above and relaxation below a segment being stimulated.
- Peristalsis is not affected by vagotomy or sympathectomy indicating that it is mediated by intrinsic nervous system.
- When the chyme enters, the mechanical distension stretches the wall, the part behind the chyme contract and the part in front relax.
- Peristalsis is neurally mediated reflex, one group of interneurons activates excitatory motor neurons above the bolus—these neurons release acetylcholine and substance P, stimulate contraction of circular muscle above the bolus.

- Another group of interneurons activates inhibitory motor neurons that causes relaxation of circular muscle and contraction of longitudinal muscle below the bolus. These neurons use nitric oxide, vasoactive intestinal peptide as neurotransmitters. Ring of contraction proceed to forward direction and propel the content towards the caudal end.

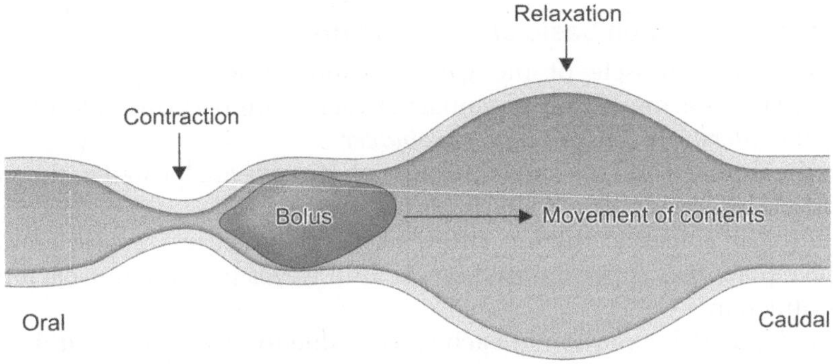

Fig. 20.5: Peristalsis.
(*Source*: Koeppen BM, Stanton BA. Berne & Levy physiology. 6th edition. Mosby, 2008)

14. Write short notes on migratory motor complex.

Ans.
- During interdigestive periods, a specific pattern of electrical and motor activity observed in the GI smooth muscles is referred as migratory motor complex (MMC).
- This pattern of motor activity migrate from stomach to distal ileum at a rate of approximately 5 cm/min
- Occur at an interval of about every 90 minutes

Each cycle consists of **(Fig. 20.6)**:
- A quiescent period (phase I)
- A period of irregular electrical and mechanical activity (phase II)
- A short phase of regular activity (phase III).

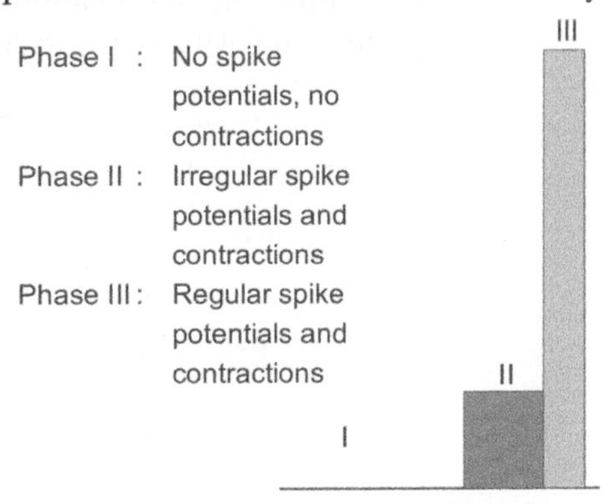

Fig. 20.6: Phases of MMC.

Several hormones may be involved in the initiation of MMCs, including motilin, opioid peptides and somatostatin.
- MMCs are believed to have a "housekeeping" function, clearing the luminal content of stomach and small intestine in preparation for the next meal.
- The bile flow, gastric and pancreatic secretion increases during each MMC.
- When a meal is ingested, MMCs is abolished and secretion of motilin is suppressed

15. Describe the movements of large intestine.

Ans.
- **Haustral contraction (segmentation contraction):** It is similar to segmentation contractions that mix the contents of the colon and also expose it to the mucosa thus facilitate absorption water and electrolyte, making the chyme as semisolid feces.

- **Peristalsis** propel the content towards rectum.
- **Mass action contraction** occurs only in the colon in which there is simultaneous contraction of the smooth muscle over large area of colon. These contractions move material from one portion of the colon to another. They also move material into the rectum, and rectal distention initiates the defecation reflex.
- It occurs 3–4 times a day.

16. Write short notes on basic electrical rhythm.

Ans.
- The smooth muscle of the gastrointestinal tract has spontaneous rhythmic fluctuations in membrane potential between -65 and -45 mV, referred as is initiated by the *interstitial cells of Cajal, pacemaker*
- In the stomach and the small intestine, these cells are located in the outer circular muscle layer near the myenteric plexus
- The basic electrical rhythm (BER) itself rarely causes muscle contraction, but spike potentials superimposed on the BER waves increase muscle tension causes contraction
- The depolarizing portion of each spike is due to Ca^{2+} influx, and the repolarizing portion is due to K^+ efflux.
- Circulating hormones and enteric neurons affect the BER.
- Acetylcholine increases the number of spikes and the tension of the smooth muscle, whereas epinephrine decreases the number of spikes and the tension.
- The rate of the BER is about 4/min in the stomach. It is about 12/min in the duodenum and falls to about 8/min in the distal ileum.
- The function of the BER is to coordinate peristaltic and other motor activity **(Fig. 20.7)**.

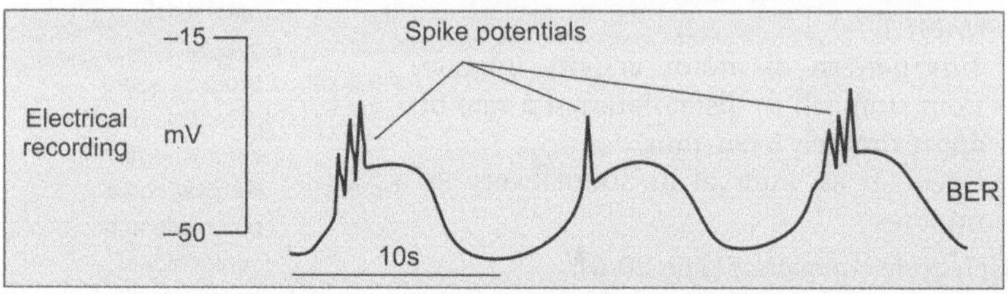

Fig. 20.7: Action potential of GI smooth muscle.

17. Describe the movements of small intestine.

Ans.
- Peristalsis
- Segmentation contractions
- Migrating motor complex
- Villus contraction

Peristalsis: When the chyme enters, the mechanical distension stretches the wall, the part behind the chyme contract and the part in front relax. Peristalsis is neurally mediated reflex response, one group of interneurons activates excitatory motor neurons above the bolus—these neurons release acetylcholine and substance P, stimulate contraction of circular muscle above the bolus. Another group of interneurons activates inhibitory motor neurons that Causes relaxation of circular muscle and contraction of longitudinal muscle below the bolus. These neurons use nitric oxide, vasoactive intestinal peptide as neurotransmitters.Wave of contraction then move in oral to caudal direction propelling the content of lumen forward at rate that varies from 2 to 25 cm/s.

Segmentation contraction: Segmentation contractions are ring-like contractions that appear at fairly regular intervals along the gut and then disappear and are replaced by another set of ring contractions in the segments between the previous contractions. Segmentation contraction move the chyme to and fro and increase its exposure to the mucosal surface. Food is grinded and thoroughly mixed with digestive secretion **(Fig. 20.8)**.

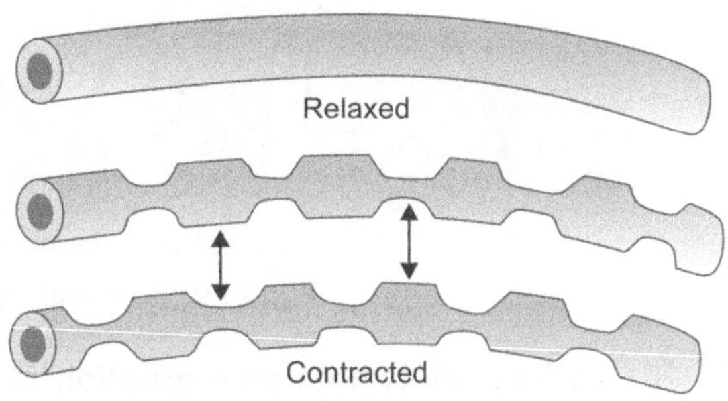

Fig. 20.8: Segmentation contraction.

Migrating motor complex: During interdigestive periods, a specific pattern of electrical and motor activity observed in the GI smooth muscles. This pattern of motor activity migrate from stomach to distal ileum. It occur at an interval of about every 90 minutes. Each cycle consists of:

- A quiescent period (phase I)
- A period of irregular electrical and mechanical activity (phase II)
- A short phase of regular activity (phase III).

Villus contraction:

- Seen in upper part of SI
- Villus contraction empty the central lacteals of the villi
- Increases the intestinal lymph flow
- Initiated by local nerve plexuses

SHORT ANSWERS 3 MARKS

18. Enumerate the functions of digestive system.

Ans. Gastrointestinal tract (GIT) is responsible for:

1. Ingestion
2. Digestion of food
3. Absorption of nutrients and water
4. Excretion of undigested food
5. Intestinal flora has many advantages to the body (synthesis of vitamin K, metabolic, immunological and gut protective functions).

19. Draw a labeled diagram of structural organization of the gut.

Ans. Transverse section of the gut shows four layers **(Fig. 20.9)**:

1. **Mucosa**
2. **Submucosa**
3. **Muscle layer**
4. **Serosa**

Two nerve plexus:

1. Submucosal plexus
2. Myenteric plexus

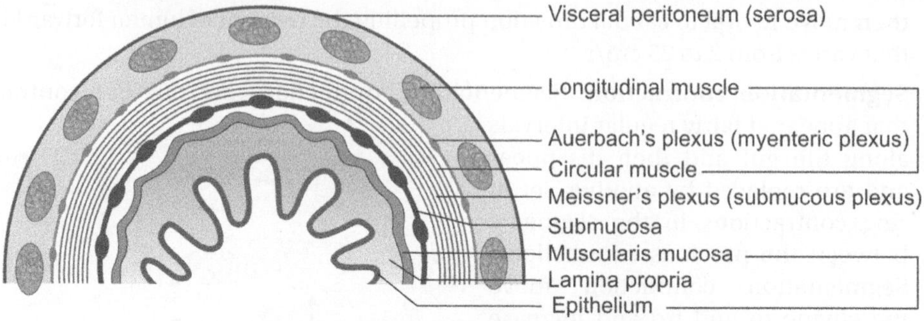

Fig. 20.9: Structural organization of the gut.

20. Write a short note on regulation of salivary secretion.

Ans. Salivary secretion is controlled by neural mechanism parasympathetic stimulation increases salivary secretion rich in enzyme **(Flowchart 20.4)**.

Sympathetic stimulation causes scanty secretion of organic constituents and mucus also cause decreased blood flow.

Reflex secretion of saliva: Contact of food in oral cavity causes salivary secretion. It is referred as unconditional reflex which is present since birth. In conditional reflex, salivary secretion occurs following smell or sight of food which occurs due to learning.

Flowchart 20.4: Regulation of salivary secretion.

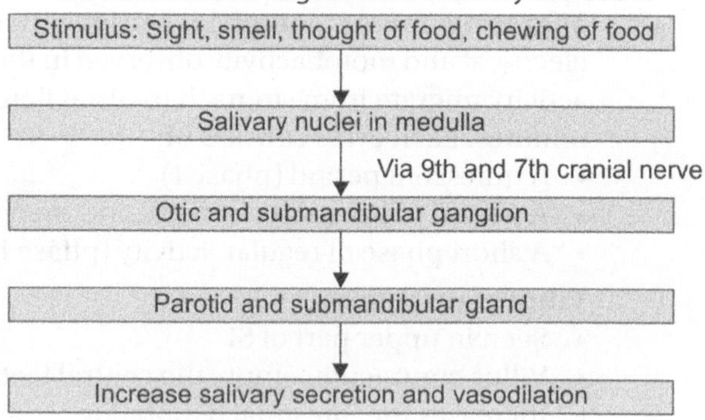

21. Describe the factors affecting HCl secretion.

Ans. Factors affecting HCl secretion **(Fig. 20.10)**.

22. Enumerate the gastric movements and its function.

Ans.
- Hunger contraction
- Migrating motor complex (MMC)
- Gastric relaxation: Receptive relaxation
- Peristalsis
- Reverse peristalsis

Functions
- Ingested food from esophagus is received by stomach and stored
- Crushed, ground and mix the food with gastric juice and made into chyme.
- To empty the contents into the duodenum at a controlled rate by the process called gastric emptying.

23. Define gastric emptying and mention the factors regulating it.

Ans. **Gastric emptying:**
- The process by which the contents of stomach is pushed into the duodenum by the coordinated activity of the gastric antrum, pyloric sphincter and duodenum

Factors affecting HCl secretion

Stimulants of gastric acid secretion
- Acetylcholine
- Gastrin
- Histamine
- Mechanical distension of stomach
- Product of protein digestion

Inhibitors of gastric acid secretion
- Somatostatin
- Acidic chyme into duodenum
- Prostaglandin E2

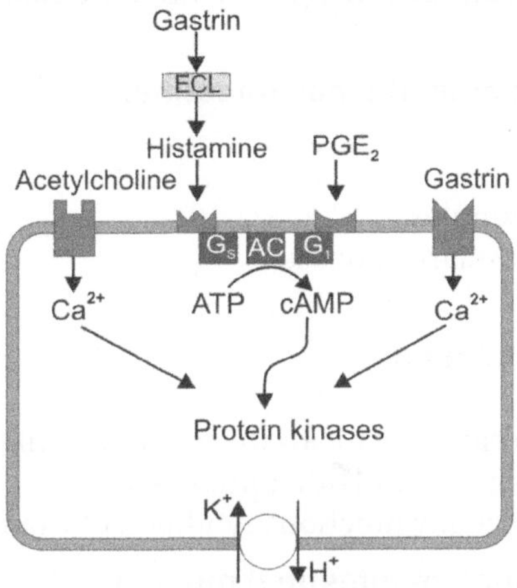

Fig. 20.10: Receptor sites for binding of various chemical substances for modulation of the activity of parietal cell.

- Gastric contents enter the duodenum in small squirts
- It is a highly regulated process.

Factors regulating gastric emptying

Factors which decrease gastric emptying are:
- Acid in the duodenum:
- Osmolality of duodenal contents: Hypertonic contents
- Products of fat digestion
- Protein digestion products: Delay gastric emptying
- Sympathetic stimulation

Factors which increase gastric emptying are:
- Vagal stimulation
- Certain hormones (thyroxine)
- Liquid content

24. List the functions of liver.

Ans.
- Secrets bile which plays a major role in metabolism of nutrients
- Synthesis of clotting factor, plasma protein, angiotensinogen
- Stores—carbohydrate, protein, fat, vitamin C, minerals (iron, copper)
- Kupffer cells and liver are involved in immunity
- Destroys endogenous and exogenous compounds
- Excretion of bilirubin, cholesterol and drugs.

25. Enumerate the functions of bile.

Ans.
- Helps in emulsification and absorption of lipids
- Helps in absorption of fat soluble vitamin
- Activate pancreatic lipase

26. What is choleretics and cholagogue?

Ans.
- Agents that increase bile secretion are called choleretics, e.g., bile salt, vagal stimulation, secretin.
- Agents that cause contraction of gallbladder are called cholagogue, e.g., cholecystokinin.

27. Mention the movements of small intestine.

Ans.
- Segmentation
- Peristalsis
- Migrating motor complex
- Movements of muscularis mucosa
- Villus contraction

28. Functions of large intestine.

Ans. Colon serves as:
- Reservoir for the residues of meals that cannot be digested or absorbed
- Absorption of water, Na^+, and other minerals.
- Colonic bacteria as many functions synthesis of vitamin K, color to the stool.

29. What are the functions of intestinal movement?

Ans.
- Mixing the chyme with digestive secretions
- Facilitate absorption of nutrients
- Propel the chyme towards rectum for excretion

30. What is paralytic ileus?

Ans.
- The term paralytic ileus denotes intestinal obstruction occurring due to loss of peristalsis (pseudo-obstruction). There is no structural defect. If it occurs after abdominal surgery, it is adynamic ileus.
- As a result, its contents are not propelled into the colon.
- This acute and reversible state of complete or partial gastrointestinal motor dysfunction is characterized by abdominal distension, anorexia, nausea, and vomiting. Gastrointestinal transit is delayed and the bowel is distended by pockets of gas and fluid.

21
CHAPTER

Endocrine System

LONG ESSAYS — 10 MARKS

1. Describe the functions of growth hormone.

Ans. **Introduction:** Growth hormone (GH) is secreted by anterior pituitary.

The functions of GH are as follows:

1. **Effects on growth:** Stimulation of linear bone growth due to its action on epiphyseal cartilage of long bone. Chondrogenesis is accelerated, and the cartilaginous epiphyseal plates widen, they lay down more bone matrix at the ends of long bones. Therefore, stature is increased.
2. **Effect on bone:** Osteoblastic activity increases which facilitate bone formation. The total bone mass and the mineral content of bone increases.
3. **Effect on skeletal muscle:** Growth hormone increases muscle mass by increasing protein synthesis.
4. **Effect on visceral organ:** GH stimulate growth of visceral organs (liver, heart, pancreas, kidney).
5. **Effect on metabolism:**
   a. **Protein metabolism**
      - Protein anabolic hormone
      - Increased amino acid, RNA and DNA synthesis
      - Increase protein synthesis

   b. **Carbohydrate metabolism**
      - Diabetogenic hormone
      - Increases liver glucose output by hepatic neoglucogenesis
      - Decrease glucose uptake in skeletal muscle and adipose tissue

   c. **Fat metabolism**
      - Lipolytic hormone
      - It activate hormone sensitive lipase and therefore plasma free fatty acid level increases.

2. Describe the steps involved in synthesis of thyroid hormones.

Ans. The steps in synthesis of thyroid hormone occurs in the follicular cells of the thyroid gland. The principal components for this are iodine obtained from diet and thyroglobulin.

1. The iodine from the capillaries is taken up by the thyroid follicular cells by active transport involving *sodium-iodine symport protein*. This is called **Iodide trapping**.

2. **Thyroglobulin synthesis and secretion:** It occurs in rough endoplasmic reticulum and Golgi apparatus. This molecule is secreted into the lumen of the thyroid follicle.
3. **Oxidation of iodide:** Iodide is converted into iodine and transported into the lumen of follicle by iodide-chloride transporter called *pendrin*.
4. **Iodination of tyrosine residues present in thyroglobulin**—and it is catalyzed by thyroid peroxidase. Binding of iodine with tyrosine molecule at 3rd and 5th position of thyroglobulin to form monoiodotyrosine (MIT) and diiodotyrosine (DIT) molecule of thyroglobulin.
5. **Coupling reaction**—2 molecules of DIT undergo oxidative condensation to form **T4 (tetraiodothyronine)**. Condensation of MIT with DIT to form **T3 (triiodothyronine)** called as *coupling reaction*, which is facilitated by *thyroid peroxidase* thyroglobulin with MIT, DIT.
6. **T3 and T4 is stored** in the colloid for several months.
7. T3, T4 are transported with thyroglobulin by endocytosis into the follicular cells. Proteases in lysosomes digest the thyroglobulin and T3 and T4 are released into the circulation. The iodide and tyrosine residues are taken up for recycling **(Fig. 21.1)**.

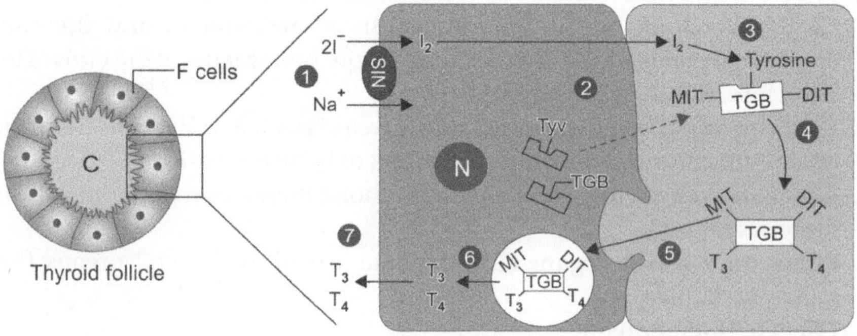

F cells – Follicular cells	❶ Iodine trapping by follicular cells
NIS – Na^+–I^- symportar	❷ Synthesis of thyroglobulin
TGB – Thyroglobulin	❸ Iodination of tyrosine residue
MIT – Monoiodotyrosine (T_1)	❹ Coupling of MIT and DIT
DIT – Diiodotyrosine (T_2)	❺ Endocytosis
T_3 – Triiodotyronine	❻ Release of T3 and T4
T_4 – Thyrozine	❼ Tranportation into plasma
tyr – Tyrosine residues	

Fig. 21.1: Steps in synthesis of thyroid hormones.

3. What are the functions of glucocorticoids?

Ans. Glucocorticoid hormones are secreted by the adrenal cortex. It includes cortisol. It performs diverse functions and are listed below:

A. **Metabolism:**
   - **On carbohydrate metabolism:** Increases blood glucose level through several mechanisms:
     - ¤ Reduced peripheral utilization of glucose in most tissues
     - ¤ Hepatic gluconeogenesis and glycogenolysis
   - **On protein metabolism:** Promote proteolysis.
   - **On lipid metabolism:** Causes lipolysis.

B. **Permissive action:** Small amount of cortisol is essential for other hormone action to occur
   - Calorigenic effect of glucagon and catecholamine
   - Bronchodilator and vasopressor effects of catecholamine.

C. **Effect of cardiovascular system (CVS)**
   - Increases myocardial contractility
   - Cortisol is needed for normal vascular integrity and responsiveness of arterioles to catecholamines.

D. **Musculoskeletal system:**
   - Increases the force of skeletal muscle contraction
   - Decreases bone mass and mineralization.

E. **Effect on central nervous system (CNS)**
   - Influence mood and behavior of the persons
   - Cortisol causes growth and maturation of CNS.

F. **Role in stress:** Help in coping up with stress.

G. **On blood:**
   - Causes neutrophilia, monocytosis
   - Eosinopenia and lymphocytosis.

H. **Anti-inflammatory effect:** High dose glucocorticoids suppress inflammation by inhibiting the synthesis of chemical mediators of inflammation

I. **Antiallergic effect:** Inhibiting the degranulation of mast cells and prevents release of histamine

J. **Immunosuppressive effect:**
   - Decrease in circulating T lymphocyte
   - Inhibit the cytotoxic effect of T8 cells

SHORT ESSAYS 5 MARKS

4. Describe the functions of somatomedins.

Ans. The effects of growth hormone on growth, cartilage and protein metabolism depends partly on the production of insulin-like growth factors (IGFs). Initially, they were called somatomedins, as they were found to mediate the somatic effects of GH:

1. The principal circulating somatomedins are IGF-1 and IGF-2
2. IGF-1 and 2 have similar actions as insulin and therefore, they called insulin-like growth factors.

A. Actions of IGF-1

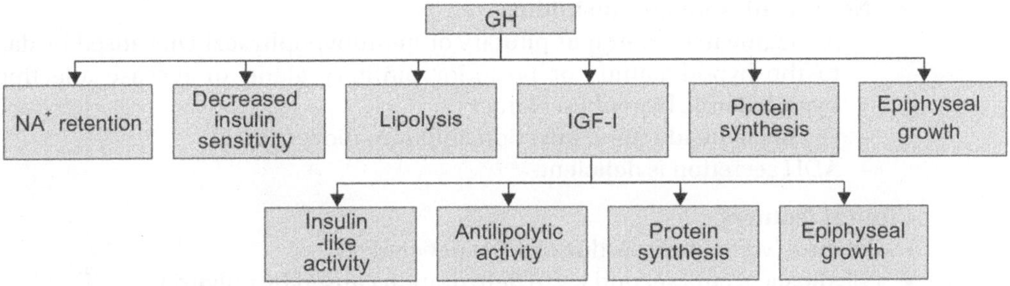

B. IGF-2: Its play a role in fetal growth.

5. Write short note on acromegaly.

Ans. Hypersecretion of GH after the fusion of epiphysis (growth plates have fused) result in acromegaly.

Etiology

- Tumor of somatotrophs of anterior pitutary
- Hypersecretion of GH due to hypothalamic tumors.

Features: The clinical features include:

- Enlargement of peripheral regions (acral parts—hands and feet)
- Prognathism (protrusion of lower jaw)
- Prominent eyebrow
- Acromegalic facies (overgrowth of malar, frontal and facial bones)
- Macroglossia
- Glucose intolerance
- Visceromegaly
- Osteoarthritis (due to skeletal changes)
- Gynecomastia and lactation
- Hirsutism
- Visual field changes

Diagnosis

- Based on the clinical presentation
- Demonstration of tumor by CT or MRI
- Raised GH level in plasma

Management

- Use of somatostatin analogue
- Growth hormone receptor antagonist
- Surgical removal of tumor

6. Write a short note on diabetic insipidus.

Ans.
- Antidiuretic hormone (ADH) deficiency causes diabetes insipidus (DI)
- Diabetes insipidus is defined as the passage of large volumes (>3 L/24 hr) of dilute urine (<300 mOsm/kg).

It is of two types:

1. **Nephrogenic diabetes insipidus:** It occurs when the kidney tubules do not respond to antidiuretic hormone. ADH secretion is normal, but kidney is unresponsiveness to it, due to receptor (V2) deficiency or abnormality. Receptor defect may be acquired or genetic cause.
2. **Neurogenic diabetes insipidus:**
   - Also known as central or pitutary or neurohypophyseal DI, caused by damage to the hypothalamus or posterior pituitary gland or disease affecting the hypothalamic hypophyseal tract
   - Occurs in head injury, infection, inflammation, tumors.
   - ADH secretion is deficient.

Clinical features

- Polyuria (water diuresis due to ADH deficiency)
- Polydipsia occurs secondary to dehydration caused by polyuria
- Pure water loss (urine osmolality is <300 mOsm/L).

7. What are the functions of insulin?

Ans. It decreases blood glucose level, it is the only antidiabetogenic hormone.

1. **Carbohydrate metabolism:**
   - Insulin promote glycogen synthesis and storage
   - Inhibit glycogenolysis and gluconeogenesis, thus decreases blood glucose level.
2. **Fat metabolism:**
   - Promote storage of fat in the target tissue
   - Stimulate lipogenesis
3. **Protein metabolism:** Promote protein synthesis
4. **Plasma potassium level:** It causes hypokalemia (decrease k^+ level) by causing rapid uptake of potassium into the cells.

8. Write short notes on diabetes mellitus.

Ans. Deficiency of insulin causes diabetes mellitus (DM).

Features

- Hyperglycemia (↑ blood glucose level)
- Glycosuria (presence of glucose in the urine)
- Polyphagia (increased food intake)
- Polydipsia (increased thirst)
- Polyuria (frequent passage of large volumes of urine)
- Weight loss

It is of two types:

1. **Type I diabetes mellitus (juvenile onset DM)**
   - It is due to autoimmune destruction of beta cells in pancreas leading to insulin deficiency
   - It occur before 40 years
   - Ketoacidosis is common
   - Small percentage of population is affected by this condition
   - Features are same as above
   - Insulin therapy is the mainstay of treatment.
2. **Type II diabetes mellitus (maturity onset DM)**
   - It is due to insulin resistance, many factors contribute to it like obesity, chronic stress, adipokines, etc.
   - Usually occurs after 40 years
   - Majority of people are affected by this condition
   - Ketoacidosis is uncommon
   - Clinical features are similar to diabetes mellitus type I.
   - Oral hypoglycemic drugs are the firstline of treatment.

9. Describe the functions of thyroid hormones.

Ans. The thyroid hormones T3 and T4 are secreted by the thyroid gland and play essential role in all the physiological activities.

The functions are listed below:

I. **Calorigenic action:** Thyroid hormone increases oxygen consumption of most of the tissues and therefore the basal metabolic rate (BMR) increases, the increased metabolism, in turn increases the heat production.

II. **Systemic effects**

a. **Central nervous system:** It is essential for normal development of CNS in intrauterine life and early childhood. It helps in formation of synapse and myelination in the developing brain.

b. **Cardiovascular system:** It increases heart rate, myocardial contractility, therefore increases the cardiac output.

c. **Gastrointestinal system:** Increases GI motility.

d. **Reproductive system:** Play an important role in regulation of reproduction

e. **Musculoskeletal system:** Promote skeletal growth and development. In the muscle it promote protein catabolism.

III. **Substrate metabolism**

a. **Carbohydrate metabolism:**

- Increases the rate of absorption of glucose from GIT
- It also stimulate hepatic glycolysis and gluconeogenesis.

b. **Fat metabolism:** Promote by lipolysis, increases the release of fatty acid and glycerol from adipose tissue thus increases the plasma concentration of free fatty acid.

c. **Protein metabolism:** Promote proteolysis.

10. Short note on myxedema.

Ans. Hypothyroidism in adult is called myxedema.

Causes
- Iodine deficiency
- Autoimmune diseases of thyroid gland
- Drug induced

Features
- Cold intolerance
- Fatigue
- Constipation
- Hoarse voice
- Coarse yellow skin
- Weight gain
- Hair loss
- Slow heart rate
- Goiter
- Poor memory
- Slow reaction time
- Puffy face
- Decreased BMR
- Edematous limbs

Diagnosis: Diagnosed by thyroid function test which shows elevated THS with decreased T3 and T4

Treatment: Thyroid hormone replacement is the mainstay of treatment.

11. Write short notes on hyperthyroidism.

Ans. Increase thyroid hormone secretion is known as hyperthyroidism.

Causes
- Autoimmune disorder
- Adenoma of thyroid gland

Features
- Increase in BMR
- Excessive sweating
- Palpitation
- Increase in heart rate
- Tremor
- Irritability
- Heat tolerance
- Hyperdefecation
- Loss of weight
- Hypertension
- Exophthalmos

Diagnosis: Estimation of thyroid function test which shows increased T3 and T4

Treatment: Antithyroid drug.

12. Short note on Cushing syndrome.

Ans. Excess secretion of glucocorticoids leads to Cushing syndrome.

Common cause: Adrenal tumors

Features
- Moon face
- Centripetal obesity (fat deposition in the abdomen with thin limb)
- Hypertension
- Prominent stretch marks in the abdomen
- Muscle wasting
- Poor wound healing
- Osteoporosis
- Hyperglycemia

13. Physiological action of parathyroid hormone.

Ans. The primary function of parathyroid hormone (PTH) is to maintain plasma calcium level by increasing it and decrease the level of phosphate. The target organ of this hormone is kidney, bone and intestine **(Flowchart 21.1)**.

14. What is tetany?

Ans. Deficiency in parathyroid hormone leads to hypocalcemic tetany.

Features are:
1. Carpopedal spasm
2. Chvostek sign (tapping over the facial muscle causes contraction of the muscle on the same side)

Flowchart 21.1: Parathyroid hormone.

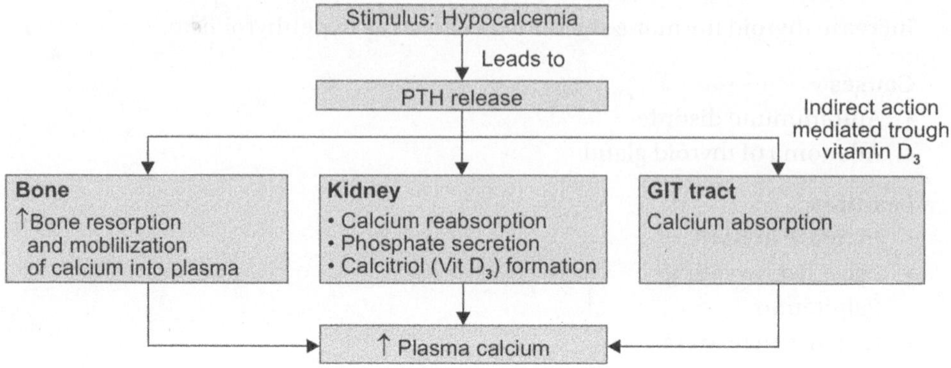

3. Trousseau's sign (to elicit the sign, a blood pressure cuff is placed around the arm and inflated to a pressure greater than the systolic blood pressure and held in place for 3 minutes. This will occlude the brachial artery. In the absence of blood flow, the patient's hypocalcemia and subsequent neuromuscular irritability will induce spasm of the muscles of the hand and forearm)
4. Laryngospasm.

15. Write a short note on milk ejection reflex.

Ans. It is a neurohumoral reflex **(Flowchart 21.2 and Figure 21.2)**

- **Stimulus**: Suckling of breast
- **Receptor**: Tactile receptors in and around the nipple
- **Afferent**: Ascending sensory pathway (neural)
- **Center**: Hypothalamus
- **Efferent**: via HPA axis, oxytocin released from posterior pituitary into the circulation (humoral)
- **Response**: Contraction of myoepithelial cells of the alveoli causing milk ejection.

Flowchart 21.2: Milk ejection reflex.

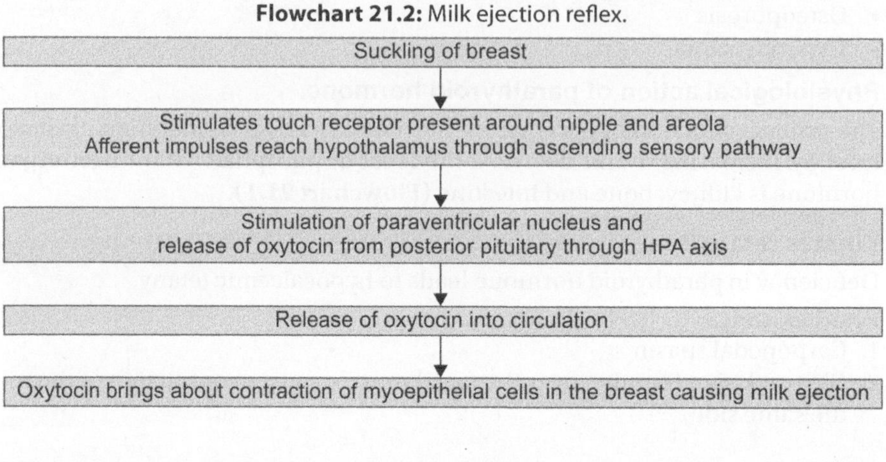

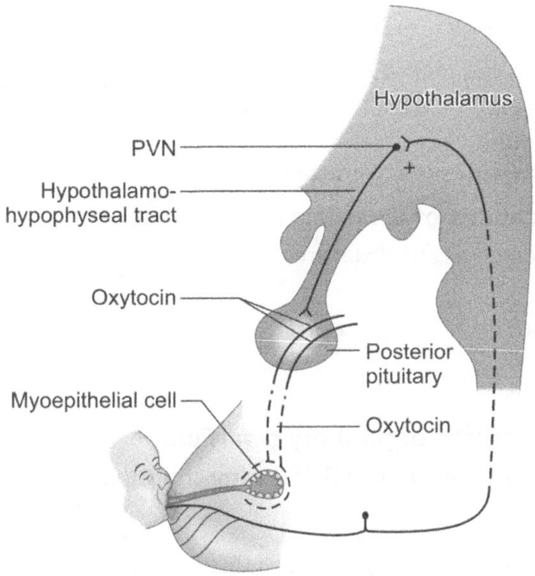

Fig. 21.2: Pathway involved in milk ejection reflex.
(PVN: paraventricular nucleus)

SHORT ANSWERS 3 MARKS

16. Name the major endocrine glands.

Ans.
- Hypothalamus
- Pituitary
- Thyroid
- Parathyroid
- Adrenal
- Pancreas
- Gonad
- Pineal gland

17. What are second messenger?

Ans. They are intracellular signaling molecule that are formed in the cell upon binding of hormone with the receptor.

Examples: Cyclic AMP, GMP, IP3 DAG, transcripted mRNA

18. Name the hormones secreted by anterior pituitary.

Ans.
- Growth hormone (GH)
- Thyroid-stimulating hormone (TSH)
- Adrenocorticotropic hormone (ACTH)
- Luteinizing hormone (LH)
- Follicle-stimulating hormone (FSH)
- Prolactin

19. What is gigantism?

Ans. Hypersecretion of GH before fusion of epiphysis.

Causes

- Childhood pituitary tumors
- Hypothalamic tumors

Clinical features

- Abnormally tall
- Other features same as acromegaly

20. What are the causes of dwarfism?

Ans. Dwarfism is referred as short stature.

Causes

- Pituitary dwarf
- Thyroid dwarf
- Genetic causes.

21. What are the features of pituitary dwarfism?

Ans. Deficiency of growth hormone (GH) during childhood causes pituitary dwarfism.

Features

- Short stature
- Delayed sexual maturation
- Decreased muscle mass, total body mass and bone density
- Mental development is normal.

22. Describe the physiological actions of prolactin.

Ans.
1. **Stimulate milk synthesis:** During lactation along with insulin and cortisol it increases milk synthesis and secretion in mammary gland.
2. **Development of mammary gland:** Along with estrogen, progesterone, cortisol and GH it causes proliferation of ducts and lobules of alveoli of mammary gland.
3. **Effects on reproduction:** Increased prolactin, inhibits GnRH release from hypothalamus, therefore LH and FSH level decreases during lactation and this prevents ovulation and causes amenorrhea in lactating mothers known as lactational amenorrhea.

23. What are neuroendocrine reflex?

Ans. Neuroendocrine reflex or neurohumoral reflex involves both neural and hormones in the reflex pathway.

Examples:

- Milk ejection reflex and
- Parturition reflex

24. What are the functions of TSH?

Ans.
- TSH promotes the growth of thyroid gland
- Stimulates thyroid hormone synthesis and secretion
- It facilitate all the steps of thyroid hormone synthesis.

25. What are functions of ACTH?

Ans.
- ACTH stimulates synthesis and secretion of cortisol from adrenal cortex
- ACTH has intrinsic melanocyte stimulating hormone (MSH) activity therefore it stimulate melanocyte growth and activity
- ACTH receptors are present in the brain, GIT where it acts as a neurotransmitter.

26. Mention the functions of FSH and LH in humans.

Ans. **FSH**

- FSH stimulate granulosa cells of ovary and Sertoli cells of testis to synthesize and secrete inhibin B.
- It controls oogenesis and spermatogenesis.

LH

- LH stimulate theca cells of ovary and Leydig cells of testis to secrete estrogen and testosterone
- LH surge causes ovulation in the middle of the menstrual cycle.

27. What are the functions of ADH or vasopressin?

Ans.
- ADH acts on the distal convoluted tubule and collecting duct of renal tubule and increases the water reabsorption. It is an important hormone for restoration of ECF volume in volume depleted state.
- ADH causes vasoconstriction and increase in BP in higher concentration.
- It acts as a neurotransmitter in few areas of the brain.
- It increases CRH release therefore increases ACTH secretion.

28. Name the hormones secreted by endocrine pancreas.

Ans. Islet of Langerhans of pancreas contain four types of cells:

1. Beta (β) cells secrete insulin
2. Alpha (α) cell secrete glucagon
3. Delta (δ) cells secrete somatostatin
4. F cells secrete pancreatic polypeptide (PP).

29. Name the hormones secreted by thyroid gland.

Ans.
- Triiodthyronine (T3)
- Tetraidothyronine (T4)
- Calcitonin
- Reverse (T3)—metabolically inactive form of T3.

30. What is goiter?

Ans. Enlargement of thyroid gland present as swelling in the neck referred as goiter.

- It is common in iodine deficiency
- Low thyroid hormone in the circulation stimulate anterior pituitary to produce TSH, which causes enlargement of thyroid gland to occur and also facilitate thyroid hormone synthesis.

31. Name the secretions of adrenal gland.

Ans.
- Mineralocorticoid—aldosterone
- Glucocorticoid—cortisol
- Sex steroid hormones called androgens

32. Write short note on Addison's disease.

Ans. Hyposecretion of adrenal gland secretions causes Addison's disease.

Features

- Pigmentation of skin
- Weight loss, hypotension
- Inability to cope up with stress

33. What are the functions of aldosterone?

Ans. Primary function of aldosterone is it act on the collecting duct and distal convoluted tubule of kidney and increase sodium and water reabsorption and promote potassium and hydrogen excretion. Therefore aldosterone increases plasma sodium and decreases potassium concentration.

34. Name the hormones regulating calcium homeostasis.

Ans.
1. Parathyroid hormone—elevate blood calcium levels.
2. Calcitonin—decreases the levels of calcium in blood.
3. Cholecalciferol (vitamin D_3)—helps in absorption of calcium and phosphorous.

All these hormones act on bone, kidney and intestine.

35. What are functions of calcitonin?

Ans. It is produced from the par follicular cell (c cells) of thyroid gland. It secreted in response to hypercalcemia, acts on bone and kidney and bring the calcium level back to normal.

Calcitonin lowers blood Ca^{2+} levels by three mechanisms:
1. Inhibits osteoclast activity in bones
2. Decreases renal tubular cell reabsorption of Ca^{2+} and phosphate, allowing them to be excreted in the urine
3. High concentrations of calcitonin causes increase urinary excretion of calcium and phosphate, via actions on the kidney tubules. Leading to marked hypocalcemia

36. Mention the functions of melatonin.

Ans. **Source:** Pineal gland.

Functions:
- Controls sleep wake cycle
- Control of circadian rhythm
- Immunomodulatory function
- Inhibit the onset of puberty

37. Name the hypothalamic hormones.

Ans.
- Growth hormone releasing hormone (GHRH)
- Somatostatin or growth hormone inhibiting hormone (GHIH)
- Gonadotropin releasing hormone (GnRH)
- Thyrotropin releasing hormone (TRH)
- Corticotropin releasing hormone (CRH)
- Prolactin inhibitory factor (dopamine)
- Prolactin releasing peptide (PrRP)

38. What is HPA axis and give its function?

Ans. Hypothalamus is anatomically and functionally connected to pituitary. The hypothalamus delivers precise signals to the pituitary gland, which then releases hormones that regulate the functions of major endocrine glands in the body is referred as HPA or hypothalamo pituitary axis.

Hormones released from hypothalamus are transported to the anterior pituitary through hypophyseal blood vessels and regulates anterior pituitary hormones.

Paraventricular and supraoptic nucleus of hypothalamus synthesize hormones (oxytocin and ADH) that are transported to the posterior pituitary through its axonal transport and stored there until the proper signal for its release arises.

Therefore both of the anterior and posterior pituitary are under the control of hypothalamus, which together creates an axis for hormone release.

39. What are functions of oxytocin?

Ans. Oxytocin is secreted from posterior pituitary. It has the following functions:

A. Oxytocin mediate two important physiologic reflexes:
   1. Milk ejection reflex
   2. Parturition reflex
B. Oxytocins facilitate corpus luteum degeneration in menstrual cycle.
C. In males at the time of ejaculation oxytocin causes contraction of smooth muscles of vasdeferens help in propelling sperms towards urethra.
D. In females oxytocin causes contraction of nonpregnant uterus to facilitate sperm transport into fallopian tube.

40. What are G proteins?

Ans. G proteins are intrinsic membrane protein, guanine nucleotide binding regulatory proteins. They can be activated by hormones, neurotransmitters and proteases. When the ligand binds to the G-protein-coupled receptor in the cell membrane, the G protein exchanges GDP for GTP. The GTP–protein complex brings about the effect of the G-protein **(Fig. 21.3)**.

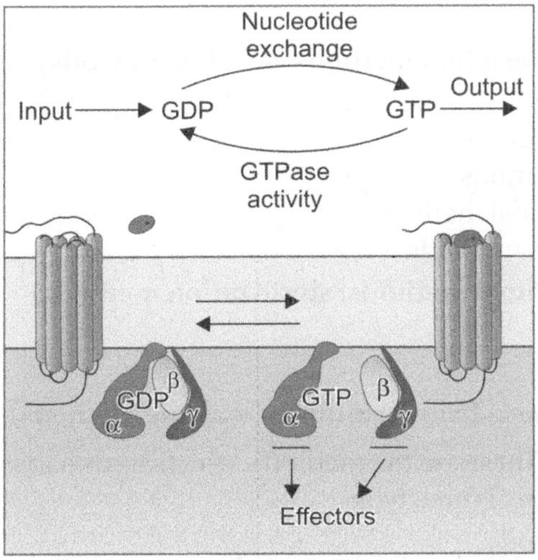

Fig. 21.3: Mechanism of action of hormone through G protein.
(GDP: guanosine diphosphate; GTP: guanosine triphosphate)
(*Source:* Barrett KE, Basman SM, Brooks HL, et al. Ganong's Review of Medical Physiology, 26th edition. McGrow-Hill Education, 2019)

22
CHAPTER

Reproductive System

LONG ESSAYS — 10 MARKS

1. Write an essay on physiology of contraception.

Ans. Contraceptive measures mean methods used to prevent conception (pregnancy). They include all temporary and permanent measures to prevent pregnancy resulting from coitus (sexual intercourse). The birth control procedures work prior to implantation of the fertilized egg. They are called contraceptives and when they work after implantation (cause death of the embryo), they are termed as abortifacients.

Classification of contraception: Contraceptive methods are classified into following categories:

Temporary (nonterminal methods: spacing methods)

1. Barrier methods
2. Intrauterine devices
3. Hormonal methods
4. Postconceptional methods
5. Miscellaneous methods

Permanent (terminal methods: sterilization methods)

1. Vasectomy
2. Tubectomy

Temporary methods (Nonterminal or spacing methods)

Barrier method: These are the methods, which act as barrier between the sperms and the ovum. They are of three types:

A. Physical methods
B. Chemical methods
C. Combined methods

Contraceptive Measures in Males

Physical methods:

a. **Condom** is a latex sheath, cylindrical shaped device measuring 15–20 cm length, 3 cm diameter, and 0.003 cm thick. It is closed at one end with a closed-end and open at the other end, with an integral rim. It is used by the male partner to cover erect penis during coitus. Condom is the most widely used barrier device in male. It prevents sperm to be deposited in the vagina. It provides protection against sexually transmitted diseases.

b. **Coitus interruptus:** In this method, during fertile period, the male partner withdraws penis from vagina before ejaculation. Thus, sperm is not deposited in the female genital tract.

Contraceptive Measures in Females

Physical methods: The devices employed for physical barrier methods are diaphragm, cervical cap.

a. **Diaphragm (vaginal diaphragm):** It is a shallow, soft rubber cup, with a stiff but flexible rim, made up of coiled spring, which helps in retention. Size varies from 5 to 10 cm in diameter. It is simple, safe and easy to use.
b. **Cervical cap:** It is thimble shaped. It is like diaphragm but smaller. It covers the vaginal portion of the cervix, thus acting as a barrier.
c. **Vault cap (dumas cap):** It fits into the vault of the vagina and occludes the cervix. This is indicated when neither diaphragm nor cervical cap is suited to the woman.

Chemical methods: These are the contraceptives that a woman place in her vagina shortly before sex. These are foams, creams, jellies, pastes. All these devices are impregnated with spermicides. They are surface active agents. They must be inserted high up in the vagina. They attach themselves to sperms and inhibits oxygen uptake and kill them.

Combined Methods

A. **Intrauterine devices:** Intrauterine devices (IUDs) are most effective contraceptive devices for a parous lady (who has borne at least one child). These are the devices which when placed inside the uterus act as a foreign body.
   Mechanism of action: they prevent implantation
   1. Presence of these small objects in the uterus interfere with the endometrial preparation for acceptance of the blastocyst.
   2. Lead to cellular and biochemical changes in the endometrium.
   3. Copper facilitates cellular reaction in endometrium, composition of cervical mucous, impairs sperm motility and impairs capacitating of sperm.
B. **Hormonal contraceptives:**
   1. *Oral contraceptive pills (OCPs):*
      a. Combined pills—both estrogen and progesterone. The pill is given for 21 days from the 5th day of the cycle. Both the hormones inhibit gonadotropin release thereby preventing ovulation.
      b. Progestin-only pill—this is also called as mini pill. It thickens the cervical mucous making it difficult for the sperms to pass through. It inhibits the estrogen-induced proliferation of the endometrium, making it inhospitable for implantation.
      c. Postcoital pill—any woman can adopt this method if she is not pregnant, and to prevent unplanned pregnancy (only as an emergency measure).
      d. Once a month pill.

      Side effects of OCPs: Cerebral thrombosis, venous thrombosis, and essential hypertension.

2. *Injectable contraceptives:* They are slow-release formulations. They are composed of depot medroxyprogesterone acetate (DMPA).

C. **Miscellaneous: Rhythm method (calendar method: safe period method):** The rhythm method is the abstinence from sexual intercourse during the fertile period of cycle. 28 days in regular cycles, normally ovulation occurs in between 12th and 16th day.

Permanent Methods

a. *Males-vasectomy:* It is bilateral ligation of vas deferens. It is a simple, safe, highly effective, cheap, permanent surgical method of family planning for men.

b. *Females-tubectomy:* This is also known as "voluntary surgical contraception", "tubal ligation".

It is simple, safe, effective, cheap, convenient, and permanent method of contraception.

2. Define ovulation. Mention the processes involved and the indicators of ovulation.

Ans. The mechanism of release of ovarian follicle from ovary is called ovulation. The Graafian follicle ruptures around 14th day in a 28 day menstrual cycle, releasing the oocyte onto the surface of ovary. Then it is taken up by the fimbriae of the fallopian tube **(Fig. 22.1).**

Mechanism

- It is triggered following mid-cycle luteinizing hormone (LH) surge. The rise in estrogen concentration provides positive feedback on LH secretion.
- Two days prior to ovulation, estrogen concentration increases and when it is maintained for about 36 hours, ovulation is initiated.

Chemical substances involved in rupture of ovarian follicle are:

1. Prostaglandins
2. Cyclin D2 (regulates cell cycle)
3. CCAAT-enhancer binding protein

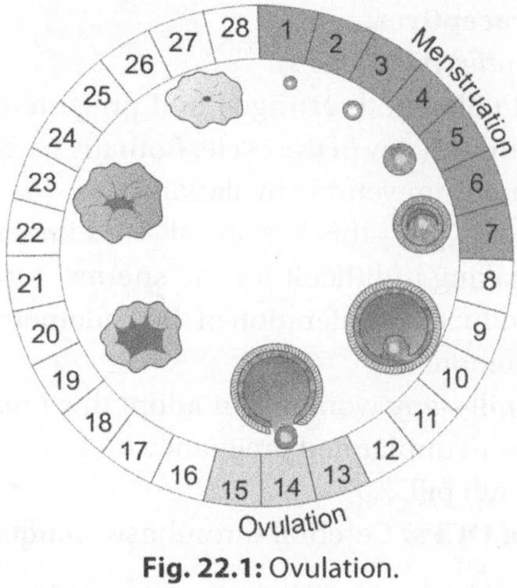

Fig. 22.1: Ovulation.

Steps in follicular release (Fig. 22.2):

Increased release of prostaglandins and bradykinin increases follicular blood flow

↓

Dominant follicle gets highly vascularized, edematous, size increases

↓

Cumulus oophorous complex gets detached

↓

Basement membrane, theca cells disintegrates due to intrafollicular pressure

↓

LH promotes synthesis of plasminogen activator, leads to conversion of plasmin

↓

Plasmin: causes proteolysis of follicular wall activates synthesis of collagenase

↓

Increase intrafollicular pressure and degeneration of follicular wall

↓

Rupture of follicle, expulsion of oocyte from follicle

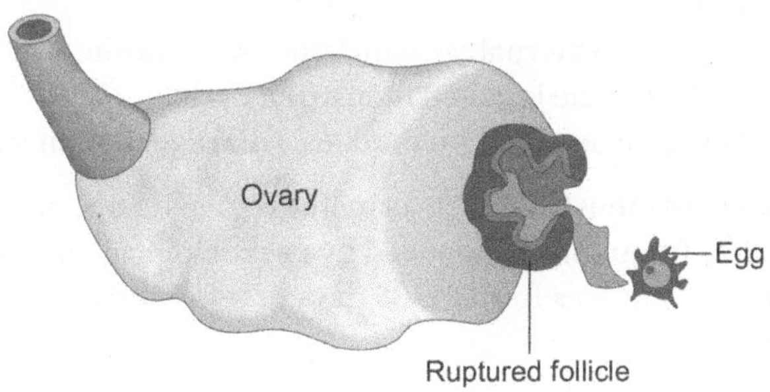

Fig. 22.2: Rupture of follicle releasing the oocyte.

Indicators of ovulation:

1. Rise in body temperature [basal body temperature (BBT)]:
   - Increases about 0.5°C
   - Early in the morning, before getting out of the bed and before drinking water
   - Due to influence of progesterone that increases with the beginning of secretory phase.
2. Fleeting lower abdominal pain (Mittelschmerz pain):
   - Bleeding occurs into antrum of the follicle
   - Small amount of blood escapes into the abdominal cavity and peritoneal irritation resulting in pain.
3. Vaginal discharge: Increase BBT associated with Mittleschmerz pain and spotting is called ovulation cascade.
4. Spinnbarkeit test:
   - Proliferative phase—estrogen makes cervical mucus thin and alkaline
   - Secretory phase—progesterone makes cervical mucus thick and tenacious

A drop of cervical mucus is collected at the time of ovulation and can be stretched as long as 10 cm more like a thread. Elastic nature of mucus called spinnbarkeit.

5. Fern test: Cervical mucus before ovulation forms an arborizing fern-like pattern when spread on slide. Following ovulation due to progesterone effect, mucus become thick and fern-like pattern not observed.
6. Laparoscopic observation: Ovum in abdominal cavity by laparoscopic observation confirms ovulation.
7. Demonstration of LH peak: LH surge occurs prior to ovulation. Daily estimation of plasma LH in preovulatory period will accurately detect the day of ovulation.

Physiological importance

- Determination of day of ovulation helps in family planning
- Life span of ovum is about 72 hours
- Helps in planning both conception and contraception.

3. Describe in detail the menstrual cycle with suitable diagram.

Ans. Menstrual cycle:

- It is the preparation of reproductive system for fertilization and implantation of fertilized ovum.
- Reproductive cycle externally manifests by periodic vaginal bleeding called menstruation. This cycle is called menstrual cycle.
- First menstrual cycle is called menarche. Usual age of menarche is 12–14 years.

Duration: Length of menstrual cycle usually averages at about 28 days. It is never fixed in all women. It is frequently influenced by psychological, environmental, nutritional and social factors. It ranges from 21–35 days. It temporarily ceases during pregnancy and lactation.

Phases

A. Follicular phase: Also called preovulatory phase. From the onset of bleeding to day of ovulation. Dominant follicle in the ovary matures in this phase to terminate in ovulation. It has two parts:
   1. Menstrual phase (phase of menstrual bleeding)
   2. Proliferative phase (phase of proliferative of uterine endometrium)

B. Luteal phase: Also called postovulatory phase. Between the ovulation and onset of menstrual bleeding. Corpus luteum is formed in the ovary which controls activities of this phase. It is also called as secretory phase.

Length of each phase of cycle: The follicular phase is of 14 days (1–14 days). Luteal phase is of 14 days (15–28 days). Once ovulation occurs, menstrual bleeding starts 14 days after ovulation. Thus the length of luteal phase remains constant irrespective of cycle length. Menstrual cycle is sometimes divided into four parts:

1. Bleeding phase
2. Follicular phase
3. Ovulatory phase
4. Luteal phase

Bleeding Phase: Bleeding phase is a part of follicular phase and ovulation is an event that occurs at the junction between proliferative and secretory phase.

Changes in Follicular Phase

a. **Ovarian changes:** Follicle is selected to become dominant follicle by 4th day. It develops into mature follicle. The granulosa and theca cells increases in size and stromal fluid increases in volume.
b. **Uterine changes**: Thickness of endometrium rapidly increase from 5th to 14th day of the cycle.
   - Endometrium increases in size and thickness. The stroma is edematous.
   - Hypertrophy and proliferation of endometrial glands.
   - Formation of more number of spiral arteries.
   - Myometrial excitability increases due to effect of estrogen.
c. **Uterine cervix:**
   - Volume, alkalinity and elasticity of cervical mucus increases.
   - Forms physiological basis of Spinnbarkeit.
   - Sperm easily passes through estrogen-dependent cervical mucus.
d. **Vaginal changes:**
   - Vaginal epithelial cells become cornified.
   - Cornification index increases from almost zero on day1 to about 100 on 14th day.

Luteal Phase

a. **Ovarian changes:**
   - Follicle rapidly filled with blood called corpus hemorrhagium. The granulosa and theca cells of follicle undergo luteinization to become granulosa and lutein cells.
   - Follicle develops into corpus luteum. If pregnancy occurs it persists, otherwise it degenerates between 26th–28th days forms corpus albicans.
b. **Uterine changes:**
   - Uterine glands become coiled and torturous.
   - Glandular cells store glycogen and carbohydrate rich mucus and fluid.
   - Vascularity of endometrium increases further. Spiral arteries become torturous.
   - Endometrial veins forms venous lake and anastomoses.
   - Myometrial excitability decreases due to effects of progesterone.
c. **Cervical changes:** Cervical mucus become thick and its elasticity decreases, sperm cannot enter through progesterone dominated cervical mucus.
d. **Vaginal changes:** Vaginal epithelium proliferates and secretes thick mucus, epithelium infiltrated with leukocytes and cornification decreases.

Mechanism of Menstrual Bleeding (Fig. 22.3)

- Decreased secretion of steroid hormone.
- Destabilization of lysosomal membranes.
- Leads to release of proteolytic enzymes and production of prostaglandins ($PGF_{2\alpha}$).
- Lysis of endometrial tissue and causes vasospasm, produces endometrial ischemia.
- Areas of local necrosis, facilitated by proteolytic damage.

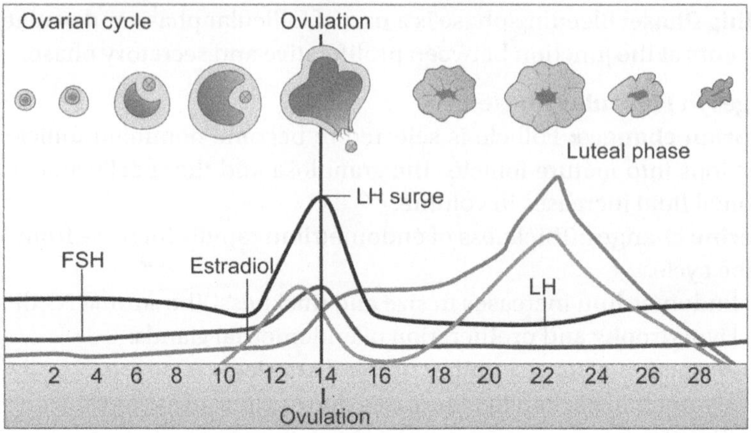

Fig. 22.3: Ovarian cycle.

- Foci of necrosis join each other.
- Sloughing of uterine endometrium.

Amount of Loss

- About 30–130 mL of blood is lost.
- Contains tissue debris, prostaglandins and fibrinolysin.
- Increase in menstrual flow is called menorrhagia, decrease in menstrual flow is called hypomennorrhea.

Hormonal Changes in Menstrual Cycle (Figs. 22.4 and 22.5):

Estrogen: Two peaks in menstrual cycle. First peak is a major peak, occur in 48 hours before ovulation. Second peak is a minor peak, it occurs in post mid luteal phase.

- The concentration rises rapidly from 8th day of cycle to reach the peak about one or 2 days before ovulation. It decreases after ovulation.
- After 2 days concentration increases slowly to reach a smaller peak.

Progesterone: Concentration is minimal in proliferative phase, rises following ovulation and reaches peaks in 4–5 days after ovulation. Peak is maintained till corpus luteum is active.

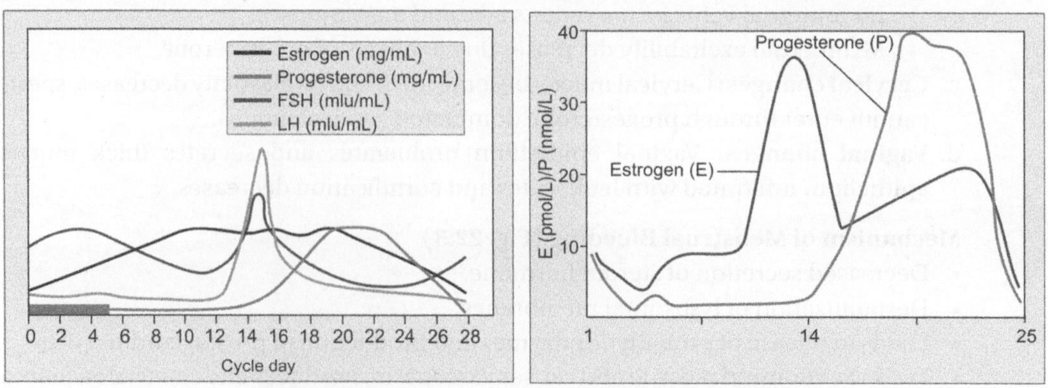

Fig. 22.4: Hormonal changes during menstrual cycle.

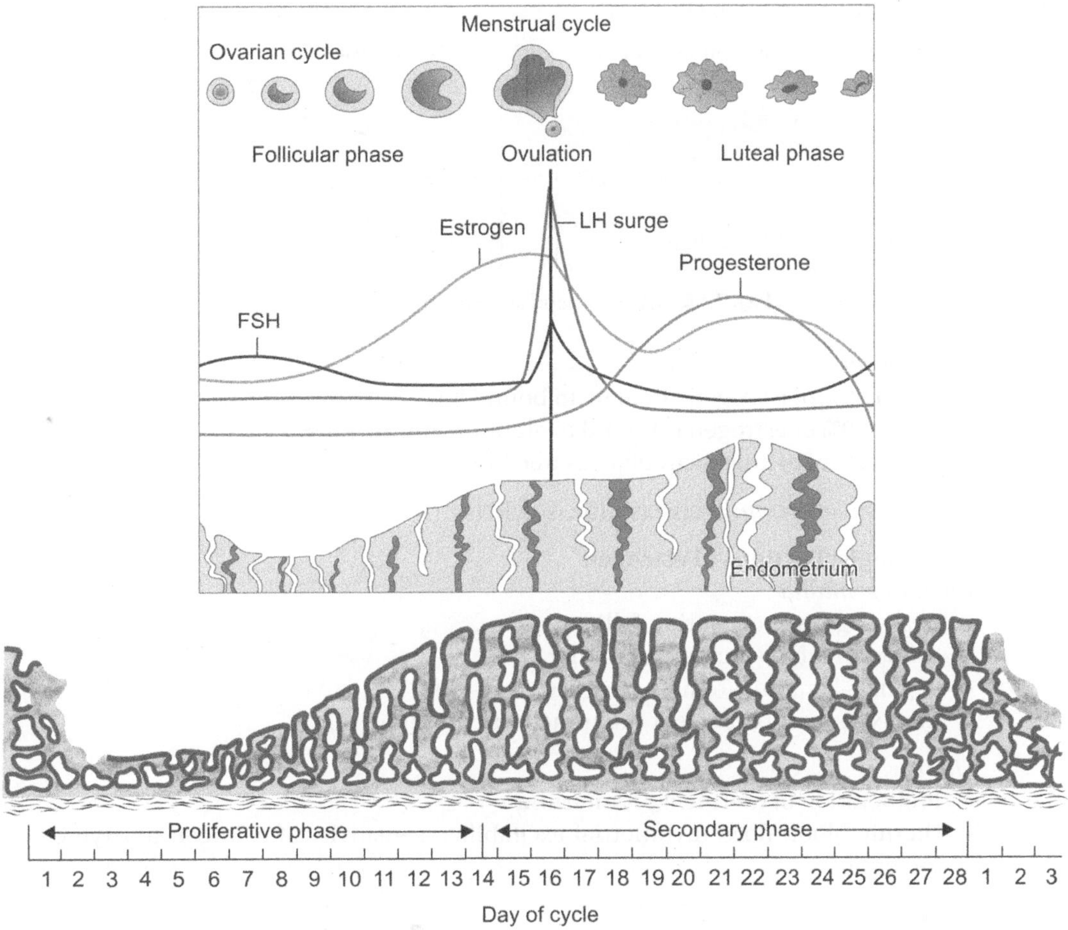

Fig. 22.5: Uterine changes during menstrual cycle.

Luteinizing hormone (LH):

- Concentration remains low almost throughout proliferative phase
- About a day before ovulation secretion of LH increases sharply to reach peak about 8–10 hours before ovulation called LH surge.

Follicle-stimulating hormone (FSH):

- Increases in early part of follicular phase, decreases slowly
- Rises towards ovulation. FSH is similar with LH pattern.

4. Describe about the female sexual hormones—estrogen and progesterone.

Ans. They are steroid hormones:

Estrogen

Source:

- Granulosa cells of ovarian follicle
- Corpus luteum
- Placenta

Naturally occurring estrogens are estradiol, estrone, and estriol.

Biosynthesis of estrogen (Fig. 22.6).

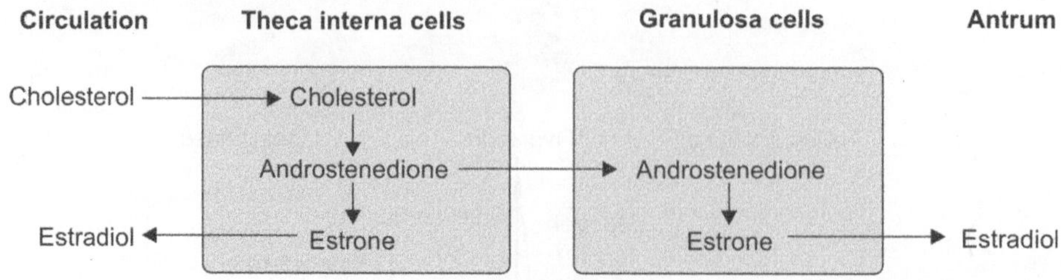

Fig. 22.6: Synthesis and secretion of estrogen.

Metabolism

- About 98% of estrogen circulate in bound form.
- About 60% of estrogen is bound to albumin and 38% to SBG.
- About 2% of estrogen circulate as free form.

Mechanism of action: Transcription of mRNA.

Physiological actions of estrogen

Internal genitalia

- Ovary—growth of ovarian follicle
- Fallopian tube—increases motility
- Vagina—keratinization
- Cervix—secretion of clear thin mucus membrane

Uterus

- Proliferation of uterine endometrium
- Uterine blood flow, myometrial excitability, sensitivity of estrogen to oxytocin is increased.

Breast

- Breast enlargement during puberty
- Causes Ductular growth
- Pigmentation of areola

Development of secondary sexual characteristics

- Narrow shoulders and broad hips, thighs that converge, and arms that diverge (wide **carrying angle**)
- Female distribution of fat in the breasts and buttocks
- Less body hair and more scalp hair
- Pubic hair generally has a characteristic flat-topped pattern (female escutcheon).
- High pitched voice.

Effects on endocrine organs

- Estrogen, inhibit's LH secretion (negative feedback) but prior to ovulation it increases LH secretion (positive feedback)
- Estrogens decrease FSH secretion
- Promotes the synthesis of angiotensinogen from liver
- Increases formation of thyroxine binding globulin
- Stimulate androgen secretion.

Effect on CNS: They increase libido in humans (direct effect on certain neurons in the hypothalamus).

Effects on musculoskeletal system

- Stimulates bone growth
- Prevent osteoporosis (by preventing osteoclastic activity.)

Effect on water metabolism: Salt and water retention.

Effect on lipid profiles:

- Cholesterol lowering activity (prevents atherosclerosis)
- Effect on sebaceous secretion and skin
- Make sebaceous gland secretions more fluid and thus one and inhibit's formation of **comedones** ("blackheads") and acne.

Progesterone

Source:

- Corpus luteum
- Placenta
- Ovarian follicle

  The principal target organs of progesterone are uterus, breasts, and brain.

  Metabolism:

  - The progesterone circulates in bound form (98%), 80% to albumin.
  - Progesterone has a short half-life and is converted in the liver to pregnanediol, which is conjugated to glucuronic acid and excreted in the urine.

Physiologic effects on uterus:

- Progesterone decreases automaticity and excitability of myometrium.
- Produce thick cervical mucus

Progestational agents are used in abortion

- Reasons: Inhibits the uterine myometrial contraction

Mechanism:

a. Progesterone **decreases** excitability of myometrium sensitivity to oxytocin reduces estrogen receptors
b. It increases—the rate of conversion of 17b-estradiol to less active estrogens
c. Causes relaxation of uterine muscles (direct effect).

Physiological actions

Effect on breast: Promotes growth of the glandular tissue

Effect on body temperature: Leads to rise in basal body temperature at the time of ovulation

Effect on respiration: Stimulate respiration.

Other effects:

- Progesterone exhibit negative feedback effect on hypothalamic pituitary axis. It decreases LH secretion therefore prevents ovulation.
- Progesterone causes vasodilation (relaxation of vascular smooth muscles). Decreases diastolic blood pressure.
- Causes natriuresis and diuresis by blocking the effect of aldosterone on kidney.

23

CHAPTER

Renal System

LONG ESSAYS 10 MARKS

1. How do you estimate renal blood flow? Explain the special features and factors regulating renal blood flow.

Ans. Renal blood flow = RPF × 1/1- Hct. (where as Hct: hematocrit, RPF: renal plasma flow)
Renal plasma flow is estimated by measuring the PAH (para-amino hippurate) concentration in urine and plasma after injecting it in the blood. Most of the PAH is removed by kidneys. Renal plasma flow is calculated by dividing the amount of PAH in urine by the plasma level known as the effective renal plasma flow. eRPF is 625 mL/min.

$eRPF = (U_{PAH} + P_{PAH}) \times V$

This represents the clearance of para-aminohippuric (PAH) acid. The PAH extraction ratio is 0.9.

Then the renal plasma flow is eRPF/extraction ratio.

Renal blood flow equals renal plasma flow

There are two mechanisms of regulation of renal blood flow. They are **(Table 23.1)**:

1. **Extrinsic**
   a. **Hormonal**
   b. **Neural**

Table 23.1: Mechanisms regulating renal blood flow.

Mechanisms regulating renal blood flow		**Factors responsible**	**Effects**
Extrinsic	Hormonal	Angiotensin II	Vasoconstriction of afferent and efferent arterioles
		Catecholamines	Vasoconstriction of afferent and efferent arterioles
		ADH	Vasoconstriction in large doses
		Prostaglandins, bradykinin, ANP	• Vasodilatation • Increase RBF, GFR
	Neural	Sympathetic stimulation (fear, anxiety, stress)	Vasoconstriction
Intrinsic		Autoregulation	• In the range—90–220 mm Hg • By tubuloglomerular feedback **(Flowchart 23.1)**

(ADH: antidiuretic hormone; ANP: atrial natriuretic polypeptide; RBF: renal blood flow; GFR: glomerular filtration rate)

Flowchart 23.1: Tubuloglomerular feedback mechanism.

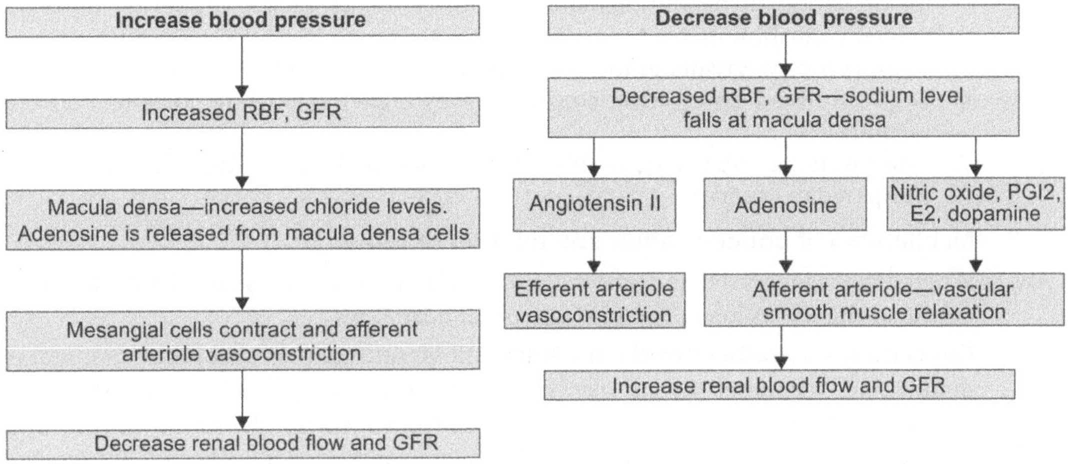

(RBF: renal blood flow; GFR: glomerular filtration rate)

2. **Intrinsic:** Autoregulation of renal blood flow is seen despite changes in systemic arterial blood pressure. The range for autoregulation is seen between 90 and 220 mm Hg.
   Myogenic theory of regulation of blood pressure states that whenever there is increase in blood pressure there is stretching of the vessel wall followed by vasoconstriction.

Tubuloglomerular feedback: It is an adaptive mechanism linking the rate of glomerular flow to the concentration of salts delivered at the tubule related to macula densa **(Flowchart 23.1).** Increased blood pressure causes increase in renal blood flow and GFR. This leads to increase in chloride concentration at macula densa causing release of adenosine from the macula densa cells. This causes contraction of mesangial cells and constriction of afferent arteriole. This leads to decrease in RBF and GFR.

When blood pressure falls, there is decrease in RBF and GFR. This leads to fall in chloride concentration. This leads to activation of vasodilator and vasoconstrictor mechanisms. There is release of angiotensin II leading to vasoconstriction and stimulation of sympathetic system further increasing the systemic blood pressure. The vasodilator mechanisms, is due to release of adenosine and relaxation of vascular smooth muscle. Due to the effect of nitric oxide, PGI_2, E_2 release and action of dopamine. This leads to greater action of the vasodilator system and return of the RBF and GFR to normal levels.

Special features of renal blood flow:

1. This is unique in a way that the renal portal system constitutes of arterioles and capillaries.
2. The renal artery is a high pressure system where the pressure in the glomerular capillaries is 45 mm Hg. The same in the peritubular capillaries is 15 mm Hg and in the systemic capillaries 30 mm Hg. This enables a better filtrate in the tubules.
3. The special features of vasa recta enable maintenance of medullary interstitial osmolarity.

4. Autoregulation of renal blood flow due to the chloride ion concentration maintenance, myogenic regulation via the smooth muscle properties makes a greater contribution.
5. Kidneys receive greater amount of the cardiac output—420 mL/100 g/min.
6. Regional blood flow—renal cortex receives higher rate of blood flow than the medulla.
7. Arteriovenous (AV) oxygen difference is not so high in the renal system as compared to others.

2. Mechanism of concentration and dilution of urine.

Ans. When there is increased or decreased intake of fluids the kidneys moderate the urine output under the influence of ADH and other hormones.

Concentration gradient in the medulla: The peritubular concentration gradient is maintained by *counter current mechanism.* This is a system in which the fluid flows in opposite direction in the parallel tubes. The Henle's loop, collecting duct (CD) and vasa recta form this system. The osmolality increases in multiples of 100 from the corticomedullary junction to the renal papillae.

There are two components:

1. Counter current multiplier
2. Counter current exchanger

Counter current multiplier: *Refer* Figure 23.1

a. **Na^{2+} and Cl^-:**
   - The *thin ascending limb of loop of Henle* is permeable to these ions.
   - In the *thick part,* the **chloride** ion is transported actively followed by sodium.
   - *K and Cl^- are co-transported* out of the thick ascending limb following active reabsorption Na^{2+} and Cl^-.
   - This leads to *decrease in tonicity of the fluid in the ascending limb* and
   - *increasing the tonicity in the peritubular fluid.*
   - The fluid concentration in the distal limb of loop of Henle increases and reaches equilibrium with that of the medullary interstitium—1,200 mOsm/kg.

b. **Na^{2+}, Cl^- or HCO_3^- ions in the collecting duct:**
   - Under the influence of *Aldosterone,* Sodium is actively absorbed by principal cells of the CD into the medullary interstitium.
   - Sodium is accompanied passively by Cl^- or HCO_3^- ions.
   - This *increases medullary osmolality* by increasing sodium and chloride ions which in turn causes **water reabsorption in the presence of ADH.**
   - These enhance the urea cycle causing the urea concentration in the collecting duct.

c. **Urea cycle:**
   - Urea is absorbed by *facilitated diffusion at the CD.*
   - It enters the medullary interstitium and then on to the ascending limb of loop of Henle.
   - Again, it is absorbed from the CD and then gets recycled.
   - About 50% of the medullary interstitial osmolality is contributed by the urea cycle.

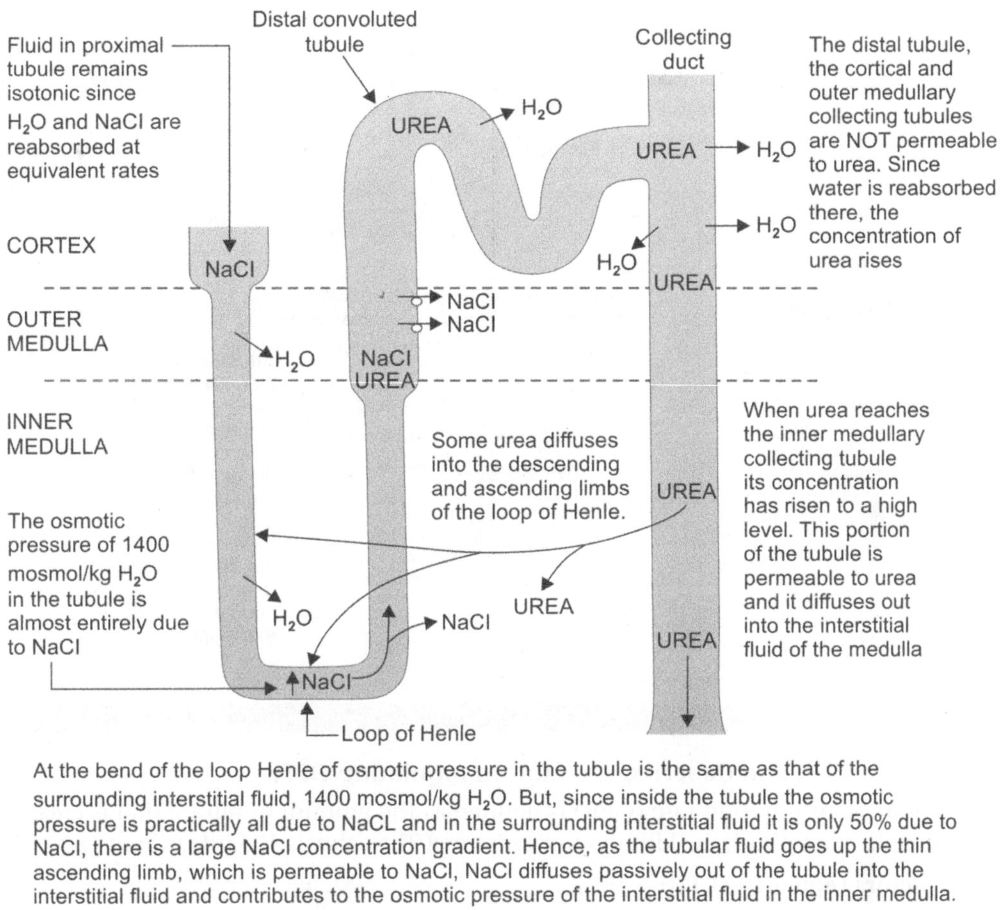

Fig. 23.1: Counter current mechanism.
(*Source*: Mackenna BR, R Callander, 6th edition)

Counter current exchanger: *Refer* Figure 23.2

- There is an exchange of ions and water between the two limbs of vasa recta, loop of Henle and medullary interstitium.
- Vasa recta descends to the renal papillae.
- Isotonic blood enters the descending limb.
- Due to the *gradient difference* water leaves and NaCl enters by a *passive mechanism* to maintain the osmotic equilibrium with the hypertonic peritubular fluid.
- When this fluid flows into the ascending limb the solutes leave the blood and water enters the medullary interstitium.
- Thus, the ions sodium and chloride recycle between the ascending and descending limbs of vasa recta.
- Urea absorbed from the inner medullary collecting duct enters vasa recta and recirculates with the other solutes.
- Water flows into the medullary tissue and then to the ascending limb of vasa recta.
- The slow blood flow into vasa recta prevents washing out of solutes.
- Thus, vasa recta act as an exchanger to maintain the osmotic gradient.

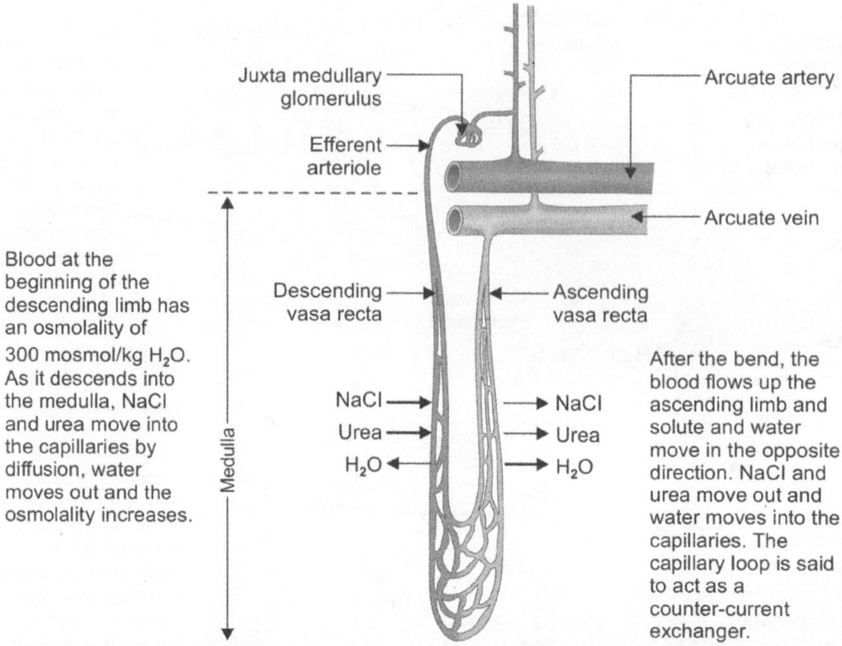

SHORT ESSAYS 5 MARKS

3. Define GFR and describe the factors regulating GFR.

Ans. Glomerular filtration rate (GFR) is defined as the amount of filtrate that is cleared of the plasma by both the kidneys per unit time. The value is 125 mL/min or 180 L/day.

Factors regulating GFR:

1. **Characteristics of glomerular capillary membrane**
   - *Structure*: Glomerular capillary endothelium has pores ranging from 75 to 85 nm in diameter. The basal lamina carry negatively charged proteoglycans.
   - Epithelial cells known as podocytes form the visceral layer of the Bowman's capillary which has a pore of 25 nm in diameter.
   - *Surface area:* In a normal person it is 0.8 m^2. GFR is proportional to the surface area. Mesangial cells contraction causes decrease in the surface area.
   - *Permeability*: Glomerular capillaries are more permeable than the systemic capillaries. Molecules up to 8 nm can get filtered, but those above 8 nm do not get filtered. Charges carried by the substance also matters. Normally no protein is present in urine and if present is taken up by pinocytosis.
   - *Filtration coefficient:* This represents the function of the surface area totally and the permeability of the membrane. K_f = 12.5 mL/min/mm Hg for both the kidneys.
2. **Forces acting across the glomerular capillary membrane**
   - Glomerular capillary hydrostatic pressure: 5 mm Hg (facilitates)
   - Colloidal osmotic pressure: 25 mm Hg (opposes)
   - Hydrostatic pressure in the Bowman's capsule: 10 mm Hg (opposes)
   - Net effective filtration pressure: 10 mm Hg

- Hence GFR = EFP × K_f = 12.5 × 10 = 125 mL/min. (EFP=effective filtration pressure; K_f = filtration coefficient)

3. **Neural mechanism:** The sympathetic activity is enhanced when blood volume decreases leading to increased catecholamines and vasoconstriction and thence decrease in renal blood flow and GFR. Sympathetic stimulation occurs in pain and emotional states. This decreases GFR.
4. **Hormonal mechanism:** Angiotensin, histamine, dopamine, ANP, nitric oxide and glucocorticoids affect GFR.
   - *Angiotensin* causes constriction of both afferent and efferent arterioles more so on the afferent arteriole causing a decrease in GFR.
   - *Histamine* causes increase in blood flow by causing arterial vasodilatation. By causing mesangial cell contraction it decreases GFR.
   - *Dopamine* increases GFR by causing renal arterial vasodilatation and stimulation of mesangial cells causes decrease in GFR. By inhibiting the secretion of renin, angiotensin II secretion is decreased.
   - *Atrial natriuretic peptide* causes dilatation of afferent arteriole and constriction of efferent arteriole causing increase in GFR.
   - *Endothelin* decreases GFR by causing constriction of both the afferent and efferent arterioles.
   - *Nitric oxide* causes profound vasodilatation of renal blood vessels and hence increases GFR.
   - *Bradykinin* increases GFR by stimulating release of nitric oxide.
   - *Adenosine* causes a decrease in GFR by constriction of afferent arteriole.
   - *Glucocorticoids* increase GFR by increasing renal blood flow.
   - *Prostaglandins* increase renal blood flow by decreasing the effects of catecholamines.
5. **Autoregulation of renal blood flow:**
   - Tubuloglomerular feedback and myogenic theory.
   - This enables maintenance of RBF and thence GFR despite changes in systemic arterial pressure between 80– 180 mmHg.
   - In myogenic mechanism stretch of the vessel wall causes constriction of the smooth muscles of the afferent arteriole decreasing GFR.
   - Based upon the tubular load, the tubular cells give a feedback to the glomerular cells to constrict or maintain a normal diameter of the afferent arteriole by releasing adenosine or nitric oxide from macula densa cells.

4. Write short notes on JG apparatus with a suitable diagram.

Ans. The juxtaglomerular apparatus (JGA) is a specialized structure located between distal convoluted tubule (DCT) and the glomerular afferent arteriole. The modified structure consists of the tubular cells, vascular components and the cells intervening between these two.

- The **DCT** passes between the afferent and efferent arteriole. The cells of DCT are different and form the **macula densa cells.** They act as sensors to monitor the ionic composition changes and gives a feedback to the renal corpuscle.
- **Juxtaglomerular cells** are the granular *modified vascular smooth muscle cells secrete renin* to regulate the activity of *renin angiotensin system.*

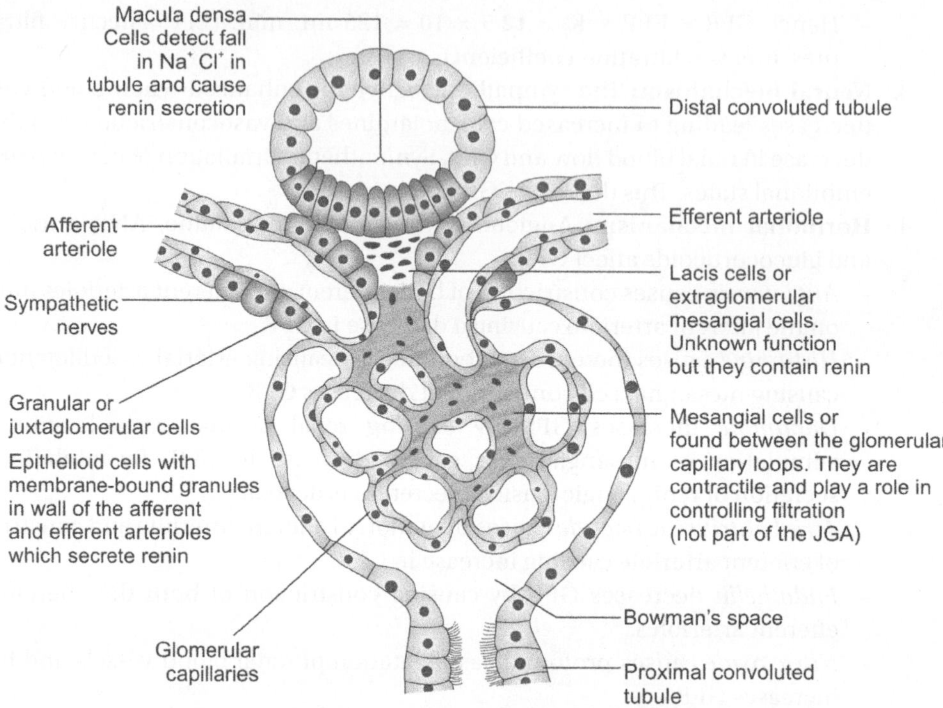

Fig. 23.3: Juxtaglomerular apparatus.
(*Source:* Mackenna BR, R Callander, 6th edition)

- The **lacis** cells which are *mesangial cells* occupy the space outside the glomerulus. All these cells help in regulation of blood volume, function to sense the rate of fluid filtration and the solute load thereby regulating tubuloglomerular feedback **(Fig. 23.3)**.
- Renin is secreted by the juxtaglomerular cells in response to a decrease in extracellular fluid volume and blood pressure or an increase in sympathetic nerve activity.
- In addition, a fall in tubular sodium and chloride is detected by the macula densa and causes an increased renin secretion.

24

CHAPTER

Cardiovascular System

LONG ESSAYS — 10 MARKS

1. Discuss the pressure volume changes that occur during the cardiac cycle.

Ans. Hemodynamic Changes

Pressure and volume changes in the atria and ventricle during cardiac cycle

- Intra-atrial pressure curve
- Intraventricular pressure curve
- Aortic pressure curve
- Ventricular volume curve

Intra-atrial pressure curve

- There are three positive waves and two negative waves that are observed in the atria.
  - 3 positive waves—a, c and v, caused by increase in intra atrial pressure.
  - 2 negative waves—x and y descent, caused by decrease in intra atrial pressure.
- 'a' wave is due to atrial systole
- 'c' wave is due to bulging of AV valve into the ventricles during isovolumetric contraction
- 'v' wave is due to filling of atria after the closure of AV valves

Intraventricular pressure curve (left ventricular pressure) **(Fig. 24.1)**

- *During isovolumetric contraction phase*—pressure rises steeply due to a rise in tension
- *Maximum ejection phase*—maximum pressure (120 mm Hg) develops as the ventricle is contracting with a maximum force
- *Reduced ejection phase*—pressure is less during this phase

Aortic pressure curve:

- During diastole of heart, the aortic pressure is maintained at 80 mm Hg
- During systole of the heart, it rises to 120 mm Hg

Ventricular volume curve:

- *End diastolic volume*: During diastole, ventricular volume increases. The maximum volume of blood in the ventricle at the end of diastole is called end diastolic volume. It is normally 130 mL.
- *Stroke volume*: Is the volume of blood ejected out from ventricle during systole. It is 80 mL
- *End systolic volume:* The minimal volume of blood remaining in the heart at the end of systole

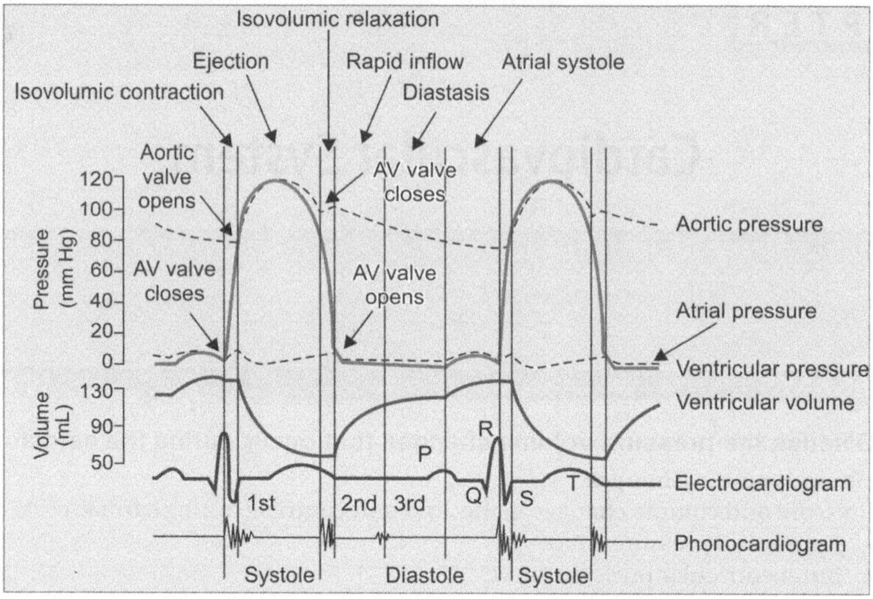

Fig. 24.1: Events of the cardiac cycle for left ventricular function showing changes in left atrial pressure, left ventricular pressure, aortic pressure, ventricular volume, electrocardiogram, and phonocardiogram.

2. Define cardiac output, its normal value and the methods to determine it.

Ans. The volume of blood ejected by each ventricle/per unit of time is known as cardiac output.

Normal values: Cardiac output: 5 L/min

Methods to Determine Cardiac Output

- Direct method
- Indirect method:
  - Fick's principle
  - Dilution principle (dye. isotope and thermodilution)

Fick's principle

The cardiac output is calculated by the following formula.

$$\text{Output of the left ventricle} = \frac{O_2 \text{ consumption by the lungs (mL/min)}}{(AO_2) - (VO_2)}$$

(AO_2): O_2 Content of arterial blood - 200 mL/L

(VO_2): O_2 Content of venous blood - 150 mL/L

$$\text{Output of the left ventricle} = \frac{250 \text{ mL/min}}{250 \text{ mL} - 150 \text{ mL}} = 5 \text{ L/min.}$$

Dyedilution technique

A known amount of dye is injected into the peripheral vein and blood samples are collected from the peripheral artery and the concentration of the dye in each sample is estimated.

Cardiac output can be calculated by using the following formula:

$$\frac{\text{Amount of the dye injected}}{\text{Mean concentration of the dye over a period of 1 minute}}$$

The commonly used dye is **EVAN'S BLUE** (T-1824).

3. Regulation of cardiac output.

Ans. The cardiac output is defined as the quantity of blood pumped into the aorta each minute **(Fig. 24.2)**.

$$\text{Cardiac output} = \frac{\text{Stroke volume} \times \text{heart rate}}{\text{Peripheral resistance}}$$

Stroke volume = Myocardial contractility × end diastolic volume (EDV)

The regulation of cardiac output is of two types: (a) Heterometric regulation, (b) Homometric regulation

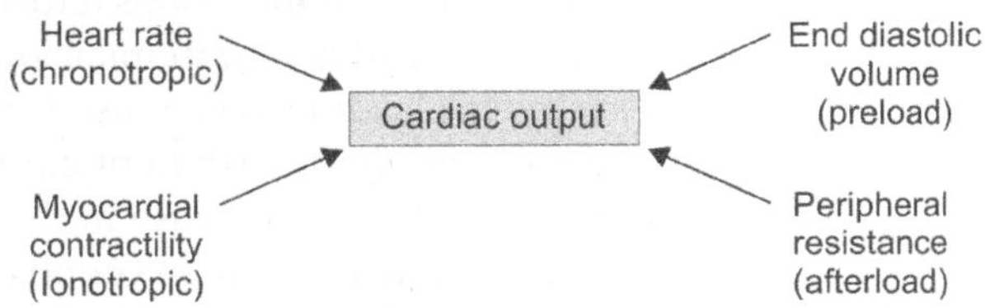

Fig. 24.2: Cardiac output regulation.

a. **Heterometric regulation:** Factors which cause an increase in the initial length of cardiac muscle before contraction.

Heterometric Regulation of Cardiac Output

I. **Intrinsic factors regulating myocardial contractility:**

Frank–Starling mechanism: The force of contraction is directly proportional to the initial length of the cardiac muscle. The initial length of the muscle depends on the end diastolic volume. Any increase in the EDV stretches the ventricular myocardium, increasing the length of the muscle fiber.

Force frequency relation: Any increase in the frequency of heart beat increases myocardial contractility within physiological limits. The increase in contractility is due to accumulation of intracellular calcium ions.

II. **End diastolic volume:** End diastolic volume is the volume of blood in the ventricles at the end of diastole. Any increase in the EDV increases the cardiac output by increasing the stroke volume.

Mechanism: Increase in EDV leads to stretching of ventricular muscle fibers that cause increase in the length of fibers. This causes a stronger muscle contraction resulting in increase in cardiac output.

Factors influencing EDV:

1. **Venous return:** The volume of blood that returns to the atria via the veins. This increases EDV and there by increases cardiac output **(Fig. 24.3)**.

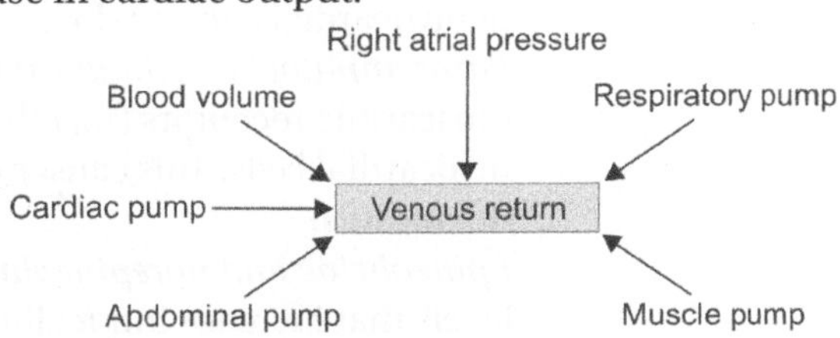

Fig. 24.3: Venous return.

Factors influencing venous return (Fig. 24.3):

- *Cardiac pump*: The pumping action of ventricles increases venous return by two forces:
  1. Vis-a-tergo (propelling force from behind): Left ventricular contraction during systole and elastic recoiling of arteries during diastole push the blood from aorta towards the right atrium
  2. Vis-a-fronte (suction force from front): Right atrial pressure - Less pressure in right atrium during diastole helps in suction of blood from the great veins into the right atrium.
- *Capacity of venous reservoir*: Venoconstriction causes a decrease in venous capacity leading to increase in venous return.
- *Blood volume*: Directly proportional to venous return, e.g., hemorrhage causes decrease in blood volume leading to decrease in venous return.
- *Respiratory pump*: Venous return increases during inspiration. Inspiration causes negative intrathoracic pressure and suction of blood into thoracic big veins leading to increased venous return.
- *Muscle pump*: Intermittent contractions of skeletal muscle squeezes the veins leading to increase in the flow of venous blood towards the heart. This leads to increase in venous return.
- *Abdominal pump*: Contractions of abdominal muscles compresses the great veins, pushing venous blood towards the heart.

2. **Ventricular compliance:**
   - Refers to the stretchability of ventricular myocardium
   - Any increase in the compliance reduces EDV and thereby stroke volume, e.g., pericardial effusion.
3. **Atrial systole:**
   - Contributes 20% of ventricular filling at rest
   - Influences EDV directly, e.g:
     - Increase in atrial systole during exercise causes an increase in EDV
     - In atrial flutter and fibrillation, the contribution of atrial systole in ventricular filling is reduced.

b. **Homometric regulation:** Factors which do not cause any change in the initial length of cardiac muscle before contraction.

Homometric Regulation of Cardiac Output

I. **Extrinsic factors regulating myocardial contractility**

a. **Neural factors:**

Sympathetic stimulation: Releases norepinephrine that binds to β_1 receptors and increases cAMP and increase in intracellular calcium causing increase in myocardial contractility.

Parasympathetic stimulation: Releases acetylcholine that binds to muscarinic receptors (M_2) that leads to hyperpolarization of SA nodal and myocardial cells. This causes decrease in myocardial contractility.

b. **Hormones:**

Epinephrine and norepinephrine: Bind to β_1 receptors, increasing in cAMP levels that increase intracellular calcium leading to increase in myocardial contractility.

Glucagon: Increases myocardial contractility by increasing intracellular calcium without binding to β_1 receptors

Thyroxine: Increases the myocardial contractility by increasing the metabolic rate.

c. **Ions:**

Sodium and potassium—decreases the myocardial contractility

Calcium—increases the myocardial contractility.

d. **Drugs:**

β-blockers, e.g., propranolol—block the β-receptors and decreases the myocardial contractility

Calcium-channel blocker, e.g., verapamil—block the calcium channel that causes decrease in intracellular calcium. As a result there is decrease in myocardial contractility

Digitalis: Blocks Na^+ - K^+ ATPase, decreasing Na^+gradient across the membrane. This leads to calcium accumulation inside the cell and increase in myocardial contractility.

e. **Coronary blood flow:**

Decrease in coronary blood flow

↓

Hypoxia, hypercapnia and acidosis

↓

Decrease in myocardial contractility

Influence of heart rate on cardiac output: Direct relationship between heart rate and cardiac output. Increase in heart rate increases intracellular calcium which in turn increases the force of contraction. This causes an increase in cardiac output.

Influence of peripheral resistance on cardiac output: Increase in peripheral vascular resistance causes decrease in the cardiac output over a period of time if the causative factor is not corrected.

Summary of regulation of cardiac output is shown in **Table 24.1**.

Table 24.1: Summary of regulation of cardiac output.

Types	Mechanism	Details
Heterometric regulation: Factors which cause an increase in the initial length of cardiac muscle before contraction	Intrinsic factors	• Frank Sterling mechanism • Force frequency relation
	End-diastolic volume	• Venous return • Ventricular compliance • Atrial systole
Homometric regulation: Factors which do not cause any change in the initial length of cardiac muscle before contraction	Extrinsic factors	• Neural: Sympathetic and parasympathetic • Hormonal: E, NE, glucagon, thyroxine • Ions: Na, K, Ca • Drugs: β-blockers, calcium channel blockers, etc. • Coronary blood flow

4. Define blood pressure and discuss the factors regulating it.

Ans. **Definition:** Blood pressure (BP) is the lateral pressure exerted by the moving column of blood on the walls of the blood vessels.

- **Systolic BP**: The maximum BP in the arteries during systole of the heart.
- **Diastolic BP**: The minimum BP in the arteries during diastole of the heart.
- **Pulse pressure**: The difference between systolic and diastolic pressure.
- **Mean arterial BP**: The average BP in the arteries. This is calculated as—diastolic BP + 1/3 of pulse pressure.

Normal values

- **Blood pressure**: 120/80 mm Hg
- **Systolic BP**: 90–140 mm Hg
- **Diastolic BP**: 60–90 mm Hg
- **Pulse pressure**: 40 mm Hg
- **Mean arterial BP**: 95 mm Hg

Regulation of Arterial Blood Pressure:

A. Short-term or rapid acting mechanisms

1. *Baroreceptor reflex:* The baroreceptors are present in carotid sinus and aortic arch which respond to stretch in blood vessel wall. It works in the range between 50–200 mm Hg of BP.

A. Increase in blood pressure

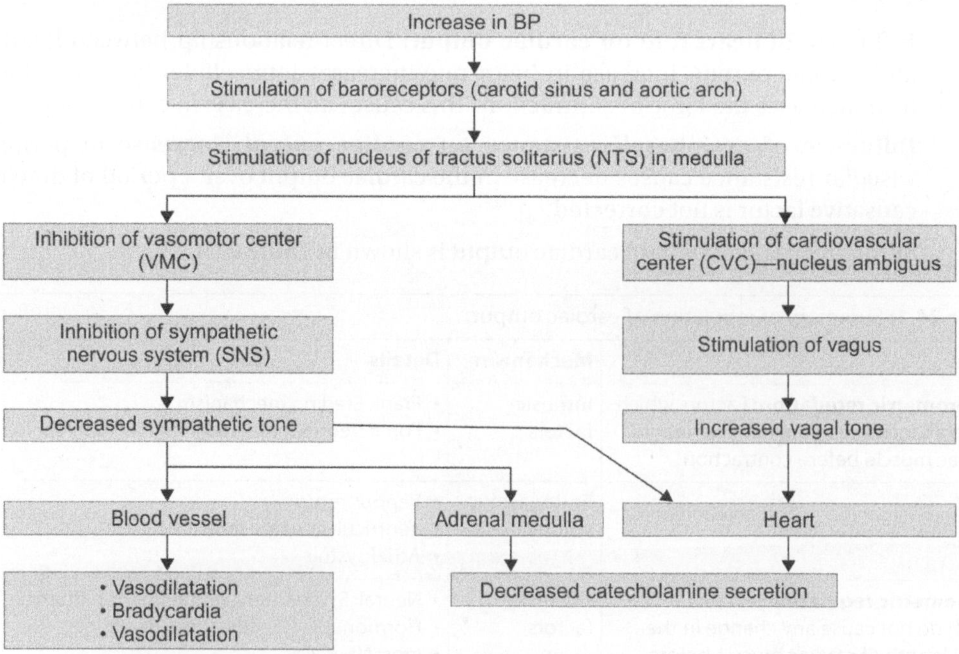

Effect: Decreased peripheral resistance, leads to decrease in BP and further decrease in cardiac output.

B. Decrease in blood pressure

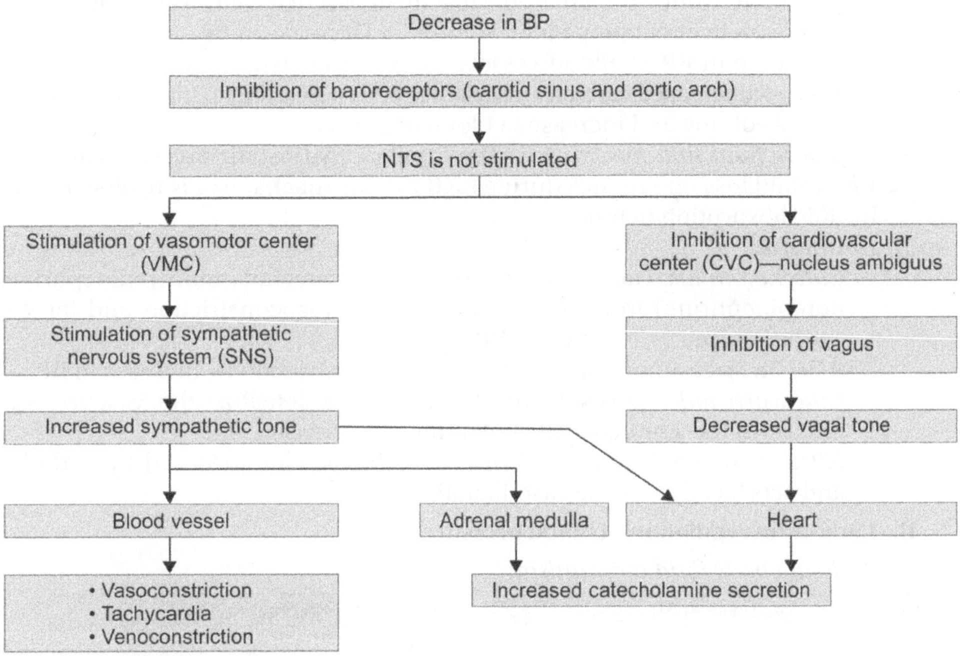

Effect: Increased peripheral resistance, increase in BP and increase in cardiac output.

C. Central nervous system ischemic response/Cushing reflex:

- This mechanism occurs due to ischemia of brain.
- This may result due to severe fall in BP below 40 mm Hg.
- If this response is specifically due to increase in intracranial pressure, it is called as **"Cushing reflex"**.
- The response is called "last ditch effort" as it tries to prevent the death of a person.
- The working range for this mechanism is 15–50 mm Hg
- It can correct 90% of the fall in BP.

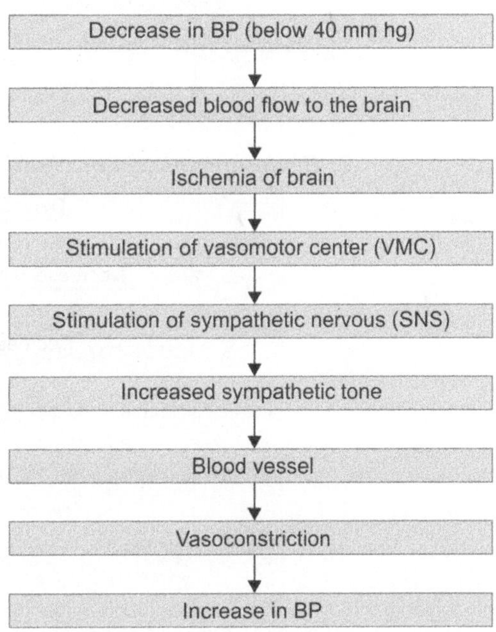

2. *Chemoreceptor reflex:* Two types of receptors—peripheral and central chemoreceptors.
   i. Peripheral chemoreceptors—carotid bodies and aortic bodies
   ii. Central chemoreceptors: Hypoxia, hypercapnia and acidosis
3. *Stress relaxation and inverse stress relaxation mechanism:*

a. Increase in BP → Stretching of blood vessels → Stress relaxation → Loss of vasomotor tone → Increased capacity of vascular bed → Pooling of blood → Decrease in circulating blood volume → Decrease in BP

b. Decrease in BP → Blood vessels are not stretched → Increase in vasomotor tone → decreased capacity of vascular bed → Leading to increase in circulating blood volume and increase in blood pressure.

4. *Capillary fluid shift mechanism:* The capillary hydrostatic pressure can influence BP by fluid loss into tissues during high BP. The mechanism is reversed if BP falls, by fluid absorption of fluid.

5. *Hormones:*
   - *Catecholamine*: Fall in BP → Release of catecholamine (epinephrine and norepinephrine) from adrenal medulla → Vasoconstriction and increase in cardiac output → Increase in BP
   - *ADH*: In large amounts ADH causes vasoconstriction → Increase in BP
   - *Glucocorticoids*: Cortisol and corticosterone sensitize the vascular smooth muscle to the action of catecholamine's (permissive role)
   - *Nitric oxide (endothelium derived relaxing factor)*: Released by endothelium and acts locally causing vasodilatation.

B. Long-term regulation of blood pressure

1. *Renal body fluid mechanism:*

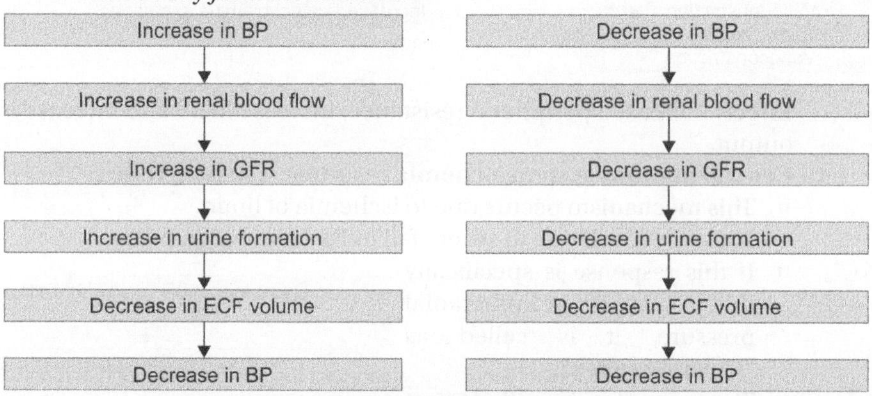

2. *Renin-angiotensin mechanism:*

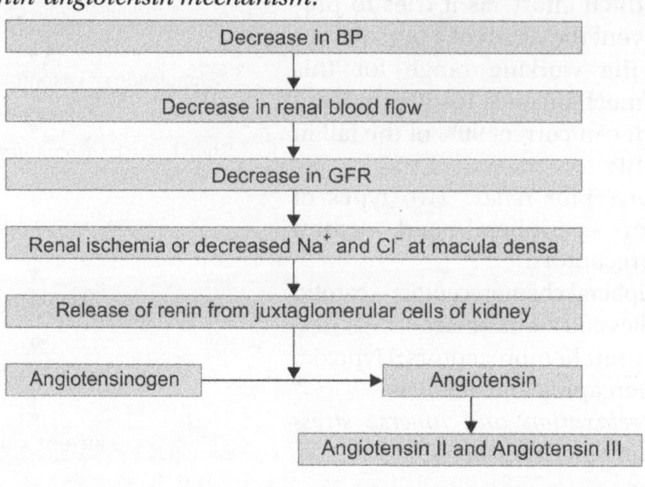

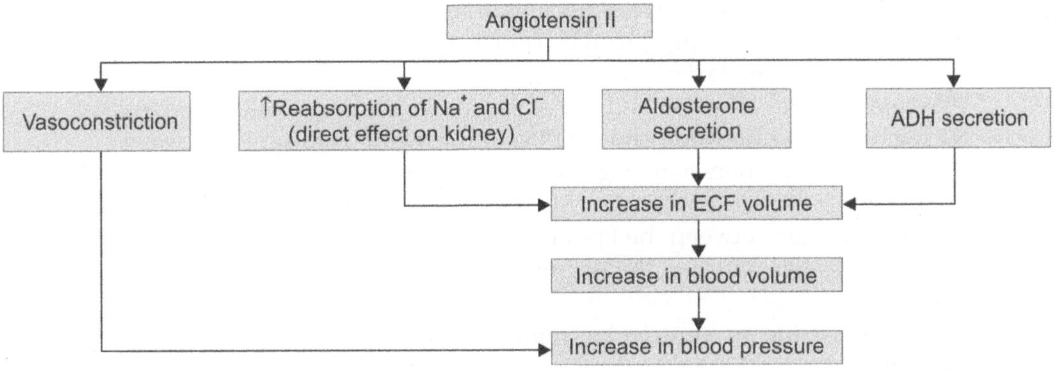

3. *Hormones regulating blood pressure:*
   - **Aldosterone**: Secreted from adrenal cortex in response to decrease in ECF volume. Increases the reabsorption of $Na^+$and Cl^- in kidney tubules. This causes increase in ECF volume and blood pressure.
   - **ADH**: Secreted from posterior pituitary. Increases water reabsorption from kidney → Increase in ECF volume and blood pressure
   - **ANP:** Secreted from atrial myocardium in response to increase in ECF volume → Facilitates Na^+, Cl^- and H_2O excretion into urine → Decrease in ECF volume and blood pressure

SHORT ESSAYS 5 MARKS

5. Draw a diagram of an electrocardiogram (EKG or ECG) and label it.

Ans. An electrocardiogram is a test used to measure electrical activity of the heart. P—atrial depolarization.

"QRS" complex = is due to ventricular depolarization which occurs before ventricular systole **(Fig. 24.4).**

Q wave—the initial negative deflection in the QRS complex.

R wave—the initial positive deflection in the QRS complex.

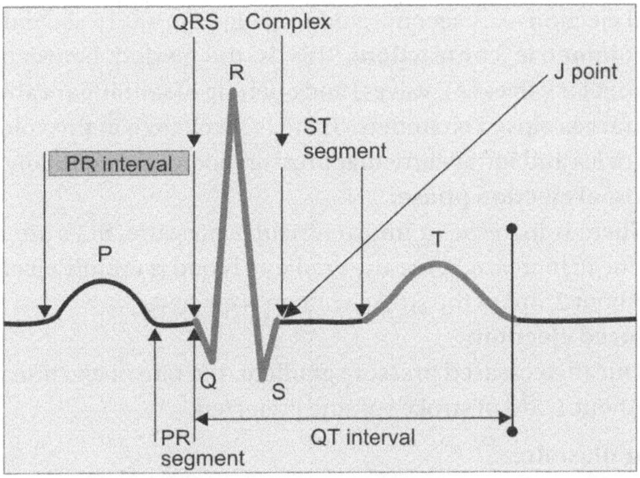

Fig. 24.4: Electrocardiogram.

S wave—the second negative deflection in the QRS complex.
T wave—positive wave produced by ventricular repolarization.
ST—ventricular repolarization.
PR segment—lies between end of P wave and beginning of QRS complex.
ST segment—lies between end of QRS complex and beginning of T wave.
PR interval—lies between beginning of the P wave and beginning of the QRS complex.
ST interval—lies between the J point and the end of T wave.
QT interval—lies between the beginning of the QRS complex and the end of the T wave.
"T" wave is due to ventricular repolarization which occurs before ventricular diastole

6. Describe about cardiac cycle.

Ans. The cyclical changes that take place in the heart during each heart beat is known as cardiac cycle.

Duration for one cycle = 0.8 seconds. **Phases: Systole and diastole.**

- Atrial systole — 0.1 second
- Atrial diastole — 0.7 seconds
- Ventricular systole — 0.3 seconds
- Ventricular diastole — 0.5 seconds

Atrial systole: Contraction of atria and movement of blood into ventricles. Contributes to 25% of the ventricular filling and forms the last phase of ventricular diastole. Produces fourth heart sound.

Atrial diastole:

Gradual filling of atria by blood that is brought by veins.

Ventricular systole:

- Contraction of ventricles and expulsion of blood into the respective blood vessels.
- It includes three phases namely—isovolumetric contraction—0.05 seconds, maximal ejection—0.1 seconds, reduced ejection—0.15 seconds.
  a. **Isovolumetric contraction:** This is the period between closure of atrio-ventricular valves (AV valves) and opening of semilunar valves (SLV). Ventricles contract as closed chambers. There is no change in the volume of blood in the ventricles and intraventricular pressure increases gradually.
  b. **Maximal ejection phase:**
     - There is increase in intraventricular pressure. SLVs are forced to open and due to increased pressure gradient, blood is rapidly ejected out of ventricles
     - About 2/3rd of the stroke volume is ejected.
  c. **Reduced ejection:**
     - Due to decreased pressure gradient, the rate of ejection of blood is reduced
     - About 1/3rd of stroke volume is ejected.

Ventricular diastole:

- Filling of ventricles by the blood flowing from atria

- Includes five phases:
  1. Protodiastolic period: 0.04 seconds
  2. Isovolumetric relaxation: 0.08 seconds
  3. Rapid inflow: 0.11 seconds
  4. Diastasis: 0.19 seconds
  5. Atrial systole: 0.11 seconds

Protodiastolic phase
- Ventricle relaxes and intraventricular pressure is less than the pressure in the aorta/pulmonary Arteries
- Semilunar valves close to prevent the back flow of blood from arteries into ventricles
- Closure of SLV produces second heart sound.

Isovolumetric relaxation
- Period between closure of semilunar valves and opening of AV valves.
- SLV and AV valves are closed and the ventricle relaxes as closed chamber. There is no change in the volume of blood in the ventricles. Intraventricular pressure decreases.

Rapid inflow phase
- Intraventricular pressure is less than intra-atrial pressure and so the AV valves open
- Blood flows from atria to ventricle at a faster rate
- Turbulence due to rapid flow produces third heart sound.

Diastasis: Increase in intraventricular pressure and blood flow from atria to ventricle is at a low rate or could remain static.

Atrial systole
- Last phase of ventricular diastole
- Contributes to additional 25% of ventricular filling.

7. Write short note on special features of coronary circulation.

Ans. Coronary circulation is important as it supplies blood to the heart.

- About 250 mL/min or 70–80 mL/100 g/min flows through the entire heart. Exercise may increase this amount (up to 2 L/min).
- Heart receives blood supply from the coronaries which are end arteries. Hence any occlusion will result in ischemic necrosis.
- The coronary arteries fill during diastole.
- However, if collateral develops there can be reduction in ischemia
- Myocardium depends largely on *aerobic metabolism.*
- The resting a-VO_2 (arteriovenous oxygen difference) is high in the myocardium being 19–7 = 12 mL/100 mL. Oxygen utilization is high.

Hypoxia is a major factor for regulating the blood flow.

Determination of coronary blood flow is by **Kety's method**.

Coronary angiography is considered as one of the standard methods for determination of coronary blood flow.

Regulation of coronary blood flow: Under resting conditions, the coronary blood flow is 250 mL/ min, but in case of exercise it can increase up to 1,000 mL/min.

1. Physical factors—the coronary vessels fill during diastole. The blood flow decreases during systole.
2. Increased O_2 demand—increased flow.
3. Hypoxia in local area (Intrinsic)—adenosine is product of metabolic reaction following hypoxia, which causes coronary vasodilation.
4. Control of vascular tone—nitric oxide from endothelium, prostacyclin, endothelin-1, etc.
5. Neural—parasympathetic is by vagus nerve and causes vasodilation. Sympathetic stimulation vasoconstriction.
6. Hormonal—thyroxin, vasopressin, etc.

25

CHAPTER

Respiratory System

LONG ESSAYS — 10 MARKS

1. Describe the neural regulation of respiration.

Ans. Two separate neural mechanisms regulate respiration:

a. *Voluntary control*—the center located in the cerebral cortex which controls the respiratory muscles through corticospinal tracts
b. *Automatic control*—the center is in the brainstem, a group of pacemaker cells in the medulla
c. Respiratory muscles are under both voluntary and involuntary control.

Impulses from these cells activate motor neurons in the cervical and thoracic spinal cord that innervates inspiratory muscles. The impulses also reach the internal intercostal muscles and other expiratory muscles.

The motor neurons to the expiratory muscles are inhibited when those supplying the inspiratory muscles are active, and vice versa **(Fig. 25.1)**.

Medullary respiratory centres can be divided into three groups:

1. Dorsal respiratory groups (DRG)
2. Ventral respiratory groups (VRG)
3. Respiratory central pattern generator (RCPG).

Dorsal respiratory groups (DRG)

- This group is within the nucleus tractus solitarius (NTS), and near reticular formation of medulla. They are *inspiratory neurons.*
- Receive input from chemoreceptor, baroreceptor, and thoracic viscera
- They emit repetitive bursts of inspiratory neuronal action potentials and reach diaphragm and external intercostal muscles.
- **Ramp signal**—it is weak in the beginning and then it steadily increases in a ramp manner for about two seconds. Then it stops for 3 seconds, which puts off the inspiratory muscle excitation and allows expiration to occur by causing elastic recoil of the lungs and chest wall.
- After expiration, next inspiratory ramp signal begins for another cycle.

Ventral respiratory groups (VRG):

- Located bilaterally in the medulla near nucleus ambiguus
- Contains both inspiratory and expiratory neurons.

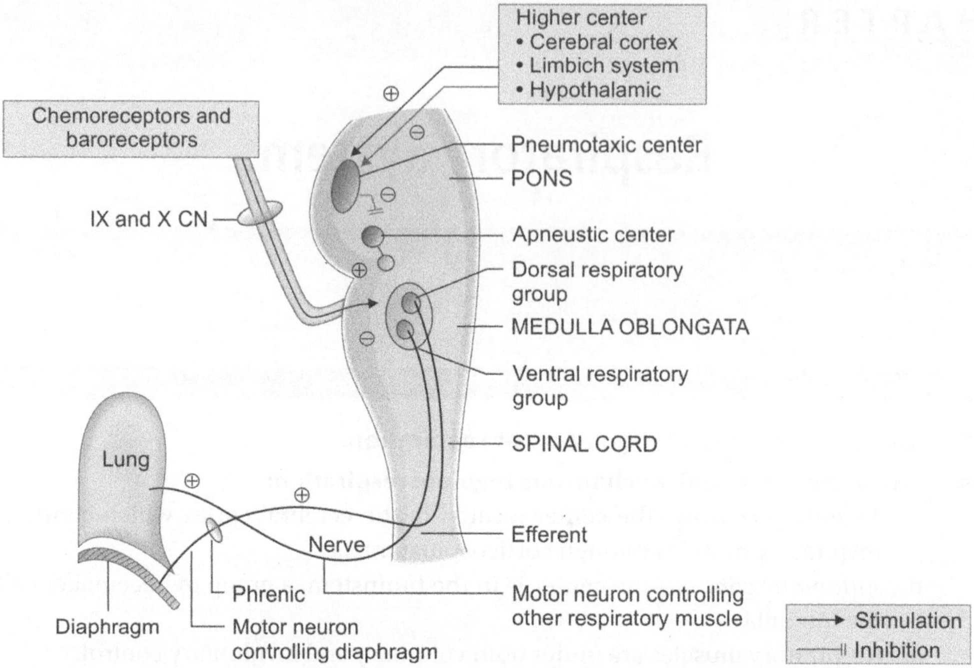

Fig. 25.1: Respiratory center and reflex controls.

- They are active during both phases of respiration especially important in providing powerful expiratory signals to expiratory muscles. This area contributes when high levels of pulmonary ventilation are required.

Respiratory central pattern generator:

- It is present in *pre-Botzinger complex* on either side of medulla
- Responsible for *normal rhythmic respiration*
- It sends projections to DRG and VRG. These neurons discharge rhythmically, and they produce rhythmic discharges in phrenic motor neurons.
- Initiate spontaneous rhythmic respiration modified by pontine respiratory centers and vagal afferent fibers.

Pontine respiratory centers: The pons has two respiratory centers are present—Pneumotaxic and Apneustic

a. **Pneumotaxic center**
   - Transmits signals to the inspiratory area and limits inspiration
   - It receives vagal afferent from lung.

b. **Apneustic center**
   - Stimulation of this center causes prolonged inspiration.
   - It is also tonically inhibited by pneumotaxic center.

These centers are responsible for modulation of respiration.

Role of vagus nerve: Vagus nerve carries afferent from the lung and airways. During inspiration, stretching of the lung increases the vagal discharge which inhibits medullary respiratory centers. Vagotomy increases the amplitude of inspiration **(Fig. 25.1)**.

SHORT ESSAYS **5 MARKS**

2. **Draw a labeled diagram of spirogram.**

Ans. Lung volume and capacity are measured by spirometry, the recording obtained by this procedure is known as spirogram **(Fig. 25.2)**.

There are four volumes and three capacities:

1. Tidal volume (TV)—volume of air inspired or expired during normal breathing.
2. Inspiratory reserve volume (IRV)—volume of air inspired maximally in excess of tidal volume
3. Expiratory reserve volume (ERV)—volume of air forcefully expired after normal tidal expiration.
4. Residual volume (RV)—volume of air remaining in lungs after a forced expiration.

Any 2 or more volumes added together is known as a capacity.

- Total lung capacity—volume of air in lungs at the end of maximal inspiration
- Vital capacity:
  - Sum of IRV, TV and ERV
  - Maximal volume of air which can be expelled forcibly from lungs after maximal inspiratory effort.
- Functional residual capacity:
  - Sum of ERV and RV
  - Volume of air left in the lung at the end of tidal or normal expiration.

Age, gender, training influence lung volume and capacities.

3. **What is timed vital capacity and mention its clinical significance?**

Ans. The fraction of the vital capacity expired in a specified time. It is also called as forced expiratory volume in the second (FEV_1) **(Fig. 25.3)**.

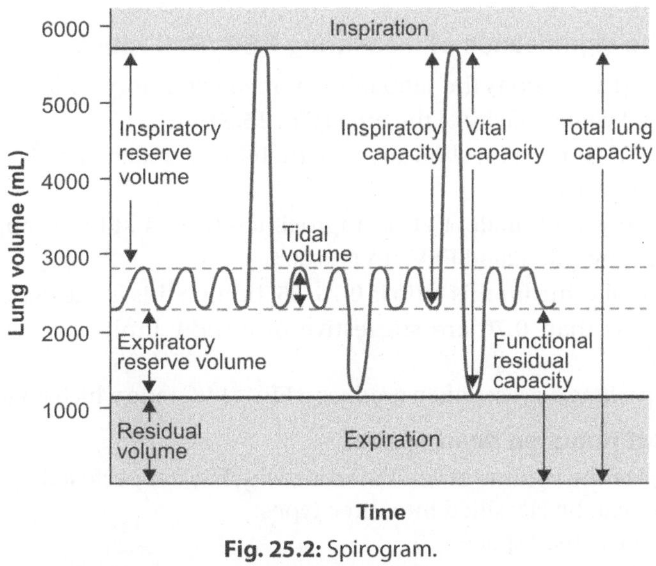

Fig. 25.2: Spirogram.

Normal value:
- FEV_1: 80%
- FEV_2: 95%
- FEV_3: 98–100%

One of the useful test to detect generalized airway obstruction.

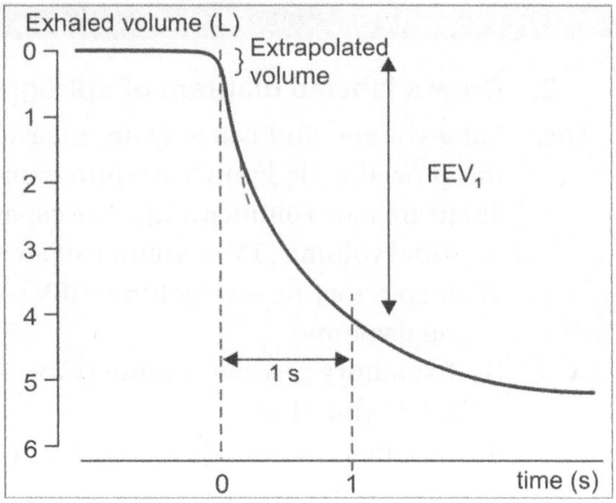

Fig. 25.3: Timed vital capacity.

4. Draw a labeled diagram showing timed vital capacity in normal and diseased patient.

Ans. The **Figure 25.4** shows forced expiratory volume in the 1 second (FEV_1) and VC

A = Normal subject

B = Patients with restrictive lung disease

C = Patients with obstructive lung disease

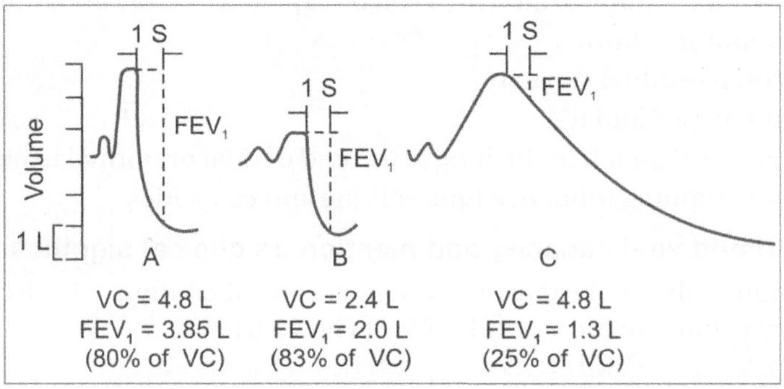

Fig. 25.4: Forced expiratory volume in the 1 second (FEV_1 and VC).

5. What is the significance of measuring FEV_1/FVC ratio?

Ans.
- The FEV_1/FVC ratio is the ratio of the forced expiratory volume in the 1 second to the forced vital capacity of the lung **(Fig. 25.5)**.
- FEV_1/FVC is important clinically than their individual measurement, in diagnosing airway diseases
- In a healthy adult male, FVC is approximately 5.0 L, FEV_1 is approximately 4.0 L, and thus, the calculated FEV_1/FVC is 80%.
- The normal value for this ratio is 0.75–85, though this is age dependent.
- Values less than 0.70 are suggestive of airflow limitation with an obstructive pattern
- Restrictive lung diseases often produce a FEV_1/FVC ratio which is either normal or high

6. Write short notes on dead space.

Ans. Dead space is the volume of ventilated air, which is not perfused by pulmonary blood. Dead space can be classified into three types:

1. Anatomical dead space

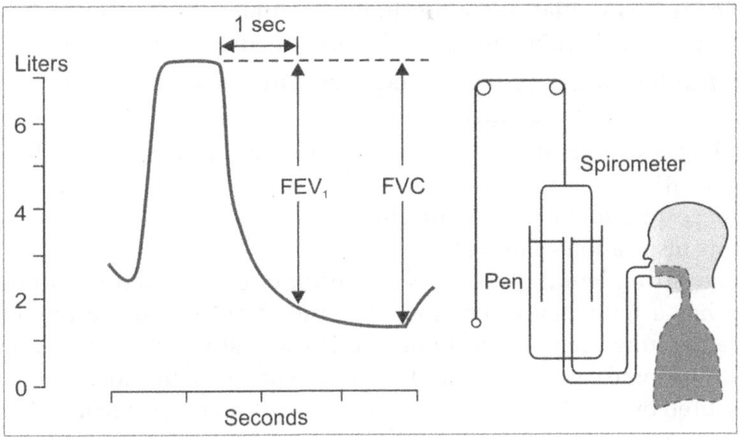

Fig. 25.5: Measurement of forced expiratory volume (FEV_1) and vital capacity (FVC).

2. Alveolar dead space
3. Physiological dead space

Anatomical dead space:

- The volume of air in the conduction zone that does not take part in gas exchange.
- Tidal volume is 500 mL, about 150 mL remains in the conduction zone, which is not used in gas exchange.

Alveolar dead space: It is the volume of inspired air in the alveoli that does not participate in gas exchange. This occurs when areas of the lung are being ventilated but not being perfused and this leads to ventilation perfusion mismatch.

Physiologic dead space: Physiologic dead space is equal to anatomic plus alveolar dead space which is the volume of air in the respiratory zone that does not take part in gas exchange. Alveolar dead space is negligible in healthy individuals.

Volume of dead space can be measured by two methods:

1. Single breath CO_2 technique
2. Single breath N_2 technique

7. What are the nonrespiratory functions of lung?

Ans.
- Lungs contain a fibrinolytic system that lyses clots in the pulmonary vessels
- Filtration of inhaled air
- Warming and moisturizing of inhaled air
- They release a variety of substances that enter the systemic arterial blood like form of prostaglandins, bradykinin, serotonin, acetylcholine, etc.
- Plays an important role in activating angiotensin. The physiologically inactive form angiotensin I is converted to angiotensin II in the pulmonary circulation due to the presence of large amounts of the angiotensin-converting enzyme (ACE) produced in the endothelium of the pulmonary vessels.

- Microorganisms that enter the lungs are phagocytosed by pulmonary alveolar macrophages, therefore lungs are involved in defense function.

8. Why intrapleural pressure is negative and what is the normal intrapleural pressure? Mention its significance.

Ans.
- It is the pressure in the pleural space between the visceral and the parietal pleura **(Fig. 25.6)**.
- During expiration: It is -2.5 mm Hg
- During inspiration -6 mm Hg
- The negative pleural pressure is the result of balance of two opposite forces. The lung has a tendency to collapse and the chest wall has a tendency to expand therefore lung recoil inward and the chest wall recoil outward, these equal and opposing force cause the intrapleural pressure to be negative.
- Measured by esophageal manometry through an esophageal balloon catheter.

Significance
- Negative in intrapleural pressure facilitate inspiration
- It maintains the normal shape of the chest wall.

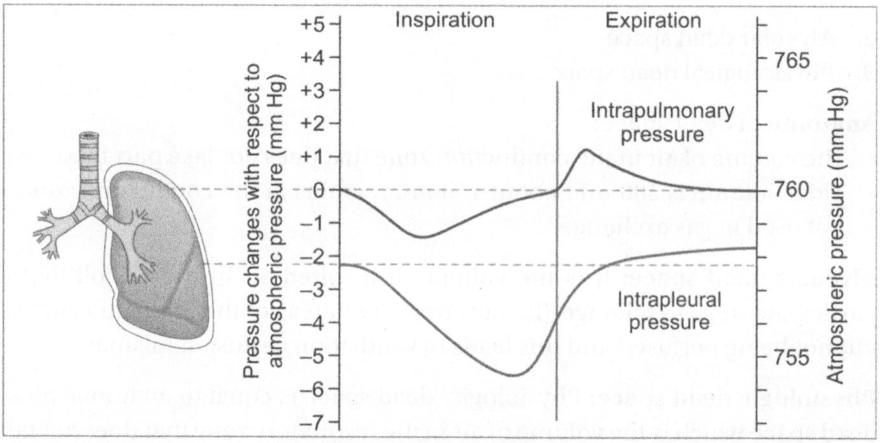

Fig. 25.6: Intrapleural pressure.

9. Mention the steps in mechanics of breathing.

Ans. **Inspiration:** Inspiration is an active process. The following sequence of events causes inspiration to occur:
- Contraction of inspiratory muscle (diaphragm and external intercostal muscles)
- Increases intrathoracic volume
- Intrapleural pressure becomes negative
- Fall in alveolar pressure
- Air flows into the airway and lungs
- At the end of inspiration, the inspiratory muscles relax and the recoiling force of lungs begins to pull the chest wall back to expiratory position.

Expiration: Expiration during quiet breathing is passive in the sense that no muscles are activated.
- Relaxation of inspiratory muscles
- Roll back of rib cage

- Intrapleural pressure become less negative
- Deflation of the lung
- Increase in alveolar pressure
- Air is pushed out of the lung.

10. What are the functions of pulmonary surfactant?

Ans. It is surface tension lowering agent. Produced from type II pneumocytes in the alveolar epithelium. It contain dipalmitoylphosphatidylcholine.

Functions

- Reduces the tendency of alveoli to collapse
- Reduces work of breathing
- Prevents pulmonary edema
- Provide stability of alveoli

Significance

- Deficiency of pulmonary surfactant leads to infant respiratory distress syndrome in newborn babies.
- In which there is increased alveolar surface tension, hence difficult to expand the lungs and work of breathing is greatly increased.
- This results in severe respiratory insufficiency.

11. Discuss the special features of pulmonary circulation.

Ans.

- The pulmonary circulation is a low-pressure, low-resistance system.
- In pulmonary artery, systolic pressure is 25 mm Hg and diastolic pressure is 8 mm Hg
- The pulmonary artery and its branches have much thinner walls due to less smooth muscle than the aorta, therefore they are highly distensible.
- Pulmonary vascular resistance is very low compared to systemic vascular resistance (decreased resistance facilitate better gas exchange in pulmonary capillaries).
- The pulmonary capillaries mesh together in the alveolar wall, so that blood flows as a thin sheet.
- Pulmonary capillaries lack resting sympathetic vasoconstrictor tone though they are richly innervated by sympathetic nerves.
- Hypoxia causes vasoconstriction in pulmonary arterioles.

12. Describe the changes in the body on exposure to high altitude.

Ans. A height, more than 10,000 feet (3,000 mts) above the sea level is defined as high altitude. The harmful effects on the body on exposure to high altitude are due to low oxygen tension.

- Exposure to high altitude causes change in respiratory system, cardiovascular system blood and tissues due to tissue hypoxia
- The primary objective of these changes is to increase oxygen supply to the tissues.

Respiratory system

- Increases ventilation
- Increase pH (respiratory alkalosis)
- Pulmonary vasoconstriction causing increase in pulmonary artery resistance
- Shifts the oxygen Hb dissociation to right.

Cardiovascular system

- Hypoxia stimulate sympathoadrenal axis therefore increase in heart rate, cardiac output (CO) and BP. Increased cardiac output increases blood flow
- Hypoxia causes vasodilation in the systemic circulation
- ↑CO and systemic vasodilation—increase blood flow and tissue oxygenation.

Tissue changes

- Increase in capillary density
- Increase in mitochondria
- Increase in the activity of oxidative enzymes (cytochrome oxidase)
- Increase in myoglobin
- Tissue angiogenesis (new blood vessels) occur

Hematological changes

Hypoxia stimulate production of erythropoietin which stimulate erythropoiesis therefore red cell mass increases which facilitate oxygen delivery to the tissues.

13. Define hypoxia and classify it.

Ans. **Definition:** Deficiency of oxygen at tissue.

Types

- Hypoxic hypoxia
- Anemic hypoxia
- Stagnant hypoxia
- Histologic hypoxia

Type of hypoxia	Hypoxic hypoxia	Anemic hypoxia	Stagnant hypoxia	Histotoxic hypoxia
	PO_2 in the arterial blood is reduced	PO_2 in the arterial blood is normal but hemoglobin in the circulation is inadequate, therefore the oxygen carrying capacity is reduced	Decreased blood flow to the tissue though oxygen content is normal	Tissue cannot utilize the oxygen despite normal oxygen supply
Causes	• Exposure to high altitude • Airway obstruction due to any cause	• Anemia carbon monoxide poisoning • Carbon monoxide poisoning	Heart failure and circulatory shock	Cyanide poisoning and diphtheria infection

Effects of hypoxia on the body

- Headache, drowsiness, mental and muscle fatigue
- Decreased mental proficiency, which decreases higher functions of brain
- Reduced performance of discrete motor movement.

14. What is hyperbaric oxygen therapy?

Ans.
- Administration of 100% oxygen at high pressure is known as hyperbaric oxygen therapy
- It increases the dissolved form of oxygen in the plasma.
- Useful for decompression sickness, carbon monoxide poisoning, diabetic gangrene.

- But 100% oxygen therapy produces side effects on prolonged use which includes:
  - Lung damage
  - Sinus damage
  - Changes in vision, and retrolental hyperplasia in newborn
  - CNS effects like irritability, disorientation, muscle twitching and seizures.
- Oxygen toxicity occurs due to hyperbaric oxygen therapy, mechanism postulated is formation of excess free radical in the body
- Free radicals oxidize the polyunsaturated fatty acids present in the cell membranes and also oxidize some of the intracellular enzymes thus damage the cellular metabolic systems.

15. Write short notes on Caisson's disease.

Ans.
- It is also called as decompression sickness (DCS).
- Occurs in individuals *who ascend rapidly to sea level* after exposure to high atmospheric pressure
- Seen in deep sea divers and workers in caisson. It is a form of gas embolism.
- Symptoms of DCS usually appear 10–30 minutes after the diver resurfaces.
- Deep-sea divers usually breathe gas mixture containing 80% of N_2 and 20% O_2 because inhalation of 100% O_2 at high pressure causes CNS depression.
- N_2 is lipid soluble. When the driver descends into deep sea N_2 dissolves in the body fluid and tissues.
- If the diver returns gradually, no harm occurs. If the ascent is rapid, nitrogen escapes from the solution, and bubbles form in tissue and blood.
- In the **mild form of DCS**, bubbles in the tissues cause severe pain in muscles and joints referred as bends.
- In **severe form of DCS** bubbles in the blood vessels, obstruct arteries and decrease the blood flow to brain and spinal cord resulting in sensory and motor deficit paralysis—also known as divers palsy.
- Gas emboli in the pulmonary circulation, produce pulmonary symptoms (dyspnea, cough, and respiratory distress) known as chokes.
- Bubble in the coronary vessel causes coronary ischemia.

Treatment
- Tank decompression: Affected individual is put in pressurized tank and recompressed.
- Quick recompression is followed by slow decompression.
- Recompression places the gases back under high pressure and forces them to dissolve again in the tissues, a process that instantly relieves many symptoms.
- Slow decompression is done so that body can get rid of N_2 slowly.
- Hyperbaric oxygen is also useful.

16. Describe the chemical regulation of respiration.

Ans. Two types of chemoreceptor plays a key role in the chemical regulation of respiration.

a. Central chemoreceptor
b. Peripheral chemoreceptor

Peripheral chemoreceptor

1. Peripheral chemoreceptors are carotid bodies and aortic bodies
2. They respond to alteration in PO_2, PCO_2, pH in arterial blood
3. Carotid bodies are located at bifurcation of common carotid and aortic bodies are located in the arch of aorta
   a. Each carotid and aortic bodies contains glomus cell and sustentacular cell surrounded by fenestrated sinusoidal capillaries.
   b. Hypoxia is potent stimuli for peripheral chemoreceptors
   c. Afferent is carried by 9th cranial nerve to medullary respiratory centers

Central chemoreceptor

- Located in the medulla therefore known as medullary chemoreceptor
- The chemoreceptors monitor the H^+ concentration of cerebrospinal fluid (CSF), including the brain interstitial fluid

Difference between peripheral and central chemoreceptor

Characteristics	Peripheral chemoreceptor	Central chemoreceptor
Location	Carotid body and aortic bodies	Ventral surface of medulla
Stimulus	• Hypoxia • Hypercapnia • Acidosis	Rise in PCO_2
Response	Rate and depth of respiration increased	Rate and depth of respiration increased

17. Draw a labeled diagram of oxygen Hb dissociation curve and factors affecting it.

Ans.
- The curve explains the relationship between PO_2 with oxygen saturation of hemoglobin.
- The oxyhemoglobin dissociation curve is an important tool for understanding how our blood carries and releases oxygen **(Fig. 25.7)**.
- The oxygen dissociation curve is sigmoid shape because of the cooperative binding of oxygen to the 4 polypeptide chains.
- It has two phases: Steep and plateau phase.
  1. **Steep slope between PO_2 of 10 and 60 mm Hg,** combination of oxygen with Hb increases rapidly. O_2 saturation of Hb is high (90% at PO_2 of 60 mm Hg)
  2. **Curve begins to plateau >60 mm Hg,** increase in PO_2 above 60 mm Hg produce minimal effect on Hb saturation

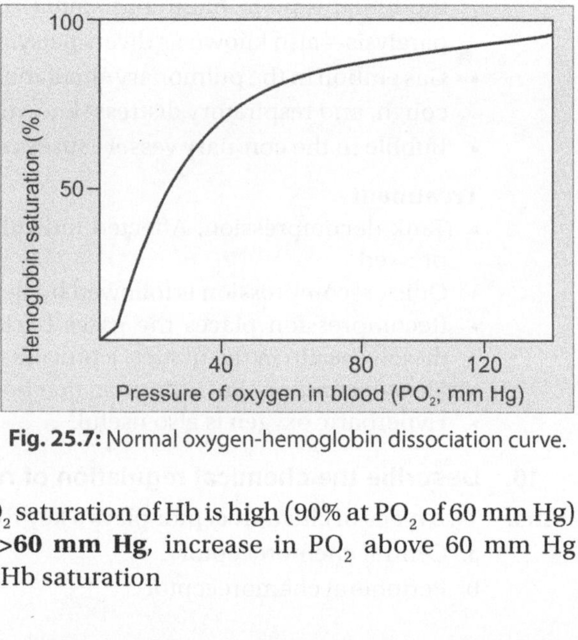

Fig. 25.7: Normal oxygen-hemoglobin dissociation curve.

The factors which affect the curve:
- Temperature
- PCO_2
- pH
- 2,3-DPG

18. What are the factors which can shift the curve to the right and left?

Ans. Rightward shift indicates (Fig. 25.8):
- Decreased affinity of Hb for oxygen
- Increased ability to release (unloading) oxygen to the tissues

Conditions
- Increased temperature
- Increased PCO_2
- Increased H^+ ion concentration (acidosis)
- Increased 2,3-DPG

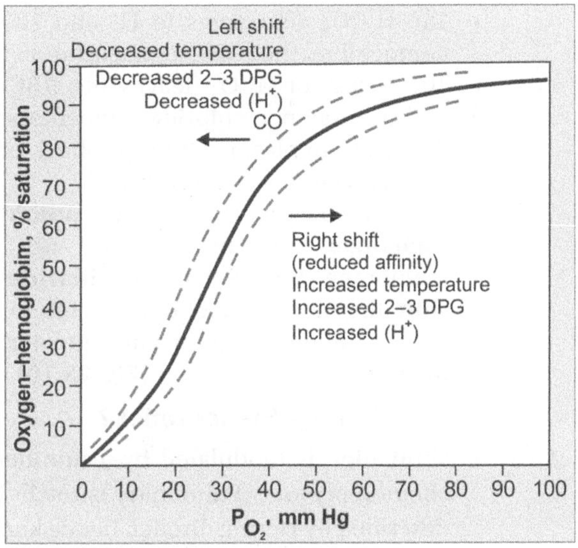

Fig. 25.8: Oxygen-hemoglobin curve shift to right and left.

Leftward shift indicates
- Increased Hb affinity for oxygen
- Decreased ability to release oxygen to the tissues

Conditions
- Decreased temperature
- Decreased PCO_2
- Decreased H^+ ion conc. (alkalosis)
- Decreased 2,3-DPG

19. What is P50?

Ans.
- P50 is the PO_2 at which the Hb is half (50%) saturated with O_2 **(Fig. 25.9)**
- It is the index of Hb affinity for oxygen
- The normal P50 occurs at PO_2 of 27 mm Hg
- High P50 signifies decrease affinity of Hb for oxygen seen in right shift of oxygen hemoglobin dissociation curve
- Low P50 indicates more affinity of Hb for oxygen seen in left shift of the curve.

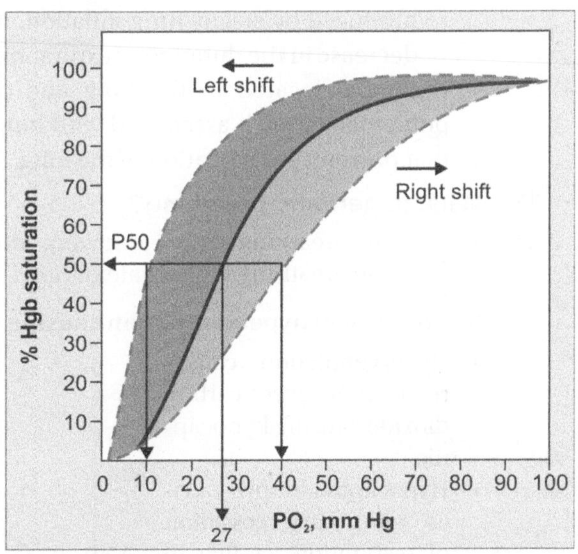

Fig. 25.9: P50.
(*Source:* Koeppen BM, Stanton BA. Bernye and Levy Physiology, 6th edition. Mosby, 2008)

20. Write short notes on chloride shift.

Ans.
- Chloride shift was first described by Hamburger
- RBC plays a key role in due to the presence of carbonic anhydrase
- The CO_2 produced due to tissue metabolism diffuses into red blood cells is rapidly hydrated to H_2CO_3 because of the presence of carbonic anhydrase.
- The H_2CO_3 dissociates to H^+ and HCO_3^-, and the H^+ is buffered, primarily by hemoglobin, the HCO_3^- concentration increases in RBC
- The excess of HCO_3^- leaves the RBC and in exchange chloride ions enters the cell from plasma (chloride shift) to maintain electrical neutrality.
- This process is mediated by **anion exchanger** present in the RBC membrane. Because of this **chloride shift**, the Cl^- content of the red cells in venous blood is significantly greater than that in arterial blood **(Fig. 25.10)**.

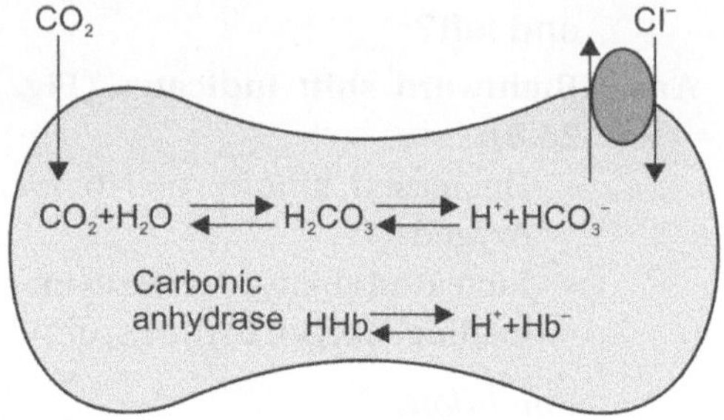

Fig. 25.10: Chloride shift.

21. What is Hering–Breuer reflex?

Ans.
- Ventilation is modulated by a number of reflexes other than those initiated by chemoreceptors. Pulmonary stretch has a profound influence on breathing, described by Hering–Breuer, hence known as Hering–Breuer reflex.
- It is of two types:
  1. Hering–Breuer inflation and deflation reflex
  2. The Hering–Breuer inflation reflex is an increase in the duration of expiration produced by steady lung inflation, and the Hering–Breuer deflation reflex is a decrease in the duration of expiration produced by marked deflation of the lung.
- Receptors located in the lung and/or pleural tissues and stimulated by the pulmonary stretch associated with lung inflation terminate inspiration in a reflex that prevents overinflation of the lung.

22. What is periodic breathing?

Ans.
- Periodic breathing occurs following voluntary hyperventilation
- Periodic breathing is alternate periods of apnea and hyperpnea **(Fig. 25.11)**.

Mechanism of hyperventilation causing periodic breathing

- Hyperventilation causes removal of excess carbon dioxide causing hypocapnia
- Hypocapnia in turn causes temporary cessation of respiration leading to apnea
- During apnea accumulation of carbon dioxide causing hypercapnia as well as hypoxia

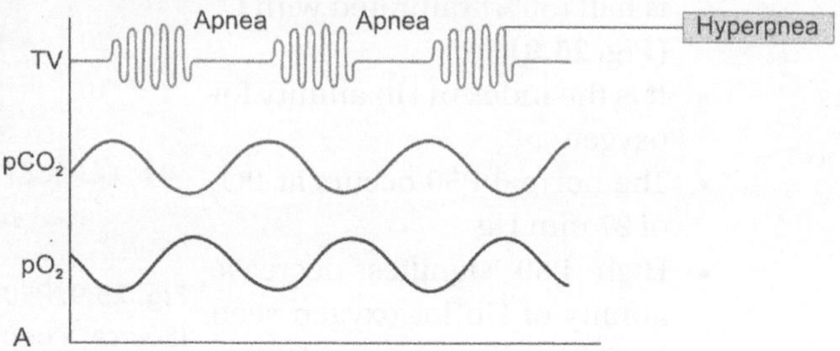

Fig. 25.11: Periodic breathing.

- Alteration in arterial gas level sensed by peripheral chemoreceptor which send information to medullary respiratory center and stimulate ventilation
- This pattern continues until gas levels returns to normal value.

23. Distinguish between Bohr and Haldane effect.

Ans.

Bohr effect	Haldane effect
• Effect of PCO_2 on the oxygen transport	• Effect of PO_2 on the CO_2 transport
• ↑PCO_2 and ↓pH shift the oxy–Hb dissociation curve to right	• ↑PO_2 shift the CO_2 dissociation curve to right
• Borh effect has mariginal impact on oxygen transport	• Haldane effect doubles the amount of carbon dioxide transport
• Postulated by Bohr in 1904	• Described by John Sott Haldane in 1936
• Loading of carbon dioxide causes unloading of O_2 in tissues	• Loading of oxygen causes unloading of CO_2 in lungs

SHORT ANSWERS 3 MARKS

24. Define vital capacity.

Ans.
- Vital capacity (VC): The maximum volume of air which can be expelled forcibly from lungs after maximal inspiratory effort.
- It provide valuable Information about the strength of respiratory muscles
- It is computed as VC = tidal volume + inspiratory reserve volume + expiratory reserve volume
- Measured by spirometer
- Normal value: Males—4.8 L and females—3.2 L.

25. Define functional residual capacity, give its normal value and clinical significance of measuring it.

Ans.
- **Definition:** It the volume of air left in the lung at the end of tidal expiration.
- **Normal value:** 2.2 -2.5 L
- **Clinical significance:**
  - It maintains the lung volume at the end of expiration
  - It keeps the small airways open
  - Prevents complete emptying of lung during each respiratory cycle
- Measured by dilution technique (helium dilution technique) or by body plethysmography

26. Mention the dynamic lung volume and capacity.

Ans.
- These are time dependent measures, represented in mL/min or L/min.
- The following measures are classified under dynamic lung volumes and capacities:
  - Timed vital capacity
  - Forced vital capacity
  - FEV_1/FVC
  - Peak expiratory flow rate
  - Maximum voluntary ventilation
  - Maximum mid-expiratory flow rate

27. Define peak expiratory flow rate.

Ans.
- Maximum velocity with which air is forced out of the lung
- Normal value is 400-600 L/min
- Measured by Wright peak flow meter
- Peak expiratory flow rate (PEFR) can be used to identify and assess airflow limitation in clinical practice and epidemiologic studies.

28. What is minute ventilation?

Ans.
- It is also called as pulmonary ventilation.
- It is the volume of air that enters the lungs each minute.
- Minute ventilation = tidal volume × respiratory rate
- If tidal volume is 500 mL and respiratory rate is 12 per minute, then Minute ventilation = 500 mL × 12 per minute = 6,000 mL/min
- Normal minute ventilation in adult is 5–10 L/min

29. What is alveolar ventilation?

Ans.
- The volume of air actually reaches the alveoli per minute
- Alveolar ventilation is important because it represents the volume of air available for gas exchange
- Alveolar ventilation = (Tidal volume - dead space) × respiratory rate
  500 mL–150 mL × 12
  350 mL × 12 = 4,200 mL/min

If anatomical dead space volume is increased due to any cause than the alveolar ventilation decreases.

30. What is alveolar pressure? Mention its significance.

Ans.
- It is the pressure inside the alveoli.
- Changes in alveolar pressure moves air in and out of the lungs
- During inspiration, alveolar pressure decreases therefore inflow of air occurs
- During expiration, alveolar pressure increases therefore air flows out of the lung
- It is -1 mm Hg in inspiration and + 1 mm Hg in expiration **(Fig. 25.12)**.

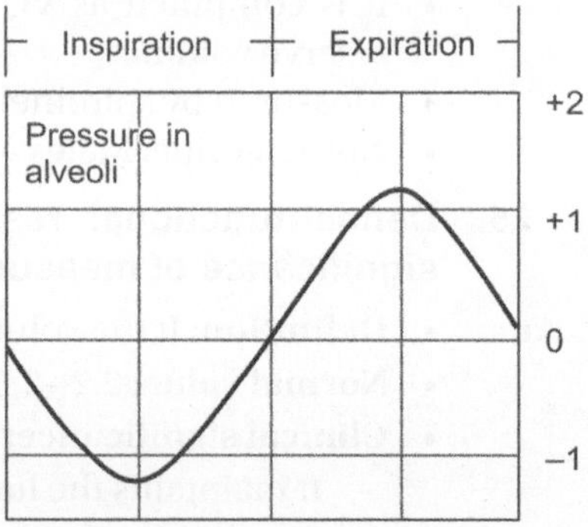

Fig. 25.12: Alveolar pressure.

31. Write short notes on ventilation: perfusion ratio.

Ans. The ratio of pulmonary ventilation to pulmonary blood flow for the lung at rest is about 0.8 (4.2 L/min ventilation divided by 5.5 L/min blood flow) **(Fig. 25.13)**.

- Differences occur in ventilation—perfusion (VA/Q ratio) in various parts of normal lung due to gravity

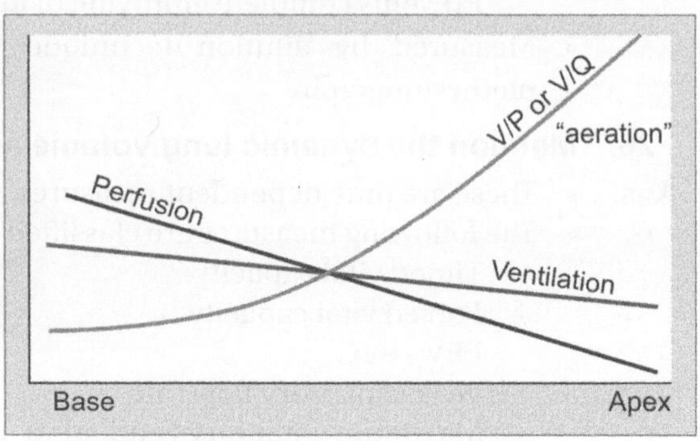

Fig. 25.13: Ventilation perfusion ratio.

- Base of the lung is better ventilated and better perfused than apex
- VA/Q ratio is high in apex of the lung
- Alterations in the ventilation—perfusion ratio of a lung affect its gas exchange and also predilection for certain diseases, for example, TB lesions occur commonly in the apex.

32. What is acute mountain sickness?

Ans. When unacclimatized individuals ascend too rapidly to high altitude, he manifest high altitude illness (HAI). Acute mountain sickness (AMS) is the milder form of HAI. Symptoms appear within 4–8 hours of exposure.

Acute motion sickness characterized by:

- Headache, fatigue, dyspnea
- Gastrointestinal tract disturbance (anorexia, nausea, vomiting)
- Insomnia and palpitations
- Dizziness or light headedness
- Loss of coordination, memory and judgment
- Euphoria and emotional changes

33. What is asphyxia?

Ans. Any condition that result in hypoxia and hypercapnia is known as asphyxia.
Seen in:

- Strangulation
- Drowning
- Foreign body occlusion of the major airways.

34. Write short notes on oxygen therapy.

Ans. The mainstay of treatment in hypoxia is oxygen therapy but it is highly beneficial to patients with hypoxic hypoxia. It is not much useful for other forms of hypoxia. It is delivered by:

- Oxygen tent
- Oxygen mask
- Through intranasal tube and mechanical ventilator.

35. What is the effect of sections at different level of brainstem and its effect on respiration?

Ans. S1 = Section below the medulla completely ceases the respiration which indicate that the respiratory centers are located in medulla and control spontaneous and rhythmic respiration.

S2 = Section between pons and medulla, do not affect basic rhythm of respiration but respiration becomes irregular which state that medullary respiratory centers generates respiration which is fine tuned by pontine respiratory centers.

S3 = Section between apneustic and pneumotaxic centers amplitude of respiration increased indicating pneumotaxic center inhibits apneustic center. Apneustic center induces inspiratory centers apneusis occurs.

S4 = Section above the PONS do not affect respiration, but if its done along with vagotomy respiration increased **(Fig. 25.14)**.

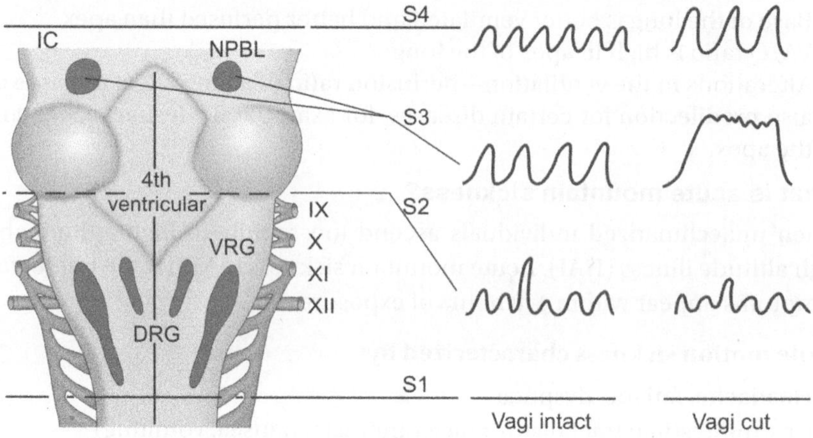

Fig. 25.14: Effects of sections at different level of brainstem.
(NPBL: nucleus parabrachialis lateralis; VRG: ventral respiratory group; DRG: dorsal respiratory group)
(*Source:* Barrett KE, Barman SM, Books HL, et al. Ganong's Review of Medical Physiology, 26th edition. McGraw-Hill Education)

36. What are the various forms by which oxygen is transported in the blood?

Ans. Oxygen is transported in the blood as dissolved and combined form:
- Dissolved in plasma = 2% (0.3 mL/dL of blood)
- Combined with hemoglobin = 98% (19.5 mL/dL of blood)

37. Why stored blood is not suitable for hypoxic patients?

Ans. The 2,3-DPG concentration in RBC decreases during storage, fall in DPG concentration shifts the oxygen-hemoglobin curve to the left. Therefore, the ability of this blood to release oxygen to the tissue is reduced. Therefore, it is not suitable for hypoxic patient. This effect is less if the blood is stored in citrate-phosphate-dextrose solution.

38. What are the various forms by which carbon dioxide is transported in the blood?

Ans.
- As dissolved in plasma: 7–10%
- As carbamino compounds: 20–30%
- As bicarbonate ions in plasma and RBC: 60–70%

39. What is Bohr and Haldane effect?

Ans.
- Bohr effect: Decrease in O_2 affinity of Hb when pH of the blood falls or pCO_2 increases is Bohr effect
- Haldane effect: Binding of oxygen with hemoglobin tend to displace carbon dioxide from blood.

40. What is Cheyne–Stokes breathing?

Ans. When periodic breathing occurs in disease it is called as Cheyne–Stokes breathing **(Fig. 25.15)**. Seen in:
- Heart failure
- Renal failure
- Brain diseases
- Poisoning by narcotics

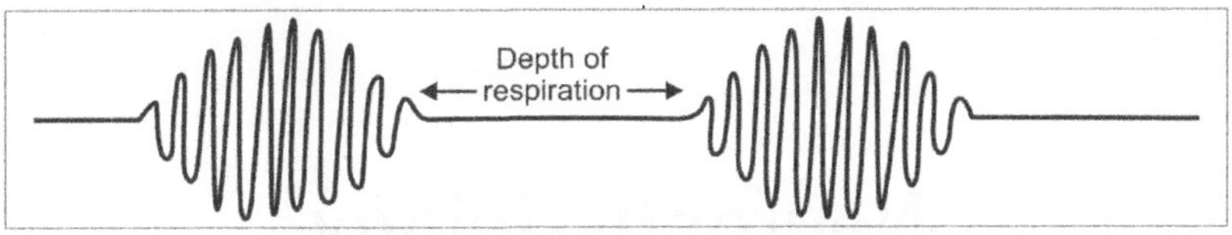

Fig. 25.15: Cheyne–Stokes respiration.

41. Write short note on artificial ventilation.

Ans. Respiratory arrest due to any cause like drowning, electric shock, certain poisoning require artificial ventilation. There are two methods:

1. Manual
2. Instrumental

Manual

- Mouth-to-mouth breathing
- Back pressure arm lift method (Holger Neilsen method)

Instrumental

- Positive pressure method
- Negative pressure method

26
CHAPTER

Neurophysiology

LONG ESSAYS — 10 MARKS

1. Trace the pathway for pain.

Ans.
- Pain and temperature sensations are carried by **lateral spinothalamic tract.**
- Fast pain is carried by A delta fibers, slow pain is carried by C fibers.
- Pain receptors are known as nociceptors they are free nerve endings.
- There are three order neuron in the sensory pathway that convey the information to the sensory cortex.
- **First-order neuron** start from receptor and enter the spinal cord through dorsal root. It terminate in second order neuron in the spinal cord.
- **Second-order neurons** cross to the opposite side of the spinal cord at the same segment and ascend up in the lateral side of the spinal cord as lateral spinothalamic tract and terminate in the specific relay nuclei of contralateral thalamus.
- From thalamus **third-order neurons** starts and terminate in sensory cortex located in the postcentral gyrus area 3,2,1 **(Fig. 26.1)**.

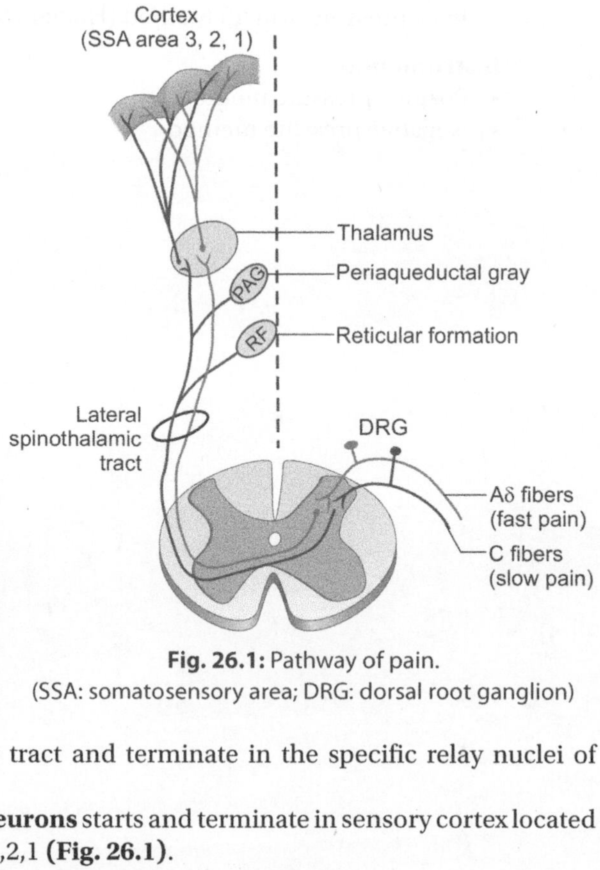

Fig. 26.1: Pathway of pain.
(SSA: somatosensory area; DRG: dorsal root ganglion)

2. Write a short note on regulation of temperature regulation.

Ans. Body temperature in humans is controlled by hypothalamus. It occurs by a feedback loop involving:
- **Receptors:** Thermoreceptor
- **Afferent:** Lateral spinothalamic tract

- **Center**: Hypothalamus
  - Anterior hypothalamus—heat loss center
  - Posterior hypothalamus—heat gain center
- **Efferent**: Sympathetic nerves to cutaneous blood vessel and sweat glands, motor nerve to skeletal muscle
- **Effector**: Sweat gland, cutaneous blood vessels and skeletal muscle.

Thermoreceptor

Cutaneous thermoreceptor	Central thermoreceptor
• Present in the skin and mucus membrane • There are two distinct thermoreceptor 1. Warm receptors(WR) 10% are WR, stimulated at 44–46°C 2. Cold receptors (CR) 90% are CR, stimulated at 40–24°C	• Located in the preoptic area of anterior hypothalamus • They collect information about temperature from both peripheral and central thermoreceptors

Center: Hypothalamus

- Heat loss center located in anterior hypothalamus
- Heat gain center located in posterior hypothalamus

Heat loss center	Heat gain center
• Increased core temperature activate neurons in anterior hypothalamus (heat loss center) and promote heat loss	• Decreased core temperature activate neurons in Posterior hypothalamus (heat production center)
• Lesions in this center cause hyperthermia	• Promote heat gain by lesion in this center leads to hypothermia

Efferent:

- Sympathetic nerves to cutaneous blood vessel and sweat glands, motor nerve to skeletal muscle.
- The hypothalamic temperature regulating center integrate information collected from thermoreceptor and the information is matched with set point for body temperature (37°C). Depending on the magnitude of deviation in body temperature, hypothalamus initiate appropriate responses and bring back the temperature to normal.

Responses activated by heat	Responses activated by cold
Cutaneous vasodilation	Cutaneous vasoconstriction.
Sweating	Shivering
Increased respiration	Nonshivering thermogenesis
Reduced physical activity	Piloerection
Reduced appetite	Increased appetite

SHORT ESSAYS — 5 MARKS

3. Classification of receptors.

Ans. Based on the location they are classified as:

- Superficial—located in the skin
- Deep—located in the muscles
- Visceral—located in the viscera

Based on the stimulus

- Mechanoreceptor—respond to mechanical stimulus
- Nociceptors—respond to pain stimuli
- Thermoreceptor—respond to temperature change
- Photoreceptor—respond to light stimuli
- Chemoreceptor—respond to chemical stimuli

4. Write short notes on receptor potential.

Ans.

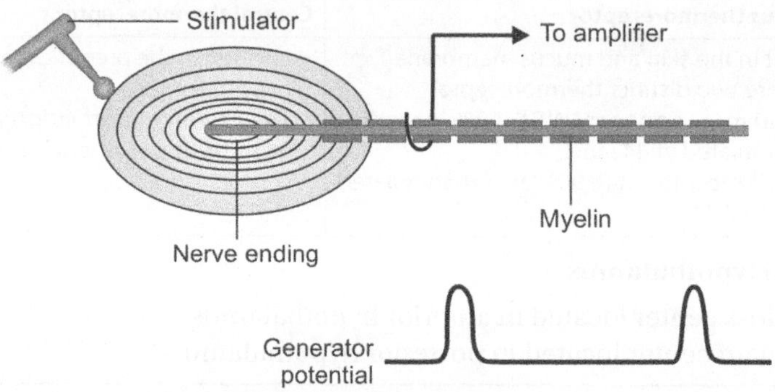

Fig. 26.2: Receptor potential.

- Receptor potential is a local and nonpropagated potential caused by a stimulus to a receptor cell.
- Receptor potential is studied in Pacinian corpuscles (mechanoreceptor) due their larger size, it is generated in the unmyelinated nerve terminal **(Fig. 26.2)**.

Application of the stimulus

↓

Activation of receptor

↓

Opens channel in the membrane causes influx or efflux of ion

↓

Resulting in generation of receptor potential (which is nonpropagated potential, when intensity of the stimulus is increased it generates an AP)

5. Write short notes on referred pain.

Ans.

- Visceral pain is not felt in the viscera, it often radiates to somatic structures away from the viscera, therefore it is known as referred pain.
- Examples of referred pain:
  - Referral of cardiac pain to the inner aspect of the left arm.
  - Pain in the appendix is felt in the umbilicus
  - Diaphragmatic irritation causes pain in the tip of the shoulder
- The basis for referred pain is convergence-projection theory and dermatomal theory.
- Convergence of somatic and visceral pain fibers on the same second-order neurons in the dorsal horn that project to the thalamus and then to the somatosensory cortex. This is called the convergence-projection theory **(Fig. 26.3)**.
- Visceral pain is usually referred to a structure that develops from the same embryonic segment this is known as dermatomal theory.

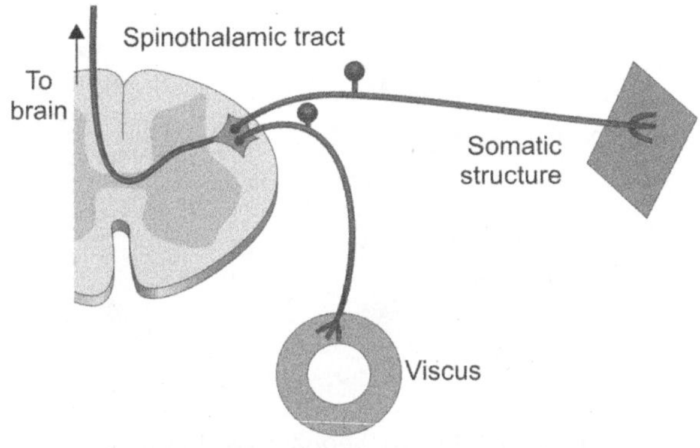

Fig. 26.3: Convergence-projection theory.

6. **Draw a labeled diagram of anterolateral system and mention the sensations carried by it.**

Ans. *Refer* **Figure 26.4**.

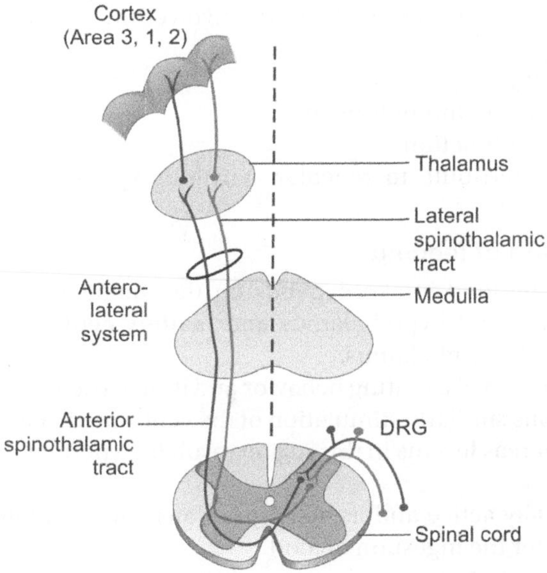

Anterior spinothalamic tract:	Crude touch
Lateral spinothalamic tract:	Pain and temperature

Fig. 26.4: Anterolateral system.
(DRG: dorsal root ganglion)

7. **What is Brown-Sequard syndrome?**

Ans.
- Brown-Séquard syndrome results from hemisection of the cord, due to injury, tumor and ischemia **(Fig. 26.5)**.
- It is manifested by ipsilateral loss of motor function, proprioception, and vibratory sensation, and contralateral loss of pain and temperature sensation.
- Ipsilateral symptoms are due to damage of the lateral corticospinal tract and dorsal column pathway.
- Contralateral symptoms are due to damage to lateral spinothalamic tract which carry pain and temperature.

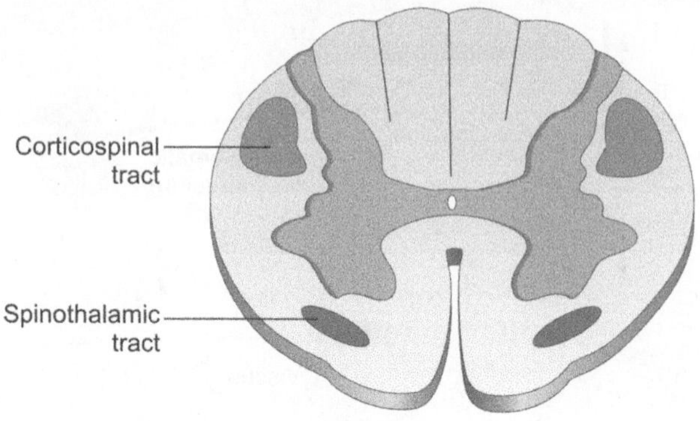

Fig. 26.5: Brown–Séquard syndrome.

8. List the functions of thalamus.

Ans.
- Major relay station for all somatic sensation
- Relay station for special sensation except olfaction
- Plays a role in sleep wake cycle
- Anterior thalamus is a part of Papez circuit therefore involved in emotion and memory.
- It plays a role in control of posture
- Plays a role in integration of sensory motor function
- Involved in language and speech function
- Thalamocortical projections contribute to reticular activating system therefore cause wakefulness and alertness.

9. Write a short note on regulation of feeding.

Ans.
- Hypothalamic regulation of the food intake depends on the interaction of two areas: A **"feeding center"** in lateral hypothalamus and **"satiety center"** in the ventromedial nucleus (VMN) of hypothalamus.
- Stimulation of the feeding center evokes eating behavior and its destruction causes fatal anorexia in healthy persons similarly stimulation of the ventromedial nucleus causes cessation of eating, whereas lesions in this region result in hyperphagia and **hypothalamic obesity.**
- The feeding center is chronically active and its activity is transiently inhibited by activity in the satiety center after the ingestion of food.

Four hypotheses has been proposed for regulation of food intake:

1. The **lipostatic hypothesis** stated that adipose tissue produces a humoral signal leptin, that is proportionate to the amount of fat and it acts on the hypothalamus to decrease food intake and increase energy expenditure
2. The **gut peptide hypothesis** postulates that food in the gastrointestinal tract causes release of one or more polypeptides GRP, glucagon, somatostatin and CCK that act on the hypothalamus to inhibit food intake.
3. The **glucostatic hypothesis** stated that VMN nucleus of hypothalamus is a glucostat, increased glucose utilization in the hypothalamus produces a sensation of satiety.
4. The **thermostatic hypothesis** stated that a fall in body temperature below a given set point stimulates appetite and a rise above the set point inhibits appetite.

10. Give the functional classification of cerebellum.

Ans. Functionally cerebellum is divided into three areas **(Fig. 26.6)**

1. **Vestibulocerebellum** consists of flocculonodular lobe, concerned with balance and eye movement.
2. **Spinocerebellum** consists of the vermis and paravermal regions, it controls posture and skilled voluntary movement.
3. **Neocerebellum** consists of the two main cerebellar hemispheres concerned with planning and programing of the movements.

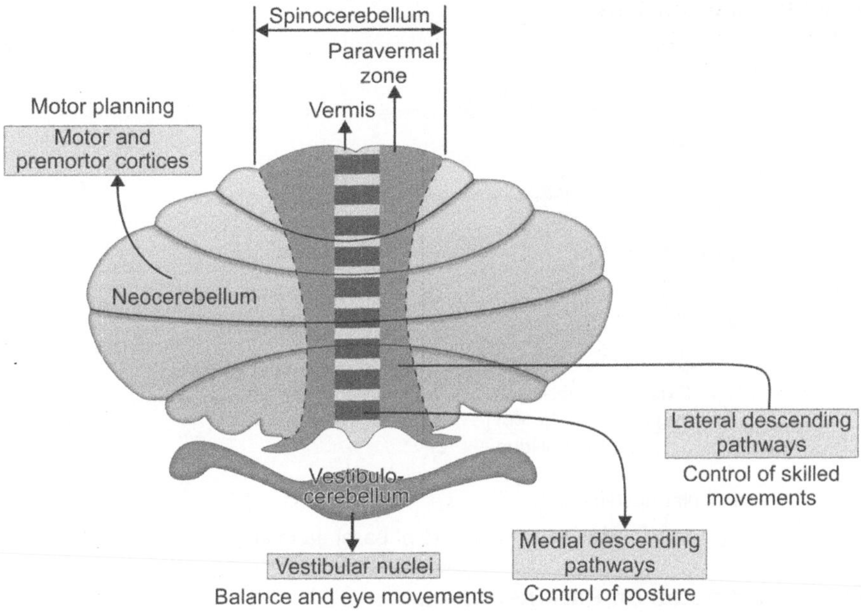

Fig. 26.6: Functional classification of cerebellum.

11. What are the functions of cerebellum?

Ans.
- Control of postural balance and equilibrium
- Concerned with vestibulo-ocular reflex
- Smoothening and coordination of ongoing movements
- Control of skilled voluntary movement
- Planning and programing of movement
- Control of eye movements
- Control of muscle tone and reflexes

12. What are the features of cerebellar disease?

Ans. Cerebellar disorders have the following features:
- **Ataxia:** It is the defect in coordination of movement. Ataxia manifests as drunken gait, scanning speech and dysmetria that is, when the patient attempts to touch an object, the hand overshoots instead of reaching the target.
- **Intention tremor:** Tremor occurs whenever the patient attempts to perform some voluntary action.
- **Rebound phenomenon:** This results due to inability to suddenly stop, the ongoing movement.

- **Adiadochokinesia**, the inability to perform rapidly repeated alternate movements, such as repeated pronation and supination of the hands
- Usually no muscle weakness, sensory deficit or alteration in the tone.

13. Name the structures in basal ganglia.

Ans. **Basal ganglia (BG) include (Fig. 26.7):**

- Caudate nucleus
- Putamen
- Globus pallidus (GP)
- Subthalamic nucleus
- Substantia nigra

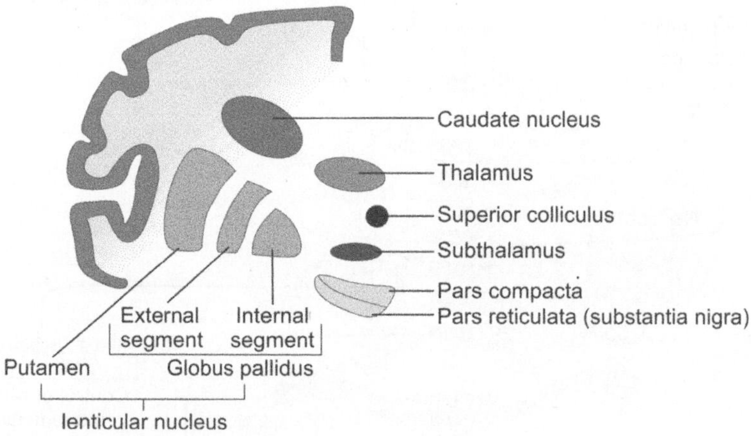

Fig. 26.7: Structure of basal ganglia.

14. Write short notes on Parkinsonism.

Ans. One of the most common neurodegenerative diseases, it occurs due to degeneration of nigrostriatal dopaminergic neurons.

Causes

1. Idiopathic: Not exactly known.
2. Drugs: Phenothiazines, risperidone, flunarizine, metaclopromide, etc.
3. Accumulation excess amount of methyl-phenylpyridinium (MPP) in the brain

Features

- Both hypokinetic and hyperkinetic movements are seen.
- Hypokinetic movements manifest as:
  - Akinesia: Difficulty in initiating movements.
  - Bradykinesia: Slowness of movement.
- Hyperkinetic movements manifest as cogwheel rigidity and resting tremor.
- Decreased associated movements: Swinging of the arms during walking or reduced facial expressions during speaking. Referred as mask-like face.
- Festinant gait: Patient walks in a way that as if he is trying to catch the center of gravity.

Treatment

Administration of L-dopa (levodopa) and anticholinergic medication.

15. Draw a labeled diagram of muscle spindle and mention its function.

Ans.
- Muscle spindles are the sense organs present in the skeletal muscles, they are the receptors that respond to change in muscle length.
- They are activated by stretch
- Stretch of the muscle causes activation of the muscle spindle, action potential is generated in the primary afferent fiber which terminate on the cell bodies of the alpha motor neuron causing muscle contraction in contracted phase of the muscle the spindle activity decreases causing relaxation **(Fig. 26.8)**.

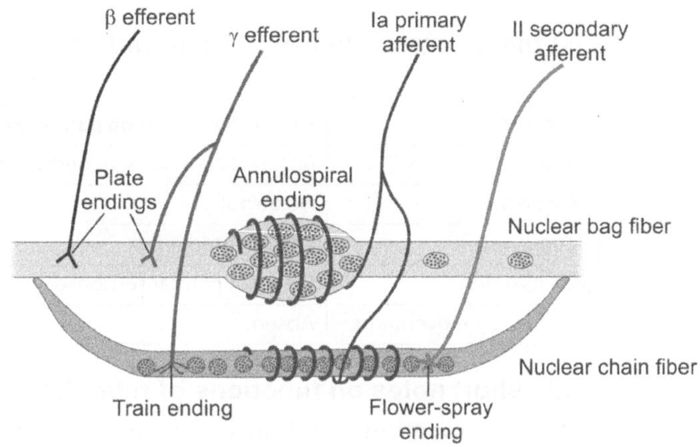

Fig. 26.8: Muscle spindle.

16. Draw a labeled diagram of corticospinal tract (*refer* Figure. 26.9).

Ans.
- The corticospinal tract originate from the *motor cortex (area 4)* and the cortical areas (premotor cortex, supplementary motor area and somatosensory cortex).
- These fibers converge through the *internal capsule* and they descend down in the brainstem.
- As they pass through the medullary pyramid, about 80% of these fibers cross the midline to form the lateral corticospinal tract. The remaining 20% make up the ventral corticospinal tract, which does not cross the midline until it reaches the level of the spinal cord at which it terminates.
- **Lateral corticospinal tract** fibers make monosynaptic connections to motor neurons in the ventral horn of the spinal cord.
- These motor neurons innervate the distal group of muscles concerned with skilled voluntary movement.
- **Ventral corticospinal tract** fibers synapse on spinal interneurons these interneuron terminate on the motor neuron that innervate proximal group of muscles concerned with postural control.

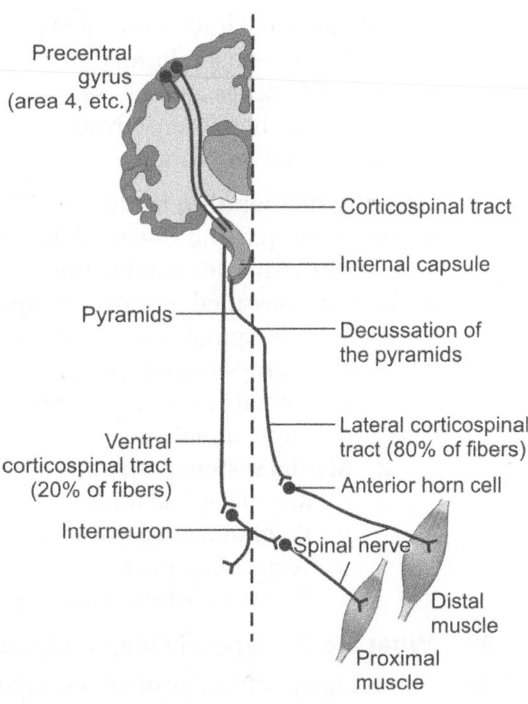

Fig. 26.9: Corticospinal tract.

- The neurons that control the motor functions of the body are divided into lower and upper motor neurons. *Lower motor neurons* refer to the spinal and cranial motor neurons in the brainstem that directly innervate skeletal muscles. *Upper motor neurons* are those in the cortex and brainstem that terminate in the lower motor neurons.

17. List the difference between UMN and LMN paralysis.

Ans.

Features	Upper motor neuron paralysis	Lower motor neuron paralysis
Paralysis	Spasticity paralysis (hypertonia)	Flaccid paralysis (hypotonia)
Muscle mass	No atrophy	Muscular atrophy
Tendon reflex	Exaggerated reflex	Hyporeflexia or areflexia
Babinski sign	Extensor plantar response	Flexor plantar response
Involuntary movements	Absent	Fasciculations

18. Write short notes on functions of reticular formation.

Ans. Reticular formation is a diffuse network of nerve fibers occupies central portion of brainstem.

Classification
- Medullary reticular formation
- Pontine reticular formation
- Midbrain reticular formation

Function
- Reticulospinal tract: Control of posture.
- Brainstem reticular formation: Controls cardiovascular and respiratory functions
- Many of the ascending sensory pathway provide their branches to reticular formation, therefore, activation of sensory pathway keeps the individual alert and aware of the sensation.

19. Classify descending tracts.

Ans.
- The fibers passing downwards from different parts of the brain to spinal cord neurons forms descending tracts
- They are classified into two groups based on their termination of the descending fibers on the spinal motor neurons.
  1. **Lateral system pathways**
     - Lateral corticospinal tract
     - Rubrospinal tract
  2. **Medial system pathways**
     - Reticulospinal tract
     - Vestibulospinal tract
     - Tectospinal tract
     - Anterior corticospinal tract.

20. What are the type of sleep and mention its features?

Ans. Sleep is temporary state of unconsciousness from which a person can be aroused with appropriate sensory stimuli. It is a physiological phenomenon.

Types of sleep

1. Nonrapid eye movement (NREM) sleep or slow wave sleep
2. Rapid eye movement (REM) sleep or paradoxical sleep

Features

Features of NREM sleep

- Decrease heart rate and BP
- Low body temperature
- Slow and regular respiration
- Increase GI activity
- Decreased muscle tone
- Nonrapid eye movement

Features of REM sleep

- Rapid eye movement
- Associated with active dreaming
- Heart rate and BP are increased
- Irregular respiration
- Penile erection seen in males
- Muscle tone is profoundly replaced
- EEG shows a pattern of brain waves similar to those that occur during wakefulness.

21. Name the limbic structures.

Ans. Limbic system consist of limbic cortex and subcortical structure

Limbic cortex consist of:

- Cingulate gyrus
- Subcallosal gyrus
- Parahippocampal gyrus
- Hippocampus

Subcortical structure:

- Hypothalamus
- Anterior thalamus
- Amygdala
- Nucleus accumbens
- Septal nuclei
- Prefrontal cortex
- Habenula

22. What are the functions of limbic system?

Ans.
- Hippocampus is involved in long-term memory
- Amygdala is and attributed to fear
- Nucleus accumbens is associated with reward and motivation
- Hypothalamus regulate autonomic nervous system, endocrine glands function, circadian rhythm, hunger, thirst, sleep-wake cycle and control of sexual behavior
- Papez circuit (comprises of hypothalamus, the anterior thalamic nucleus, the cingulate gyrus, the hippocampus and their interconnections) is concerned with emotional response and memory
- Septal nuclei contribute in sexual activity
- Maternal behavior, appetite, discriminative feeding are other functions of limbic system.

23. Define memory and its type.

Ans. **Definition:** Memory is defined as retention and recall of the information.

Types:

Explicit memory or declarative memory

- It is knowledge about facts and events
- Associated with consciousness
- Depends on the integrity of hippocampus, other parts of the medial temporal lobe of the brain for its retention.

Implicit or nondeclarative memory

- Important for training reflexive motor skill
- Does not involve awareness
- Depends on integrity of amygdala, cerebellum, striatum and neocortex.

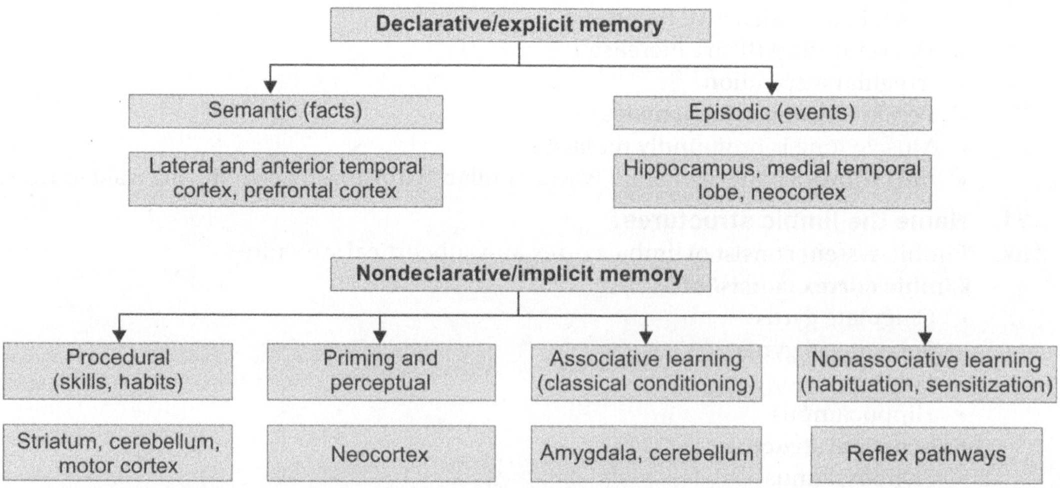

(*Source:* Barrett KE, Barman SM, Brooks ML, Jason KJ,Yuan. Ganong's Review of Medical Physiology, 26th edition. McGraw-Hill Education)

24. What is significance of cerebral dominance?

Ans.
- Human language functions depend more on, one cerebral hemisphere than on the other.
- Language means understanding the spoken and printed word and expressing ideas in speech and writing.
- The hemisphere concerned with language function is called the categorical hemisphere or dominant hemisphere.
- Lesions in the categorical hemisphere produce language disorders
- The representational hemisphere or nondominant hemisphere is involved in the identification of objects by their form and the recognition of musical themes and in facial recognition.
- Lesions in the representational hemisphere produce astereognosis—the inability to identify objects by feeling them.
- Majority of human is right handed, in them, the left hemisphere forms the categorical or dominant hemisphere.

- In left handed persons also left hemisphere is dominant in 70% of cases and right hemisphere in rest of them.

25. Write short note on aphasia.

Ans.
- Aphasia is an impairment of language, affecting the production or comprehension of speech and the ability to read or write.
- They are caused by lesions in the categorical hemisphere
- The most common cause is embolism or thrombosis of a cerebral blood vessel.
- It is broadly divided into four types:
  1. Sensory aphasia
  2. Motor aphasias
  3. Global aphasisa
  4. Anomic aphasia
- In **motor or nonfluent** aphasia, the lesion is in Broca's area, speech is slow, and comprehension of speech is preserved.
- **Sensory or in fluent aphasia,** the lesion is in Wernicke's area. In this condition, speech is fluent but irrelevant comprehension of speech is impaired.
- In **global aphasia** the lesion involves both Broca's and Wernicke's area .
- All aspects of speech and language are affected. Global aphasia may often be seen immediately after the patient has suffered a stroke.
- In **anomic aphasia**, the lesion is in the angular gyrus in the categorical hemisphere, speech is fluent but irrelevant comprehension of speech is impaired.
- They understand speech well, and in most cases, read adequately. But there is difficulty in understanding the written language.

26. Give the composition and functions of cerebrospinal fluid.

Ans.
- Cerebrospinal fluid (CSF) is the fluid that circulate in the ventricles of the brain.
- It is formed from choroid plexuses of the ventricle.

Composition and functions of CSF

Comparison of CSF

Component	CSF
CSF Volume	~150 mL
Protein (mg/dL)	15–50 mg/dL
Glucose (mg/dL)	40–70 mg/dL
Lactate (mg/dL)	10–20 mg/dL
Osmolarity (mOsm/liter)	295
CSF Pressure	50-180 mm/H_2O)
Na^+ (mEq/L)	138
K^+ (mEq/L)	2.8
Ca^{2+} (mEq/L)	2.1
Mg^2 (mEq/L)	2.3
Cl^- (mEq/L)	119
pH	7.33

Functions

- Maintain constant external environment for neurons and glia
- Acts as cushion between the brain and the cranium thus Protect the CNS from trauma
- CSF provides buoyancy effect that allow the brain to float in CSF
- Remove harmful brain metabolites through one way flow of CSF from ventricular system into venous sinuses
- Distributes neuroactive hormones throughout nervous system.

SHORT ANSWERS — 3 MARKS

27. Define synapse and classify it.

Ans.
- These are the junctions where the axon or some other portion of one cell (the presynaptic cell) terminates on the dendrites, soma, or axon of another neuron (the postsynaptic cell).
- Transmission at most synaptic junctions is chemical.

Types of synapse

- Axodendritic
- Axosomatic
- Axoaxonic
- Dendrodendritic

28. Draw a labeled diagram of synapse and mention the steps involved in synaptic transmission.

Ans. *Refer* **Figure 26.10.**

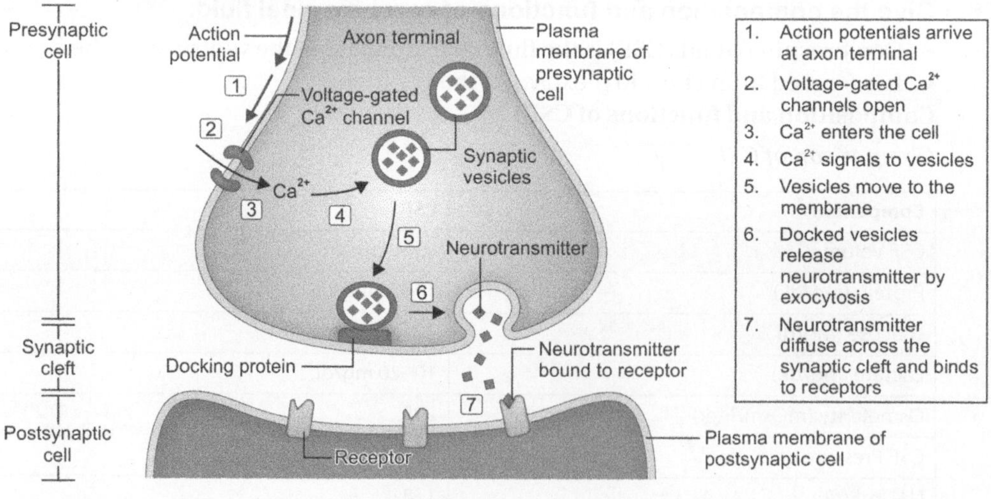

Fig. 26.10: Synapse.

29. List the properties of synapse.

Ans. The properties of synapse are:
- Forward conduction
- Law of convergence and divergence
- Synaptic inhibition

- Synaptic facilitation
- Synaptic delay
- Synaptic plasticity

30. What are receptors and classify it?

Ans. They are specialized structures which respond to specific stimulus and they act as transducers and convert various forms of energy into action potential in the afferent neuron.

31. Mention the properties of receptor.

Ans.
- Specificity
- Adequate stimulus
- Adaptation
- Law of projection

32. Name the ascending tracts.

Ans.
- Anterior or ventral spinothalamic tract
- Lateral spinothalamic tract
- Posterior column pathway

33. What are the features of visceral pain?

Ans.
- Dull, diffuse pain (poorly localized)
- Associated with autonomic symptoms (alteration in BP, sweating).
- Causes muscle spasm and rigidity
- Often referred to some other areas of the body.

34. Name the sensations carried by posterior/dorsal column and draw-labeled diagram of posterior column pathway.

Ans. *Refer* **Figure 26.11**.

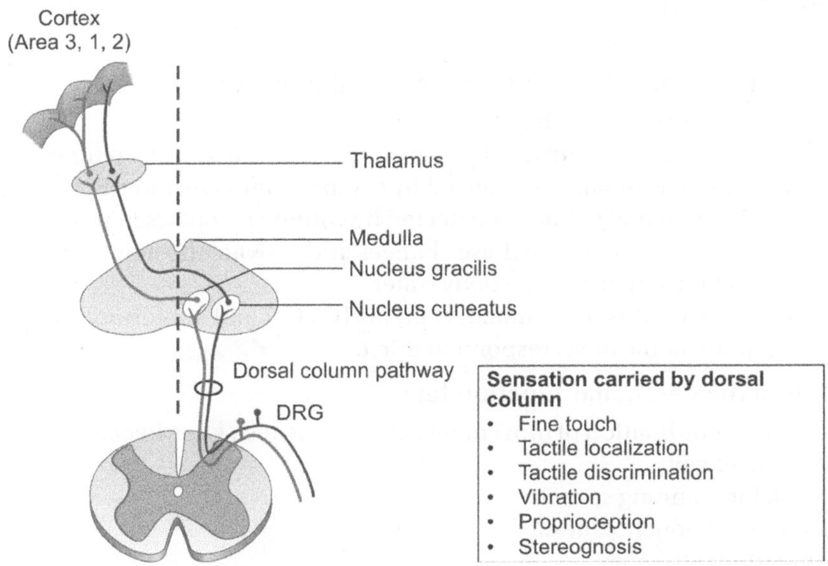

Fig. 26.11: Dorsal column pathways.
(DRG: dorsal root ganglion)

35. What is dissociation anesthesia and Romberg's sign?

Ans. **Dissociation anesthesia:** Damage to the gray matter surrounding the central canal is associated with this condition. There is loss of pain and temperature with preservation of touch. Seen in conditions like intramedullary tumors, syringomyelia and syrinobulbia.

Romberg's sign: It is also called as sensory ataxia, suspected patient is asked to stand with feet together and arms by the side with eyes first open and then closed. With eyes open he can balance and with eyes closed he sways, known as Romberg's positive, which is a test for position sense.

36. What is thalamic syndrome?

Ans. Thrombosis of posterior cerebral artery leads to thalamic syndrome. The features of this syndrome is profound muscular weakness, decreased muscle tone, ataxia, loss of discriminative aspects of sensation (loss of sensation of light touch, tactile localization and discrimination), loss of appreciation of small movements of the joints. All the features occur on the opposite side of the body.

37. Enumerate the functions of hypothalamus.

Ans. Hypothalamus is involved in control of following body functions:
- Endocrine function
- Autonomic function
- Circadian rhythm
- Temperature regulation
- Regulation of food intake
- Regulation of water intake
- Reproductive function
- Influence on emotion
- Regulation of sleep
- Immunological function

38. Describe the role of hypothalamus in water intake.

Ans.
- Hypothalamus control thirst.
- Drinking of fluid is regulated by plasma osmolality and ECF volume.
- Alteration in osmolality is detected by osmoreceptors in anterior hypothalamus
- Alteration in blood volume is detected by volume receptors in the atria
- Hypothalamus respond to these changes and activate the neural areas that induce thirst and thus maintain the body water
- Organum vasculosum lamina terminalis (OVLT) and subfornical organ (SFO) are the hypothalamic areas respond to thirst.

39. Mention the cerebellar function test.

Ans.
- Test for coordination of movement (finger nose test, knee heel test)
- Check for gait
- Look for scanning speech
- Test for adiadochokinesia
- Intentional tremor

40. What are the functions of basal ganglia?

Ans.
- Basal ganglia is involved in planning and programing of motor activities
- Controls posture
- Caudate nucleus of basal ganglia plays a role in cognitive functions.

41. Draw a labeled diagram of stretch reflex.

Ans.
- The stretch reflex is also called as myotatic or stretch reflex **(Fig. 26.12)**.
- It is a monosynaptic reflex
- When a skeletal muscle with intact nerve supply is stretched, there occurs reflex contraction of the muscle known as stretch reflex or myotatic reflex:
  - Stimulus: Stretch of the muscle
  - Receptor: Muscle spindle
  - Afferent: Ia fiber
  - Center: Spinal cord
  - Efferent: Alpha motor neuron

  Response: Contraction of the muscle being stretched
- Play an important role in maintaining posture and mediates tendon reflex.

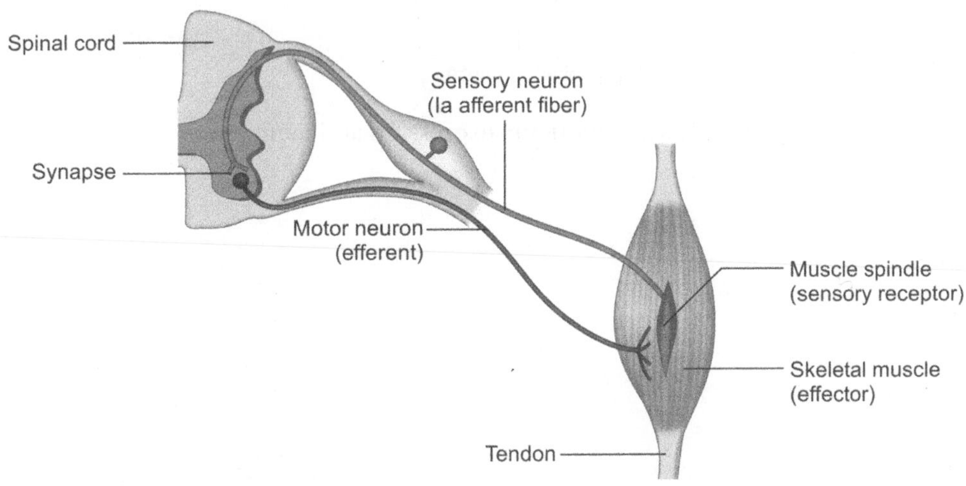

Fig. 26.12: The reflex pathway for stretch reflex.

42. Write short notes on EEG.

Ans.
- Electroencephalogram is the record of spontaneous electrical activity of the cerebral cortex that are picked up from brain surface through electrodes placed on the scalp.
- It represent the summated postsynaptic potentials (PSPs) of cortical neuron (pyramidal cells).
- These PSPs are generated as a result of electrical potentials caused by ions flow into or out of these neurons in response to binding of neurotransmitters on specific receptor.

EEG waves	Frequency	Amplitude
Alpha	8–13 Hz	50–100 μv
Beta	13–30 Hz	5–10 μv
Theta	4–7 Hz	100 μv
Delta	<4 Hz	20–200 μv

43. What is a Papez circuit and mention its significance?

Ans. Papez circuit is a neural circuit consist of cingulate gyrus, hippocampus, mammillary body of hypothalamus thalamus and anterior thalamus.

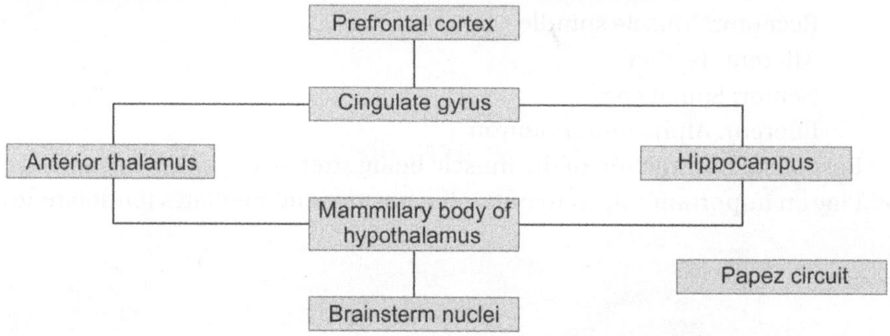

Function: Associated with emotional expression and memory.

27
CHAPTER

Special Senses

VISION

LONG ESSAYS 10 MARKS

1. Draw a labeled diagram of visual pathway.

Ans. *Refer* **Figure 27.1**.

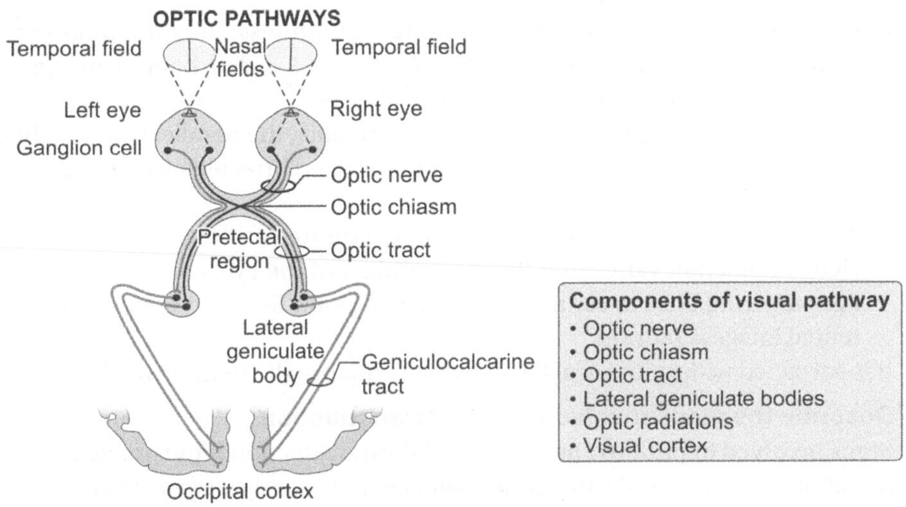

Fig. 27.1: Visual pathway.

Visual Pathway

Image falls on retina

↓

Fibers of the ganglion cells form optic nerve

↓

Optic nerve travel to optic chiasma in which nasal fibers of each eye cross over to opposite side

↓

The temporal fibers travel on the same side without crossing and both fibers terminate in lateral geniculate body

↓

From LGB fibers reach the same side primary visual cortex 9 area 17)

SHORT ESSAYS **5 MARKS**

2. Write short notes on errors of refraction.

Ans. Emmetropia is a state of refraction, wherein the parallel rays of light coming from infinity are focused at retina **(Fig. 27.2)**.

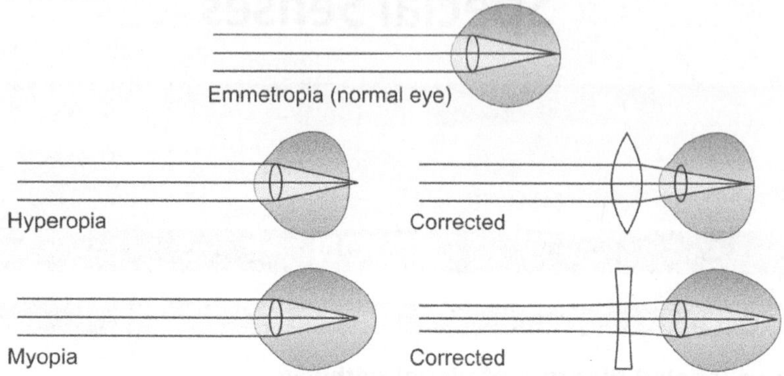

Fig. 27.2: Errors of refraction.

The errors of refraction is classified into:

- **Hyperopia or hypermetropia or long-sightedness:** In this abnormality, the parallel rays of light coming from infinity are focused behind the retina. It is corrected by wearing appropriate convex lenses.
- **Myopia or near sightedness:** In this abnormality, the parallel rays of light coming from infinity are focused in front of the retina. It is corrected by wearing appropriate concave lenses.
- **Astigmatism:** In this abnormality the curvature of the cornea is not uniform. Hence refraction varies in different meridian of the eye, consequently the rays of light entering the eye cannot converge to a point focus, therefore that part of the retinal image is blurred.

It is corrected with cylindrical lenses which equalize the refraction in all meridians.

3. Describe the steps involved in phototransduction.

Ans. **Steps involved in phototransduction:** Phototransduction is the process that occur in the photoreceptors (rods and cones) that *converts light energy into nerve impulse* in the neural structures.

- *Rhodopsin,* the photosensitive pigment, is composed of opsin and retinal (an aldehyde of vitamin A).
- When light strikes on the retina which initiates isomerization of retinal. (11-cis retinal is converted to all-trans retinal).
- From there, a series of conformational changes occur in the opsin that results in the production of metarhodopsin II.
- Metarhodopsin II activates a G-protein that is called *transducin* which stimulates a phosphodiesterase that catalyses the conversion of cyclic guanosine monophosphate (GMP) to 5'-GMP.
- Leads to *decrease in cyclic GMP* which leads to closure of the ion channels, preventing the influx of positive ions.

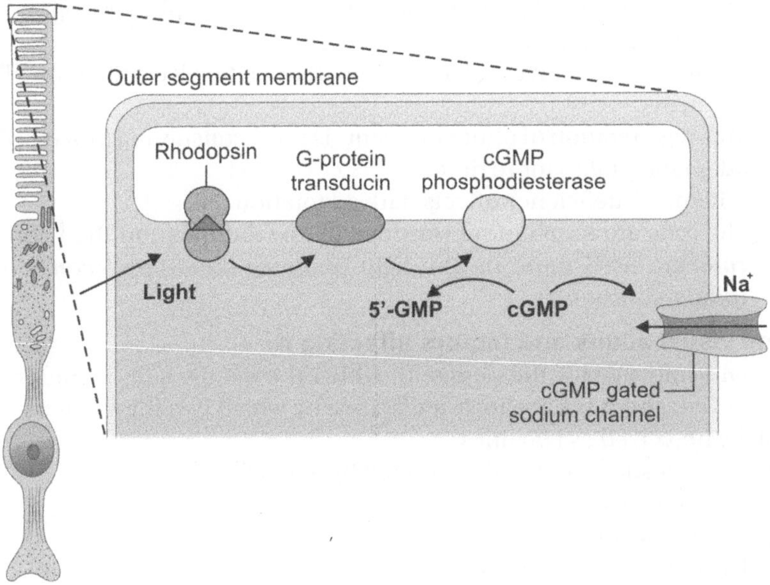

Fig. 27.3: Steps involved in the phototransduction.

- Causing *hyperpolarization* of the photoreceptor membrane, which decreases the release of glutamate (an excitatory neurotransmitter), from the synaptic terminals of the photoreceptor that results in inhibition of the bipolar or horizontal cell (i.e., decreased excitation) **(Fig. 27.3)**.

4. Write short notes on visual adaptation.

Ans. The human eye is capable of functioning normally over a wide range of illumination by a complex process termed as the *visual adaptation.*

Visual adaptation is of two types:

1. **Light adaptation (adjustment to bright illumination):**
   - The process by which retina adapts itself to the bright light is called light adaptation.
   - When a person enters from *dimly lighted area to bright light* the eyes adapt to the increased illumination and the visual threshold rises.
   - It is very quick and occurs in 5 minutes and it is merely the disappearance of dark adaptation.
   - The sensitivity of the photoreceptor decreases, rhodopsin in photoreceptor reduced to retinal and opsin, this is referred as *bleaching effect.*
   - Retinal is further converted into vitamin A, therefore rhodopsin concentration decreases and the sensitivity of the eyes to light also reduced.
2. **Dark adaptation (adjustment in dim illumination):**
   - It is the ability of the eye to adapt itself to a decreasing illumination.
   - When a person goes from a *bright lit into dim lit room,* initially one cannot perceive the objects in the room for some time and subsequently he gets optimal vision.
   - The time taken to see in dim illumination is called *dark adaptation time.*

- During this period, the retinal and opsins in the photoreceptor are converted back into rhodopsin.
- Vitamin A is converted back into retinal to give still more light-sensitive pigments.
- This regeneration of photo pigments is time-consuming process, therefore dark adaptation takes more time.
- Vitamin A deficiency affects dark adaptation.
- The rods are much more sensitive to low illumination than cones. Therefore, ***rods*** are used more in dim light (*scotopic vision*) and ***cones*** in bright light (*photopic vision*).

5. Define visual acuity and factors affecting it.

Ans.
- Visual acuity (VA) is the degree to which the details and contours of objects are perceived, and it is the shortest distance by which two lines can be separated and still be perceived as two lines.
- Clinically, visual acuity is determined by Snellen's chart
- **VA is affected by:**
  - Size of the object
  - Distance of the object from eye
  - Concentration of photoreceptors (more in the fovea and less in the peripheral retina)
  - Image forming mechanism.

6. Write short notes on light reflex.

Ans. When light is thrown at the eye the pupils of both eyes constrict. This is known as light reflex. Response of eye to light is classified as:
- **Direct light reflex**—constriction of pupil in the eye to which light is directed
- **Consensual reflex**—pupillary constriction seen in the other eye.

Pathway for direct light reflex

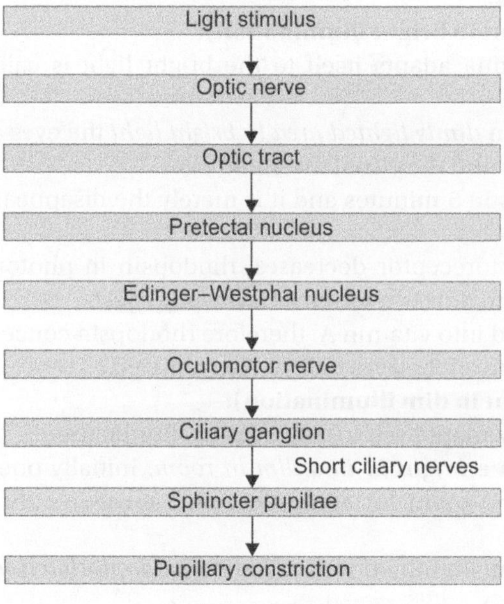

7. Write short note on accommodation reflex.

Ans. When the eyes are focused from a distant to near object. Three adjustments occur to focus include near object

1. Increased convexity of lens
2. Pupillary constriction
3. Convergence of the eye.

Pathway of accommodation reflex

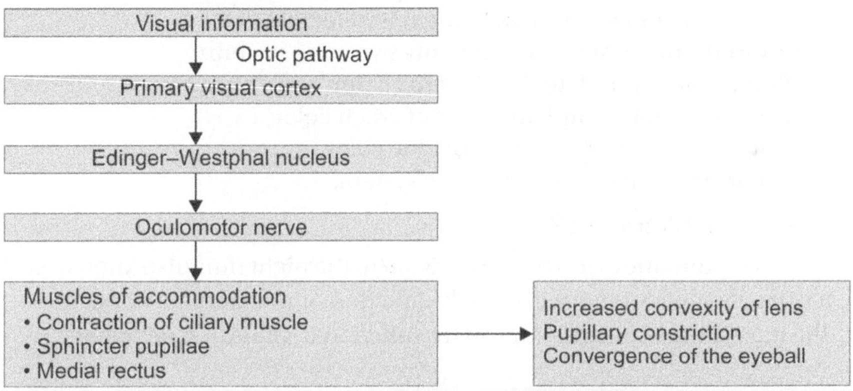

SHORT ANSWERS — 3 MARKS

8. Draw a labeled diagram of eye.

Ans. *Refer* **Figure 27.4**.

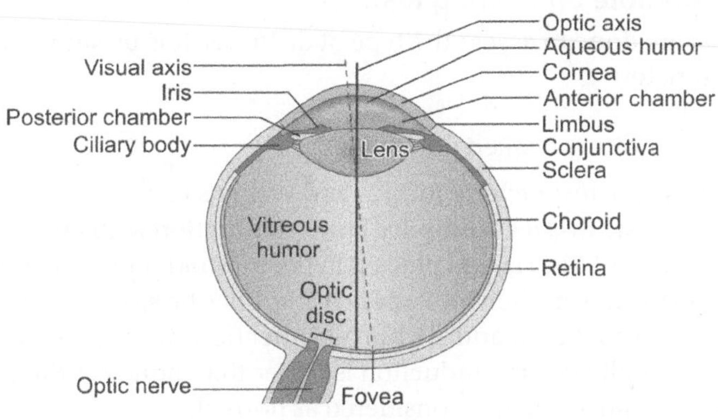

Fig. 27.4: Eye.

9. What is presbyopia?

Ans.
- Presbyopia is a visual defect, noticeable for most people beyond 40 years of age.
- With age, the lens loses its ability to focus adequately. Therefore the near point of vision recedes beyond normal working distance
- It is corrected by using bifocal lens.

10. What are the test for color vision?

Ans. The test for color blindness are:

- Ishihara charts are the most commonly used method (it is lithographic plates containing figures made up of colored spots against a background of similarly shaped colored spots)
- Edrige green lantern test
- Holmgren's wool matching test.
- Farnsworth-Munsell 100 hue test.

11. Classify color blindness.

Ans.
- **Trichromatic:** The affected person appreciate all three primary colors due to intact 3 cone system, but one or two of them is defective
- **Dichromats** are individuals with only two cone systems;
  - Protanopia, complete defect of red color
  - Deuteranopia, complete defect of green color
  - Tritanopia, complete defect of blue color.
- **Monochromats** have only one cone system.

12. What is night blindness?

Ans.
- It is a symptomatic disturbance of vision in the night time also known as Nyctalopia.
- It can occur in patients with rod dysfunction or ocular media opacities.
- The most common cause for rod dysfunction is vitamin A deficiency.

HEARING

LONG ESSAYS 10 MARKS

13. Write a short note on hearing test.

Ans. Hearing test are done to assess the type of deafness. It is broadly classified as:
- Tuning fork test
- Audiometry
- Brainstem auditory evoked potential

a. The tuning fork test include Rinnes and Weber's test
   - **Rinnes test: This test compare bone conduction with air conduction** strike the tuning fork of 512 Hz and place it in the mastoid process of one side and ask the person to inform when he stops hearing, once he stops perceiving it immediately put it close to the ear and ask him whether he is hearing the sound, if he hears the sound it indicate air conduction is better than bone conduction which is called Rinnes positive and it is considered as normal.

     In conductive deafness bone conduction is better than air conduction and in total nerve deafness no sound is heard **(Fig. 27.5)**.
   - **Weber's test:** This test compares the bone conduction of both the ear. The vibrating tuning fork is placed on the vertex of the skull or on the forehead of the subject, ask whether he hears equally on both side of the forehead or better heard in one ear, normally it is equally heard on both the side if it is lateralized to any one side it indicate conductive deafness on that side **(Fig. 27.5)**.

b. **Audiometry:** It is an accurate method to assess *hearing sensitivity*. There are various types of audiometry, which include *pure tone, speech, impedance*

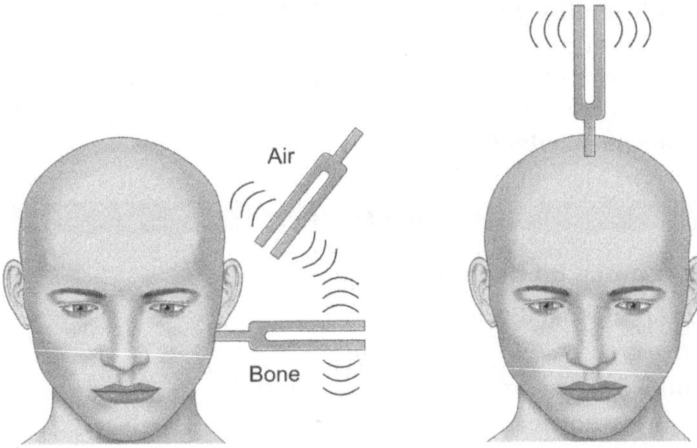

Fig. 27.5: Rinne's test and Weber test.

audiometry. This measure involves integrity of the peripheral and central auditory systems. In pure tone audiometry the electronic device, the audiometer provides pure tone of different frequency, at each frequency the threshold intensity is noted for both air conduction and bone conduction.

Then the hearing sensitivity is plotted on an audiogram which is a graph displaying intensity as a function of frequency. The test is done in the sound proof room **(Fig. 27.6)**.

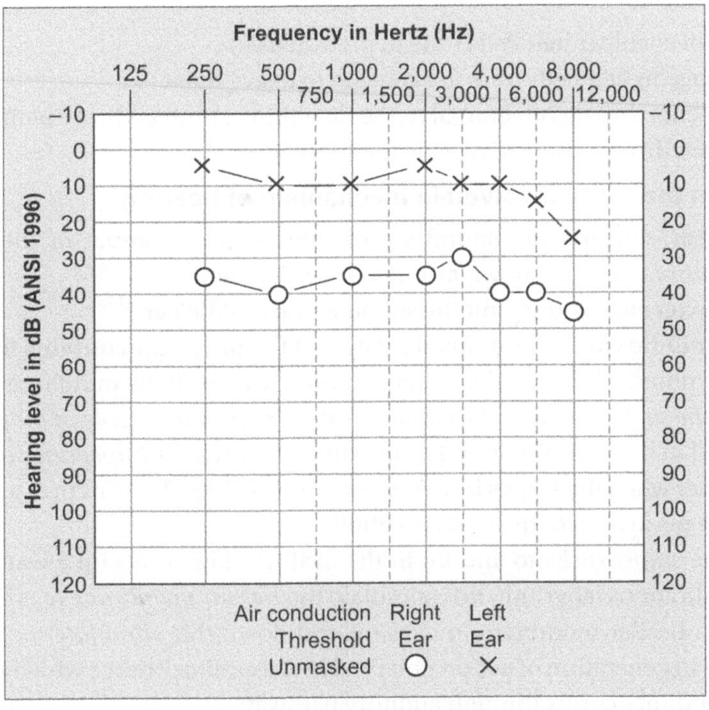

Fig. 27.6: Audiometry.

c. **Brainstem auditory evoked potential (BAEP):** It is sophisticated test to measures how our brain processes the sound waves. Brainstem auditory evoked potential test, assess the *functional status of the auditory pathway* and help to diagnose hearing loss, especially in newborns, young children, and others who do not cooperate for standard hearing test.

SHORT ESSAYS 5 MARKS

14. Write short notes on deafness.

Ans.
- Deafness is the inability to hear
- It is of two types:
  1. Conductive deafness
  2. Sensorineural hearing loss

Conductive deafness is due to impaired sound transmission in the external or middle ear.

Causes

Wax (cerumen) or foreign bodies in the external auditory canals
- Otitis externa (inflammation of the outer ear)
- Otitis media (inflammation of the middle ear)
- Osteosclerosis

Sensorineural deafness is due to defect in the auditory receptor or pathway.

Causes
- Loss of cochlear hair cells (due to prebyacusis)
- Damage to hair cells (due to exposure to heavy noise)
- Problems with eighth cranial nerve or within central auditory pathways
- Certain drugs (Aminoglycoside antibiotics).

15. Mention the steps involved in mechanism of hearing.

Ans.
- The ear converts the sound waves into action potential in the afferent nerve (auditory nerve) is known as *sound transduction.*
- The **external ear** transmit the sound to the middle ear
- The **middle ear** is the air filled cavity and the **inner ear contains fluid**, so sound is transmitted to the fluid by increasing the pressure in the middle ear, the *ear ossicles and the surface area of the tympanic membrane plays a role in amplification* of the sound in the middle ear by 22 times this is referred as *impedance matching.*
- Further when the stapes is pressed into the oval window this pressure is transferred to the perilymph of the scala vestibuli.
- As the *stapes* rocks to and fro in the oval window it sets up a wave motion in the membranous labyrinth, this stimulate the *basilar membrane to vibrate*
- When basilar membrane moves up and down this *stimulate the hair cell,* which leads to generation of action potential in the auditory nerve which is transmitted to the auditory cortex through auditory pathway.

16. Trace the auditory pathway.

Ans.

Hair cells (receptors) are innervated by cochlear division 8th cranial nerve

↓

Cochlear nuclei

↓

Superior olivary nuclei

↓

Inferior colliculus

↓

Medial geniculate body

↓

Auditory cortex (area 41 and 42)

17. Draw a labeled diagram of the taste pathway.

Ans.

- The sensory nerve fibers from the taste buds on the anterior two-third of the tongue travel in the *chorda tympani branch* of the facial nerve, and those from the posterior third of the tongue reach the brainstem via the *glossopharyngeal nerve*. The fibers from areas other than the tongue (e.g., pharynx) reach the brainstem via the *vagus nerve*.
- Taste fibers in these three nerves unite in the gustatory portion of the **nucleus of the solitary tract (NTS) in the medulla oblongata**.
- From there, axons of *second-order neurons* ascend in the same side and terminate in ventral posteromedial nucleus of the thalamus.
- From the thalamus, the axons of the third-order neurons pass and terminate in the ipsilateral postcentral gyrus (sensory cortex).
- Humans perceive five basic tastes: Sweet, sour, bitter, salt, and umami **(Fig. 27.7)**.

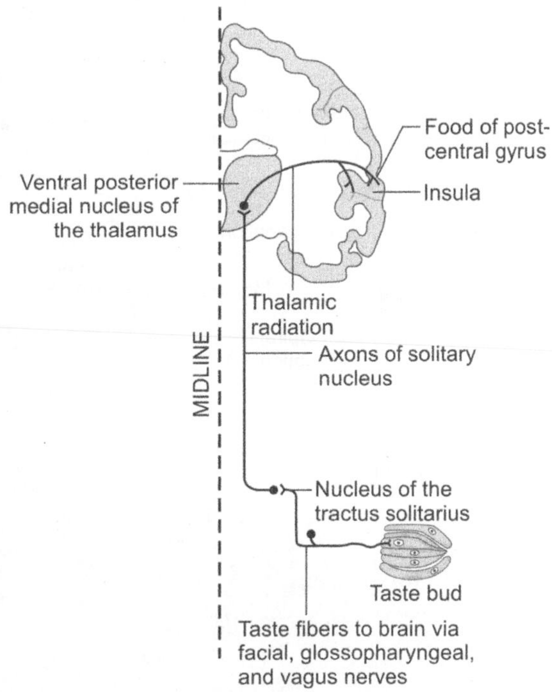

Fig. 27.7: Taste pathway.

18. Write short notes on organ of Corti (*refer* Figures 27.8A and B).

Ans.

- The organ of Corti is located on the basilar membrane of scala media.
- It contains *auditory receptors* (hair cells) whose processes pierce the tough, reticular lamina which is supported by the pillar cells or rods of Corti.

- The hair cells are arranged in four rows: Three rows of outer hair cells lateral to the tunnel formed by the rods of Corti, and one row of inner hair cells medial to the tunnel. There are 20,000 outer hair cells and 3,500 inner hair cells in each human cochlea.
- The rows of hair cells is covered by a thin, viscous, elastic *tectorial membrane* in which the tips of the hairs of the outer hair cells are embedded.
- The cell bodies of the afferent neurons arise from the base of the hair cells and its cell bodies are located in the *spiral ganglion within the modiolus,* the bony core around which the cochlea is wound.
- About 90–95% of these afferent neurons innervate the inner hair cells, the axons of the afferent neurons that innervate the hair cells form the auditory (cochlear) division of the 8th cranial nerve.

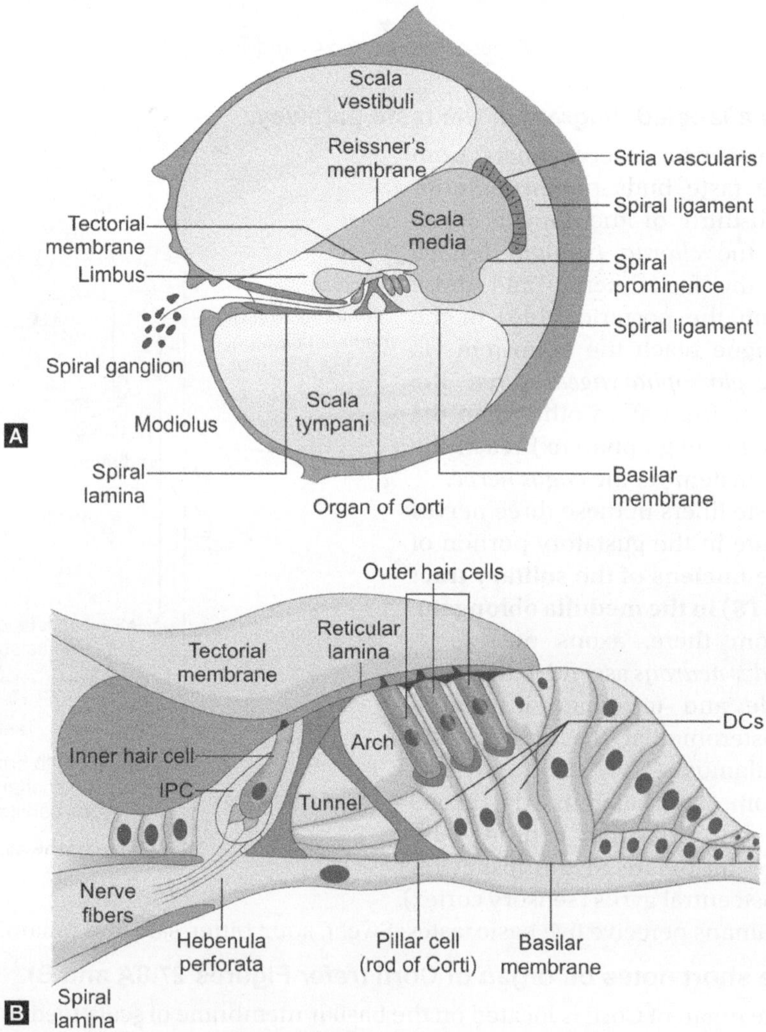

Figs. 27.8A and B: (A) Overview of organ of corti-in modiolus; (B) Detailed structure of the cells in organ of Corti.
(IPC: inner pillar cell)

SHORT ANSWERS 3 MARKS

19. What are functions of ear?

Ans.
- Ear is concerned with hearing and equilibrium of the body
- External ear (involved in receiving the sound)
  Consist of:
  - Pinna
  - Auditory canal
  - Tympanic membrane.
- Middle ear involved (transmission of the sound to inner ear)
  Consist of ear ossicles (malleus, incus and stapes)
- Inner ear (auditory transduction)
  Consist of:
  - Cochlea
  - Vestibular system

20. What are the functions of middle ear?

Ans.
- Receives sound waves from external ear. It consists of utricle, saccule and semicircular canals.
- transmission of sound waves to inner ear through tympanic membrane.
- Impedance matching (amplification of sound waves)
- Keeps the air pressure on the two sides of the eardrum equalized through Eustachian tube
- Protection of inner ear from loud sounds through tympanic reflex.

21. What are the functions of vestibular apparatus?

Ans. Vestibular apparatus is located in the inner ear.

Function:
- Maintenance of equilibrium at rest and balance during movement.
- Vestibular reflexes (vestibulo-ocular reflex, postural reflex) plays a key role in postural stability and visual fixation during movement.
- Vestibular apparatus contains otolith organs (in saccule and utricle) and crista ampullaris (in semicircular canals).
- The hair cells in these receptors respond to change in equilibrium **(Fig. 27.9)**.

Note:

a. Utricle and Saccule—static equilibrium
b. Semicircular canals—dynamic equilibrium

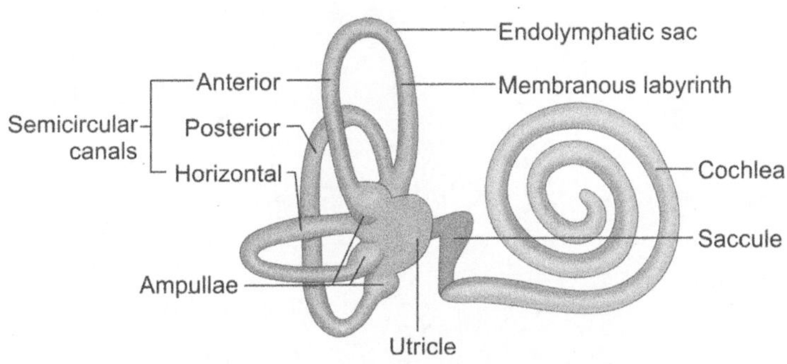

Fig. 27.9: Membranous labyrinth with utricle, saccule and semicircular canals.